MW00426500

BRAINSPANNERS

What have you done for your ***brain*** today?

BRYCE **WYLDE**

TABLE OF CONTENTS

ISBN 978-1-7351137-0-8
Self Published 2020, Canada

DEDICATION

To my dearest mother. A most terrible day is now only around the corner, the day when you will no longer recognize who I am. When this day comes, I promise to always remember and honour the ***real*** you, your love, and your most incredible spirit — long, long after your own memories have faded.

ACKNOWLEDGMENTS

In the classic American musical fantasy film, The Wizard of Oz — which some regard as one of the greatest films in cinema history — Dorothy asks the Scarecrow: "How can you talk, if you haven't got a brain?" To which he replies, "I don't know. But, some people without brains do an awful lot of talking, don't they?" Later on, when he meets up with the Wizard, he is told "A baby has brains, but it doesn't know much. Experience is the only thing that brings knowledge, and the longer you are on earth the more experience you are sure to get." When the Wizard hands him his diploma (instead of a brain), he blurts out: "The sum of the square roots of any two sides of an isosceles triangle is equal to the square root of the remaining side". There is a lot of innuendo there. Where most of us can probably sing the Scarecrow's song "If I Only Had a Brain" or at the very least, whistle it, it might make us happy that we own one ourselves. What most of us need to do is better use the brain we have. Perhaps even more important is to cherish and protect it so that we can keep using it throughout our lives.

I want to express my sincere appreciation to all of my Brainspanner experts including Dr. Julian Bailes, Dr. Andrew Weil, Dr. Dale Bredesen, Dr. Mehmet Oz, Brent Bishop, Dr. Mansoor Mohammed, Dr. Rollin McCraty, Robb Wolf, Dr. Daniel Amen, Chris Kilham, Dr. Mark Gordon, Dr. Bill Sears, Dr. David Jenkins, James Aspey, Dr. Guy Chamberland, Yanjaa Wintersoul, Nelson Dellis, and JJ Virgin. They have all dedicated some or all of their life's work to brain health and I consider them the first official group of Brainspanners. They gave me their precious time and some wonderful insights.

I also want to thank my peripheral brain, wordsmith, and editor, Robert Buckland of Encompass Editions. Without the incredible outputs of this gentleman's remarkable neurocircuitry, resourcefulness, and his attention to detail, this book would not have been possible.

And a warm shout-out to Joe Paonessa, my one-in-a-million cover and interior designer, a rare creative mind who believes that a picture speaks a thousand words and that people do indeed judge a book by its cover. Thanks, Joey. Awesome!

Lastly, I want to thank Tony Pallante, CEO of Brain Armor and a brainspanner himself, for seeing and trusting in my vision. Our similar experiences — we each have experienced a parent with Alzheimer's — and our desire to improve the health and wellness of others by focusing on the importance of the brain, was the catalyst that brought this book to life.

PART I

THE BRAIN: AN OPERATING MANUAL

We've evolved massive brains. That's clear.
The questions now are: what can we do with them and how do we care for them?

THIS BOOK AND THE BRAIN

Several paths have led me to this book and it's possible, had I missed any one of them, I might not have embarked upon the project at all.

My mother determined the first path. She's a highly intelligent woman and throughout her career as a teacher was always a busy and well-organized person whose spot at the kitchen table was littered every morning with a dozen "to-do" notes. As far back as I can recall, she'd sometimes forget the name of a person she knew in the middle of a story and she was never any good with new technologies. That's just who she was and continued to be, perhaps compounded by the normal processes of ageing. Over this last decade, she's struggled with pain due to arthritis and eventually had to undergo knee replacement surgery. She also suffered from minor glaucoma and cataracts that impacted her vision. These are the disabilities that can accompany normal aging.

In early 2018, I stopped by her condo to take her out for lunch. Over the months prior to that, our routine was that I'd pick her up outside the lobby, but on this occasion she warned me ahead of time that her knees hurt too much. I went up to the apartment and she let me in. I looked around. On the refrigerator, on the lampshades, on the sofa and the walls – scattered and posted everywhere – were notes, but they weren't her famous "to-do" notes. These were carefully handwritten reminders that said things like "Ask Bryce how to take money out of my bank account" and "What is Tonya's daughters name?" But my sister's name is Tanya, not Tonya, and my mom's granddaughter was already three years old.

I was uneasy but hesitant. Her cataract surgery was coming up. "How much," I wondered, "might this be simply her degenerative joint disease and her inability to see? Maybe it's just old age." She was 75.

Cataract surgery came and went. When she'd fully recovered, I fit her with brand new glasses. She looked around without expression, staring through me and into the distance.

My mother was at stage 4 on the Alzheimer's disease scale of 1 to 7. A complete medical evaluation revealed that the cerebellum and the occipital lobe of her brain – the areas together responsible for balance, coordination, fine muscle control, and vision – were the most affected. Her memory was in a sharp decline and her poor gait and poor vision and inability to pick up the phone and call me had very little to do with joint pain or cataracts or lack of technological skill: it was the relentless progression of Alzheimer's and I had missed the signs. The discovery that my friend and colleague Dr. Mehmet Oz (whose interview I include in this book) missed his mother's diagnosis of Alzheimer's at the same time gave me some very small solace.

I visit my mom often in her retirement home. She smiles and is quite happy there. She's met a boyfriend, an ex-military pilot and humorous conversationalist who believes chivalry still lives, and when they first met, her mental and physical health improved across the board: memory, alertness, concentration, mobility. By then I understood enough to know she was experiencing a surge of dopamine, the feel-good hormone, and we can sometimes call such a surge "falling in love." My awed respect for the complexity of the human brain, even in the grip of a terrible disease, only grew, so it should come as no surprise that over the last few years I've redoubled the time and energy spent researching the brain along with the nutrition and lifestyle interventions that may improve or even prevent dementia.

The second path leading to this project was my own professional path. I'm a clinician whose education is rooted in natural medicine and functional medicine. Throughout my career, my focus has been on clinical nutrition, supplementation, and botanical medicine. I strive to stay abreast of the latest in biological and genomic screening and medical science and technology, blending them with traditional and ancient remedies. I'm part of a team of allied health professionals at P3 Health in downtown Toronto. There, I work closely with my patients, informed by their genetic make-up, to customize care, lifestyle and functional therapeutic interventions for health promotion, disease prevention and longevity.

According to the New York Times, we spend more than $30 billion a year on dietary supplements — vitamins, minerals and herbal products, among others — many unnecessary or of doubtful benefit to those taking them. From my earliest days in clinical practice, I grew mistrustful of the supplement reps who liked to take me out to lunch and educate me on the latest and greatest. I worried that these people were beginning to cloud my objectivity. Clinicians and patients inevitably experience supplement brand loyalty, just as medical doctors and their patients do with prescription medication. I needed to learn more about what was inside the bottles that crowded the shelves of health food stores and that I myself was recommending to my patients. Over the following years, I visited dozens of high quality manufacturers throughout the U.S., Japan, India, Malaysia, Italy, Switzerland, Greece, France and elsewhere. I documented countless operations whereby plants were micropropagated, farmed, and turned into herbal remedies. I saw how probiotics are cultured and freeze dried, how fish and plant oils are refined into omega-3 essential fatty acids, how the byproducts of various food and beverage industries (the wine and egg industries, for example) are used to make nutraceuticals, how agriculture transforms select beans to make supplemental fiber and proteins, how the marijuana and hemp industry works, and how exotic mushrooms are harvested and powdered for encapsulation. As this investigation has progressed I've become increasingly confident in my ability to share what works (and what doesn't) in this burgeoning world of natural medicine — and most importantly, what is safe and what isn't. Nootropics, affectionately referred to as "smart drugs" or "cognitive enhancers" are the latest wellness supplement sold by top retailers and health food stores and promoted through social media. This ingredient category alone is projected to reach $6 billion in North America over the next four years. So it was only to be expected that this class of supplement and the organ their promoters aspire to address would fall under my purview.

The third path to this book was a public one. The number of people with diagnosed dementia is rising at a staggering rate. There are nearly 50 million people worldwide living with this condition, with about 8 million new cases diagnosed every year and an estimated 136 million by 2050. Currently, worldwide healthcare costs associated with dementia are reported to be well over $900 billion. There isn't a single country on earth whose current health-care system is well equipped to deal with these costs.

On January 1, 1990, then-President George H. W. Bush announced the start of "the decade of the brain." The U.S. federal government committed significant and overdue financial support for neuroscience and mental health research. This has formed a part of an extraordinary explosion in scientific knowledge about the organ that most of us have cheerfully admitted is important — indeed indispensable — but about which we have had little knowledge or interest. When it comes to our health, we've been inclined to know our weight and maybe our cholesterol levels and blood pressure. We might even know our Vitamin D status. But until very recently, who has known how healthy their brain might be or even how this might be measured? And who has known until recently what to do about it? The question I'm now asking all my patients is: "What have you done for your ***brain*** today?"

Finally, I've contributed considerable time as a member of the medical advisory board of Brain Armor, a company dedicated to making a positive impact on the health and wellness of the brain. More recently I've taken the position of chief innovations officer for that company, overseeing the formulation of new products able to improve brain health. I work closely at Brain Armor with Dr. Julian Bailes, former team physician of the Pittsburgh Steelers and for twenty years a team physician in the NFL or NCAA Division I. Dr. Bailes is chairman of the NorthShore Neurosurgery Department and co-director of the NorthShore Neurological Institute. He was portrayed by Alec Baldwin in the movie "Concussion," based on actual events and starring Will Smith as the pathologist Dr. Bennet Omalu. Dr. Omalu uncovered the truth about brain damage in football players who suffer repeated concussions in the course of normal play. I'll have more to say about Brain Armor towards the end of the book.

So if a convergence has led to this book, I certainly don't intend it as an encyclopedia, a textbook, or something to be read by specialists. I think of it as a conversation such as I might have some evening with a friend who knew of my interest in the brain and wondered what I might share based on my clinical practice and the wisdom of those who have devoted their lives to the field.

HOW TO READ THIS BOOK

If you're reading this book, it's probably because like me you realize two things: first, that the health of the physical brain inside our heads is supremely important; and second, there are things we can do to preserve that health,

Since the health of the brain is our foremost concern, for much of ***Part I: An Operating Manual,*** I address brain health issues and jump right into nutrition, lifestyle, and accessible supplements that have been shown effective in preventing and healing brain disorders.

In ***Part II: Talking to the Thinkers,*** I interview some of the world's most renowned researchers and practitioners for their seasoned perspective on these same issues.

I recognize that many of you won't be intimately familiar with the brain's anatomy and functions, nor with the remarkable story of the billion-year evolution that's shaped its structure and chemistry, and neither would you necessarily know much about the workings of the human genome that plays so critical a role in brain health and medicine. But I couldn't stand the idea of starting this book off with dozens of pages that might only remind you of high school biology class. Instead, I'll tuck it neatly into the back of the book and offer you the choice. If you want to learn about the critical roles of the brain's hippocampus, the profound importance of gene expression, or how we think the whole brain thing came about, I offer ***Part III: The Nuts and Bolts of Brains***. Some of you may even choose to read it first.

Finally in ***Part IV: The Bookends.*** I talk about my personal association with the Brain Armor company and present some useful tests and studies that supplement its message.

BRAINSPANNERS: THE TITLE

The title of this book is a play on "lifespan". We all know that lifespan is the number of years we'll spend on this planet. "Healthspan" is the term now used to describe the number of years we live in actual good health. But "brainspan" is the number of years we will live in good health with optimal cognitive faculties. And a "brainspanner" is a person who avails themselves of the fruits of contemporary brain research to assure that their brainspan is as long as possible.

In the past, we didn't know enough about the brain to be more than somewhat interested. Now we're overawed to realize that at last there are many simple things we can do for this overwhelmingly personal organ. I think we'd be literally crazy not to do them.

1

A DAMAGED BRAIN

All the NFL players I have examined pathologically, I have not seen one that did not have changes in their brain system with brain damage.

~ ***Bennet Omalu***

Let's begin by considering what we ***don't*** want to happen to our personal brain and our first step is to recognize that a damaged brain is a damaged brain. You might very reasonably wonder what a skier who hits her head against a tree and survives has to do with a seventy-eight year old just diagnosed with Alzheimer's disease. But by the end of this chapter, I hope you'll notice how, at the molecular and cellular level, they have something in common. And not surprisingly, their prevention and treatment also have something in common.

Along the way, I'll occasionally reference the brain's exquisite complexity. From its very atoms — the ions that are the units of neural messaging — though the delicate and dazzling structure of the neurons with their feathery dendrites and long axons, the extraordinary circuitry that wires it all together, to the scores of billions of supporting cells, membranes, fluids and blood vessels — an integrated, flexible, responsive intricacy that boggles our attempts to grasp it all — and if we ever do, it will be through the use of that very brain we're trying to understand.

Then, suddenly, rupture: injury or disease.

A DAMAGED BRAIN:
IN THE EVENT OF EMERGENCY

The skull that houses the brain is moving swiftly forward. Abruptly, it meets an obstacle — a wall, a ball, a paving stone. The brain inside continues forward and sloshes against the inside front of the skull. The skull rebounds from impact and the brain is shunted backwards to rebound off the back of the skull, twisting, turning, contorting and stretching. The dense cortical surface separates in places from the softer grey matter beneath, shearing or tearing the long connecting axons. This diffuse axonal injury disrupts their ability to communicate. The damaged axons begin to degenerate and in doing so release toxins. Neighboring neurons die. Deeper in the brain, the tearing force of impact move down the ***falx***, the fibrous tissue separating the two hemispheres, to stretch or tear the ***corpus callosum*** that connects them. Not pretty, and possibly the most common of the serious outcomes. This is concussion.

Of course not every injury to the head and brain follows this catastrophic course. But a new diagnostic technology, diffuse tension imaging, allows scientists to look at the brain's large axon bundles and observe how even mild blows repeated over time may alter them structurally. Studies of soccer players, notorious for "heading" the ball, show what appears to be significant damage to the structural integrity of these bundles, as though they were ropes that begin to fail when individual fibres start to fray. Even when there is no record of them having suffered full-blown concussion, these players often perform much worse than average on short-term memory tasks. There has been what is called an "overload of sub-concussive hits." Sadly, this overload has been linked to a degenerative brain disease known as "chronic traumatic encephalopathy" or CTE, which I'd like to look at more closely later.

Needless to say, you don't have to play in the NFL, fight in the ring, or head balls every day in a premier soccer league to be at risk of traumatic brain injury. Many of us have been involved in a car accident and many more of us have fallen and bumped our head. In fact, experts think the majority of the population has been mildly to moderately concussed at least once in their life.

Even a mild concussion, however, is considered a traumatic brain injury, and is termed an "mTBI". As published in the prestigious medical journal JAMA, a recent research paper, ***Prevalence of Concussion Among US Adolescents and Correlated Factors,*** over 5% of adolescents reported being diagnosed with more than one mTBI. In children, biking is the leading cause, more than hockey or soccer. That's why it's so surprising to learn that the helmets worn for football and biking were never designed or tested for their ability to protect a child against concussion by slowing the impact of the brain against the skull. They were in fact simply designed to protect against skull fracture and I'm bound to say that many experts believe it may not be possible to prevent concussion other than to avoid the activity in the first place. But there is at last some innovation underway. After seven years of research, development and testing, the Hövding was launched in Sweden in November 2011. This airbag bicycle helmet technology contains accelerometers that detect unusual movement and deploy an airbag if the movement matches the profile of a crash. And when I spoke to Dr. Julian Bailes portrayed by Alec Baldwin in the movie "Concussion", he described another development of great potential. My interview with him appears in Part II.

IF IT HAPPENS

Mild to moderate traumatic brain injuries can have a far deeper impact on our overall health than we previously believed. Protecting our brain from injury — even mild to moderate injury — is the best advice I can offer and one of the most powerful things we can do to for our brain health.

The symptoms of a mTBI may not appear immediately after the trauma and can take weeks to kick in. They often present as feeling "off", a general "brain fog", loss of cognitive ability and memory, a headache, a shift in personality — particularly short-temperedness, and a strong sensitivity to light and noise. And though there is greater awareness today about the risk of brain injury, the recommended solutions are not always grounded in the latest research. The most common advice doctors give in the case of a mTBI is simply to rest. Good advice as far as it goes, but there is much more you can do to support your brain during recovery from a mild to moderate traumatic brain injury.

If you think you might be suffering from such an injury, seek medical attention immediately. Don't second guess yourself. One of the most important things to do is to catch brain injury as early on as possible.

Avoid strenuous activity, including anything physically, mentally, or emotionally taxing. Rest your eyes and your brain. That means little to no reading or even watching TV.

If you've had a mild to moderate trauma to the head, a brain scan is advisable although research has shown that often no visible differences show up at first. To minimize radiation exposure, opt for an MRI over a CT whenever possible.

You may experience a range of symptoms over the following days, such as difficulty concentrating, dizziness, or trouble falling asleep. These symptoms can be part of the normal healing process, and most go away over time without any treatment. Return immediately to the emergency department if you have worsening or severe headache, lose consciousness, experience vomiting, confusion, seizures, numbness, or any symptom that concerns you, your family, or friends. In any event, always tell a family member or friend about your head injury and ask them to help monitor you for more serious symptoms. Get plenty of rest and sleep, and return gradually and slowly to your usual routines. Don't drink alcohol. Avoid activities that are physically demanding or require a lot of concentration. If you don't feel better after a week, see a doctor who has experience treating brain injuries and never return to sports before getting cleared by a doctor. A repeat blow to your head — especially before your brain has time to heal — can be very dangerous and may slow recovery or increase the chance for long-term problems. Avoid bright lights and loud sounds. Ideally, remain in a dark room and get as much sleep as possible. After a mTBI, there's a higher risk of a secondary brain injury. Avoid airline travel and high impact activities in the 6 weeks or so following your brain injury.

Meanwhile, assuming all has gone well, there are active steps on the road to recovery that may be beneficial in your case.

Pulsed electromagnetic field (pEMF) can be therapeutic. Discovered decades ago and studied by scientists around the world, pEMF directly increases capillary blood flow and reduces inflammation in the brain. There are over 2,000 published clinical studies of the benefit of pEMF, not just in cases of mTBI but as an intervention in cases of depression, insomnia, Parkinson's disease, attention deficit disorder, anxiety, conduct disorder, and posttraumatic stress disorder. It appears to work because your heart pumps blood through the main arteries but relies on the additional pumping power of "microvessels" in the brain. Nearly all blood vessels in the brain are in fact microvessels. If placed end-to-end, they would extend more than 74,000 miles (that is, about three times around the planet) and it is these tiny vessels that reach the majority of our 86 billion neurons. Red blood cells carry oxygen and nutrients through them to the cells, and the cells in turn transfer carbon dioxide and waste products to the blood cells, which travel through the microveins and out of the brain. Many brain and neurological dysfunctions are directly related to diminished circulation and excess inflammation. Exposure to select pEMF technology can result in a better supply of oxygen, a better supply of brain nutrients, and better disposal of metabolic waste and inflammation.

Contrast hydrotherapy — submersion or showers in alternating cold and hot water — can also be effective support for recovery from brain injury. A steam or infrared sauna followed by the latest cold devices such as a Cryohelmet or a fancy ice vest may work well, or you can simply use the shower at home or at the gym. Start with a very hot shower — as hot as you can handle for five minutes — until you're uncomfortably, feverishly hot — though careful not to burn yourself. Then turn the shower to the coldest setting possible for one minute. Yes, it's uncomfortable — on purpose. Then back to hot for five minutes, then back to freezing cold for another 60 seconds. Don't worry. The discomfort ends there and — although scientists have yet to crack the code on the mechanism of action — this brief "thermal stress" is probably a great way to biohack a quick boost of BDNF, the potent brain enzyme I'll discuss in a minute.

Diet can play a significant role in recovery from brain injury. Perhaps the healthiest way to eat while your brain is in recovery mode is a ketogenic diet consisting of about 75% fat, 20% protein and 5% (or less than 50 grams) of carbs per day. Focus on high amounts of healthy fat, low-carb foods such as eggs, meats, dairy and low-carb vegetables, as well as sugar-free beverages. The leading theory is that ketones formed as the main energy source from a ketogenic diet provides an alternative and more readily usable energy source for the brain and reduces its dependence on glucose metabolism, which is impaired following trauma to the brain.

The omega-3 essential fatty acid DHA is particularly important to brain recovery following trauma and some experts – including myself – suggest supplementing as high as 10g daily. A clean algal omega-3 formula that's high in DHA such as that found in "Brain Armor Daily" is ideal.

BDNF is the specialized protein (brain derived neurotrophic factor) expressed by the BDNF gene and it governs neuroplasticity – the ability of brain cells to disconnect and reconnect. It also governs neurogenesis – the ability to create new brain cells – and plays a role in mood, behaviour, and the growth of new blood vessels as well as our individual ability to recover from trauma. The more BDNF we produce, it seems, the more ***armored*** our brain becomes against damage, and the better it recovers after damage. Research has shown that curcumin significantly reduces inflammation, boosts BDNF, enhances neuroplasticity, improves cognition, and counteracts the effects of traumatic brain injury. When brain cells die, BDNF works to bring replacement connections and even new cells back to life! If you've experienced any level of head trauma, in addition to taking a hefty dose of DHA consider adding a curcumin supplement to your regime, preferably in a liquid micelle form for optimal absorption. There are a lot of curcumin supplements on the market claiming various levels of absorption. The reality is, curcumin is very poorly absorbed (i.e. it has a low bioavailability). The best bioavailability I've seen is from a product called CoreCumin that you can find at **www.nurish.me**. This curcumin is formulated in nanoparticulate complexes so as to be more usable. Being encapsulated in nanoparticles also means that you do not need to take a mega-dose of curcumin to get the same level of benefit.

Another ingredient clinically shown to significantly increase the BDNF vital to learning, memory, and higher thinking, is an extract of whole fruit of the ***Coffea arabica*** plant. I'll talk later about this product, "NeuroFactor", and in a little more detail.

A DAMAGED BRAIN:
THE TOXINS

MERCURY

Nutritionists advise us to eat more fish for good health but there is a significant "bad in the good" that comes with that advice. Conclusive evidence on the toxic effects of mercury found in seafood recently prompted national health organizations in Canada and the U.S. to suggest limiting consumption of certain fish: fresh and frozen tuna, shark, swordfish, escolar, marlin and orange roughy. There's a helpful link that advises as to what seafood we can safely consume on a regular basis.

https://www.canada.ca/en/health-canada/services/food-nutrition/food-safety/chemical-contaminants/environmental-contaminants/mercury/mercury-fish.html

University of Calgary's Faculty of Medicine, Department of Physiology and Biophysics has published conclusive evidence that there is no safe level of mercury in the body. Very simply, any level of mercury is actively destroying a few of our precious 86 billion brain cells every hour.

As you may know, "silver" dental amalgam is made up of 25% silver, a 25% to 35% blend of copper, zinc and tin, and a shocking 40% to 50% mercury. If we grind our teeth in the process of chewing our food (or even in our sleep), mercury is being released into our system and may be killing hundreds of our neurons every hour.

Another, seemingly more exotic way of exposing ourselves to mercury is breathing mercury vapor. But many people have told me how, as kids, they played with mercury from a broken thermometer. If the mercury is not immediately contained or cleaned up, it will spread over everything and then evaporate, becoming an invisible, odorless, toxic vapour. The bad news is that mothers who are exposed to mercury (and nearly 100% are) expose their infant children through their breast milk it seems that all of us have mercury in our body, though most below the levels associated with major health effects. The good news: alpha lipoic acid is a potent antioxidant synthesized in the body that protects the brain and nervous system from the harmful effects of mercury and helps expel it from the body. Taking it in supplement form at about 300 to 600mg daily will boost the rate at which mercury and most heavy metals are removed and will also help your system to make more glutathione – the most important detoxification molecule in your body.

THE ELECTRIC FILLINGS

As though the effects of mercury on our 86 billion little friends wasn't bad enough, amalgam fillings present another hidden danger. Saliva acts as an electrolyte to create an unnaturally high electric current that flows through the head of the trusting dental patient.

There are in fact two types of electrical activity on the surface of a filling. One, as in a regular battery, is called 'bimetallic'. Bimetallic activity happens when two or more dissimilar metals are in an electrolyte solution that conducts electricity. This bimetallic activity produces a current or a flow of electrons through the medium of an electrolyte. The other type of electrical activity is called differential aeration. This occurs between saliva and areas that contain differing amounts of oxygen. This can be seen in the saliva covering a filling, where there is less oxygen than in the saliva covering unrestored enamel. This differential aeration produces a current.

Essentially, mercury fillings are like having a living battery proximal to your brain. It is in fact quite easy to measure oral electrical currents with medical equipment sensitive enough to measure very low voltage. The body's normal electrical (bioenergetic) reading is about 450 millivolts, but when saliva mixes with amalgam fillings a measurable electric current of up to 1,000 millivolts is detected. The brain is bioelectric and this kind of electrical current is suspected of interrupting the brain's normal neuronal communication.

Meanwhile, the electric currents and ionic flows between various dental alloys have been shown to cause irritation in the trigeminal nerve, the main cranial nerve system. Electro-galvanism can also cause or contribute to such physical delights as seizures, hearing loss, vision problems, sleep disturbances, depression, ringing in the ear, lack of concentration and memory, and headaches.

If you have amalgam in your mouth, put the pedal to the metal. Find a "biosafe" dentist trained to safely transition you out of the metal headspace.

DIACETYL

Microwave popcorn with "butter flavoring" contains the additive diacetyl, a molecule able to cross the blood-brain barrier that prevents harmful substances from entering the brain, as we'll discuss further in a few pages, when we look at lectins. Diacetyl causes beta-amyloid clumping, a significant indicator of Alzheimer's, but you won't see the word diacetyl on the label. Instead, look for "artificial butter flavor" or "natural flavors" and just assume your popcorn "butter" contains diacetyl.

MSG

Monosodium glutamate (MSG) is in many processed foods and made its claim to fame in the 80s as synonymous with Chinese food syndrome. MSG breaks down in the body into glutamate, which appears to stimulate brain cells to death. What is most alarming is that it is found in everything, but is not required to be listed on product labels unless the product is 100% pure MSG. Spices, flavourings, and "natural flavourings" can all contain up to 99% MSG with zero mention on the label. And shopping at a "health food" store doesn't protect us. Refined soy products such as soy burgers are heavy in MSG.

Look for and avoid these ingredients that are synonymous with MSG:

- ◊ Hydrolyzed vegetable protein (HVP)
- ◊ Hydrolyzed plant protein
- ◊ Hydrolyzed protein
- ◊ Plant protein extract
- ◊ Calcium caseinate
- ◊ Sodium caseinate
- ◊ Yeast extract
- ◊ Textured protein
- ◊ Autolyzed yeast

ASPARTAME

Besides the evidence that it makes people fat, aspartame is terrible for the brain. Early animal studies showed aspartame caused seizures and brain tumors but the FDA approved it anyway. Aspartame is made up of three brain-damaging chemicals: aspartic acid, phenylalanine, and methanol. Formerly known as Nutrasweet, it now also goes by "AminoSweet". It is an easy chemical to avoid since it is always clearly labelled.

SUCRALOSE

Sucralose is branded as Splenda and is the sugar (sucrose) molecule bonded to a chlorine atom. As a "chlorocarbon", it is toxic to the brain. Some common side effects of using it are headaches, migraines, dizziness, brain fog, anxiety, depression, and ringing in the ears. Sucralose also prevents nutrient absorption and throws off the balance of your microbiome, causing a disruption in the brain-gut connection.

If you're trying to avoid the notoriously unhealthy sugar, consider using one of the naturally occurring "sugar-alcohols" derived from many plants, fruits, and vegetables. Xylitol is an example, a healthy sugar alternative extracted from birch wood. You'll find it in "sugar-free" chewing gums, mints, and other candies. It is extremely low on the glycemic index (5/100 vs sugar at 100/100) and you can use it in one-to-one ratio as a sugar substitute. As a bonus, a study has shown that it can inhibit the growth of bacteria responsible for cavities.

RED DYE #40

The food industry dumps 15 million pounds of artificial dyes into our food every year. About 40% is Red Dye #40, a petroleum-based substance that is brain toxic and known to contribute to ADHD, migraines, jitteriness, nervousness, and an inability to concentrate. It also goes by "Allura Red AC" and is found in candy, condiments, snack foods, baked goods, soda, juice, salad dressings, toothpaste, mouthwash, and medicine. Unfortunately it is also used to make brown, blue, orange, and even white things too. For example, without Red Dye #40, instant chocolate pudding would actually present itself as green because, shockingly, there is so little real chocolate in instant chocolate pudding.

Even though there are safe and natural alternatives available, artificial food dyes are a cheap way for manufacturers to make food even brighter and more appealing. Red dye #40 has been banned in many countries.

LECTINS:
NATURE'S TWO-EDGED NUTRIENTS

Most of us have been made very aware of the connection between diet, inflammation, and poor health. Most of the disease-causing chronic inflammation that plagues our society can be traced back to bad fats, sugar, and refined foods prominent in junk and fast food. But there are also "healthy" foods that are found showcased in the produce section of your grocery store that can significantly contribute to inflammation. These are foods high in lectins.

Lectins are a kind of protein that are referred to as "anti-nutrients", since they are notorious for causing inflammation and can reduce the body's ability to absorb nutrients. Lectins are thought to have evolved as a natural defence in plants, essentially as toxins that deter animals from eating the plants.

One way lectins wreak havoc in the body is to cause inflammation in the gut lining that results in hyper-permeability, especially for those who have an immune sensitivity to them. The condition is termed "leaky gut syndrome" and the unfortunate reality is that it's very common. Studies have shown that depressed patients and persons suffering from chronic fatigue syndrome often have leaky gut syndrome as well as excessive gut-derived Gram-negative bacteria in their blood and lymph systems. These elevated levels are strongly related to inflammatory, oxidative, nitrosative, and autoimmune processes in the body — and none of these are good. Some years ago researchers discovered a protein they called zonulin that regulates gut permeability and "can be used as a biomarker of impaired gut barrier function for several autoimmune, neurodegenerative, and tumoral diseases." Zonulin, more accurately called haptoglobin 2 precursor, was discovered in 2000 by Alessio Fasano and his team at the University of Maryland School of Medicine and is the gate keeper of intestinal cells responsible for absorption. When zonulin is elevated in the blood, it means too many unsolicited proteins, carbohydrates, toxins, and bacteria are being allowed into general circulation. In response, the immune system sounds the alarm in the form of inflammation as it works to attack and neutralize what it interprets as harmful infections.

The lactulose-mannitol intestinal permeability test is probably the gold standard. for the detection of leaky gut. These sugars are very different in size, actulose being a very large molecule and mannitol very small. The person being tested ingests measured amounts of both and urinary concentrations of both are then measured. As we'd expect, if a greater concentration than normal of the large lactulose molecule is found in the urine, a leaky gut is suspected.

GLUTEN

One lectin most of us are already familiar with — and perhaps with some annoyance — is the famous "gluten". High levels of gluten are present in wheat, barley, rye, and spelt and research has suggested that eating gluten can increase the risk of memory loss, dementia symptoms and even Alzheimer's disease. A true pathological reaction to gluten is called celiac disease and has more than quadrupled in the last thirty years for reasons that are not crystal clear. Other kinds of gluten intolerance now affect more than ten percent of the population. But what is known is that it's not necessary to have celiac disease or even gluten intolerance for gluten and other lectins to shrink memory performance. It's notorious for causing "brain fog" and in many people often induces a temporary, sometimes severe, inability to think clearly and perform tasks. If you haven't already tried this, remove gluten from your diet for six weeks, then purposely reintroduce it for a week and judge for yourself.

Besides gluten, a high lectin content is also found in red kidney beans, soy beans, peanuts, tomatoes, and potatoes. If these are some of your favourite foods, don't worry. The good news is that lectins are nearly completely eliminated by they way you prepare your food. Here's how:

The classic method of preparing legumes, beans, and grains is to soak them for twenty-four hours, changing the water as often as every few hours or as you can. Drain and rinse again before cooking. Adding sodium bicarbonate (baking soda) to the soaking water may help neutralize the lectins further.

Sprouting seeds, grains or beans also decreases the lectin content. Generally, the longer the duration of sprouting, the more lectins are deactivated. The lectins in some grains and beans are in the seed coat and as the seeds germinate, the coat is metabolized, thereby eliminating the lectins.

Fermentation is an excellent way to eliminate lectins. It works by allowing beneficial bacteria to digest and convert many of the harmful substances. It appears that the healthiest populations – including many of the centenarians who seem to live in various pockets around the globe – generally stick with fermented soy products like miso, tempeh, tamari and natto. Even some vegetables, such as cabbage, may have fewer anti-nutrients when fermented. Cultures with a history of grain eating traditionally have used some form of fermentation to treat grains. For example, if you've had sourdough bread or beer, you've consumed fermented grains.

Not all lectins are completely eliminated by these methods, and some particularly stubborn lectins – especially in beans – remain no matter how lengthy the treatment. So regardless of your sensitivity to grains and legumes, consuming a "paleo" diet – eating as our ancestors did in the pre-agriculture era 10,000 and more years ago and deriving our carbohydrates from fruits and vegetables rather than grains and beans, is an excellent strategy for developing an optimal memory. Check out the interview I had with Robb Wolf in Part II. Wolf is a former research biochemist and a two times New York Times Best Selling author, for *The Paleo Solution* and *Wired To Eat*.

A DAMAGED BRAIN:
THE PLAGUES

As we get closer, brain injury, brain toxicity, and brain disease often look unexpectedly similar. Many experts writing in this field now agree that inflammation, whether chronic or acute, is what links them. To make the point, let's briefly look at several well-known neurological diseases.

ALZHEIMER'S DISEASE

The list of neurological diseases is a long and painful one, but there are several I find particularly relevant to this book. I started its writing by recounting the story of my mother's recent diagnosis of Alzheimer's disease (AD), and then my father-in-law's diagnosis. In Part II, I interview my friend and colleague, Dr. Mehmet Oz, about how he missed his own mother's diagnosis and the genes his own brain wears, genes relevant to his risk for Alzheimer's. As the population ages, it seems that few of us will be spared at least knowing an Alzheimer's sufferer.

A great deal of research is focused on this miserable disease and much is written on the subject. It is sometimes confused with the term "dementia" but dementia is a collection of symptoms; Alzheimer's appears to be an actual disease, for which "dementia" describes associated symptoms. The seven stages of Alzheimer's are usually described as:

Stage 1: No Cognitive Decline
Stage 2: Age Associated Memory Impairment
Stage 3: Mild Cognitive Impairment
Stage 4: Mild Dementia
Stage 5: Moderate Dementia
Stage 6: Moderately Severe Dementia
Stage 7: Severe Dementia

Scientists are able to accurately identify the condition at a molecular and cellular level as characterized by tangles of brain proteins that formerly were part of the functioning brain network. But to date little is agreed in respect to its underlying cause and therefore its treatment. The genes unquestionably play a role at some level but fall short of a full explanation. The cholinergic hypothesis, once popular, proposes a reduced synthesis of the neurotransmitter acetylcholine as a critical step in the process, but treatments based on the cholinergic hypothesis have gone nowhere. The so-called amyloid plaques composed of tangled peptide chains are a clear markers for the disease and a genetic basis for their occurrence is a popular basis for several theories, though actually clearing the plaques has so far provided no relief from symptoms. Tau proteins are critical components of the internal structure of neurons and a theory holds that it's their malfunctioning that initiates the cascade of AD. Numerous other mechanisms have been proposed, all with some supporting evidence. Spirochete infections, chronic periodontal infection, and gut microbiota (the last two I discuss elsewhere in this book) have attracted attention, and dysfunction of the oligodendrocyte glia cells has been considered. Air pollution and smoking are fairly well established as risk factors.

Still, for all this wonderful work, no magic bullet has so far appeared and to a non-specialist such as myself, even these theories leave us with a sense that they are not ***ultimate*** causes. It's curious, though, how often chronic infection and chronic inflammation come up in the literature. My own clinical experience and reading has led me to a strong suspicion of chronic inflammation as the underlying cause of so many conditions, I wouldn't be at all surprised if Alzheimer's turns out to be one of them.

Dr. Dale Bredesen is the professor of neurology at UCLA and the best-selling author of ***The End of Alzheimer's***. He is internationally recognized as an expert in the mechanisms of neurodegenerative diseases such as Alzheimer's disease and I have him weigh in on the topic in Part II of this book. He has some game-changing insights and protocols and many of us believe that he may one day be a recipient of one of the most prestigious awards in science: the Nobel Prize in Physiology or Medicine.

PARKINSON'S DISEASE

Parkinson's is among the best known of the incurable neurological diseases, having been described in the early nineteenth century. I witnessed the father of a good friend of mine live with this disease for well over a decade and its insidious decline is as horrific as Alzheimer's. It is characterized neurologically by a depletion of the neurotransmitter dopamine and symptomatically by shaking, rigidity, slowness of movement and difficulty walking, with emotional, cognitive and mood disorders often occurring at later stages. The underlying cause is unknown but appears to a be a combination of genetic and environmental factors. I'm including it in this chapter because current research is pointing to exercise in middle age and the use of anti-inflammatory drugs as tending to lower the risk of Parkinson's. We don't have much else to go on, so as with Alzheimer's, I think the reduction of chronic inflammation is a protective bet.

CHRONIC TRAUMATIC ENCEPHALOPATHY

Here's where brain trauma and brain disease so obviously intersect. People diagnosed with chronic traumatic encephalopathy (CTE) suffer from changes in mood and behaviour that begin appearing in their 30s or 40s followed by problems with thinking and memory that can in some cases end in dementia. The culprit is a protein called ***tau***, whose task is to support tiny tubes — ***microtubules*** — inside our axons. Unlike Alzheimer's and Parkinson's, the ultimate cause of CTE is ***not*** controversial. Repeated sub-concussive hits cause damage to these microtubules; the tau proteins dislodge and clump together and so disrupt transport and communication within the neuron. A chain reaction develops as more clumps form and spread throughout the brain long after the athlete has retired and the repeated head insults have stopped. Studies of football players suggest that, because it's difficult to tell if a concussion has occurred in the first place, between 50% and 80% of concussions go unreported and untreated. And of course the athlete is under pressure — his or her own and pressure from others — to keep going for the sake of their careers and the team.

I've had the privilege of interviewing two of the world's preeminent doctors in this field. Whether you immediately recognize them by name or not, you'll want to read my interview with Dr. Julian Bailes and Dr. Mark Gordon in Part II.

ALL THE REST

I intend *Brainspanners* as a guide to the choices I hope will contribute to your greatest possible brainspan. I don't intend it to be a guide to serious neurological disease and I won't extend the above list to include multiple sclerosis, ALS, autism, schizophrenia, Creutzfeldt–Jakob disease, or any of the other dreadful afflictions that involve the brain. But I do suggest that, in the course of your own reading or watching, you keep an eye out for how the mechanisms of these diseases so often overlap with the drivers of everyday brain health — and its opposite.

While writing this book, I spoke to renowned psychiatrist and brain disorder specialist Dr. Daniel Amen, director of the Amen Clinics, located throughout the United States. That interview appears in Part II of this book. Dr. Amen works with many leading figures in American sports, so I intended to talk only about sports injury, but his real interest is in the brain itself and he had much to say about the common ground shared by traumatic injury, mental illness and preserving health in our more ordinary brains. So as does Dr. Amen, I'll now broaden our discussion to include the health of the brain for those of us who aren't suffering from a serious head trauma or a fatal brain disease.

Aspects of these catastrophic conditions seem often to lie along a spectrum that encompasses the brain's role in our daily and ostensibly healthy lives. I see evidence of this in my clinical practice, so much so that I'll devote the rest of this book to just that: our daily brains.

2

SHARPENING OUR FOCUS

Brain studies of mental workouts in which you sustain a single, chosen focus show that the more you detach from what's distracting you and refocus on what you should be paying attention to, the stronger this brain circuitry becomes.

~ *Daniel Goleman*

The benefits of focused attention — the ability to bring our powers of mental concentration to bear on a specific subject to the exclusion of other stimuli — are so obvious they hardly need recounting. Nonetheless, considerable research has been devoted to "multitasking" — performing two or more tasks simultaneously or switching rapidly between them — as a possible alternative to exclusive focus, since modern folklore often elevates multitasking to a virtue. That research has almost universally found multitasking to be inefficient compared to executing the same tasks successively. Focused attention, which we often (not always) find hard work, gets the job done right.

It's possible that the frequent references to multitasking may arise from a desperate effort to make a virtue of necessity. We live in a society in which our environment promotes attention deficits, even in persons of quite normal psychological make-up. We have more things to do in less time than we have to do them in, and more external stimuli than our nervous systems were ever equipped to deal with. A tendency to hyperactivity might seem adaptive, even though its consequences are frazzled nerves and a failure to sustain focus that results in diminished quality of life and workplace inefficiency. So we strive to be better focused, to improve our productivity, to perform better, faster, more energetically, and work longer days, improve our attention span, our alertness, our concentration. And yet, at the same time, we yearn for a calm and collected mind, less frazzled and distracted. Resolving the two is not a trivial problem for many.

For a small but significant number of people, failure to focus as expected manifests as an actual pathology, or at least an affliction, that goes by the name of "attention deficit disorder" (ADD) or "attention deficit and hyperactivity disorder" (ADHD). So much has been written and said on these conditions, I won't add more here except to point out how they highlight the milder but more widespread condition of the society at large.

THE ILLUSION SOLUTIONS

Perhaps because we often assume the cause to be chemical, we often seek chemical solutions. Sugar is not generally regarded as a medication, but its effects on the brain and other organs are as real as the effects of many drugs. Evolution has programmed us to love the stuff — a source of energy so hard to come by in our distant past — but increasingly advanced technologies over recent centuries have made it abundant. More recently still, equally advanced food industry sophistication has wrapped sugar in a thousand guises including savories such as breads, tomato sauces, crunchy snacks and "protein bars." The secret to sugar's great success is its ability to release a huge burst of the "feel good" neurotransmitter dopamine. Dopamine is of course a critical molecule in the operation of our brain and nervous system, but we have not evolved as a species to handle it in such overwhelming bursts. Our first response is a delightful wave of satisfaction and a perception of increased physical energy. This after all is why we ate the sugar. But no brain exposed repeatedly to this surge can fail to crave more and the results, if much milder, are similar to the habituation famously associated with powerful drugs such as cocaine. Of course sugar is cheap enough that, unlike cocaine, supply is no problem. But sugar's effects don't stop with a craving for dopamine highs. Like all stimulants, its overabundance in our systems is followed by a depletion, which we may experience as an unpleasant "sugar crash." And many studies have linked the chronic ingestion of too much sugar to true depression. But no matter which way the cause-and-effect arrow flies in the case of depression, sugar's other effects are not in its favour, as we'll see when we talk about diet.

It's a bit fanciful to think of sugar as a food, but almost everyone who drinks coffee recognizes caffeine to be a stimulant. To be sure, there's little evidence to support the notion of toxicity when coffee is drunk in moderation — say, two or three cups a day. But like many good things, excess changes coffee's character. Like sugar, it has addictive qualities normally found in more powerful drugs and too much for too long can produce symptoms such as heartburn, insomnia, anxiety, panic attacks, and over the long term, impaired learning and memory. And what goes for coffee goes for energy drinks, which needless to say usually contain caffeine ***and*** way too much sugar.

Ratcheting up the stakes several notches are the drugs over-prescribed for attention deficit disorder. There are of course patients who meet the criteria for ADD prescription medication, but the ready availability of these "smart drugs" is creating an epidemic that threatens the health of millions. ***The Journal of Attention Disorders*** reports that more than 1 in 10 prescribed medications such as Adderall are taken by people who have no diagnosis of attention deficit disorder and are simply misusing the drugs recreationally for their stimulant effects. But these "schoolastic steroids", affectionately referred to as "study buddies", commonly circulate on campuses and many taking them are quite unaware of the risks they are running: serious addiction, psychosis, stroke, and even death.

I won't delve further into the scourge of street drugs, whose reputations for destructive effects on the human mind and body are known to all my readers. Currently the non-stimulating opioids are stealing the headlines, but close behind are those that produce a stimulating effect on the central nervous system: the infamously expensive cocaine and the infamously cheap methamphetamine (crystal meth). They offer a sort of hyped-up version of the mental energy and focus we seek, but if sugar and caffeine in excess require us to pay a price for an unearned psychic boost, these two magnify that effect to a dreadful degree, as recovered addicts will unhappily testify.

WORKING WITH WHAT WE'VE GOT

In our discussion of genetics in Part IV, we'll see how research over the last century has allowed scientists to close in on the fundamental role genes play in so many of our brain's functions. It won't surprise you to learn that this extends to our ability to remain positive and focused. The DRD2 gene, for example, regulates the levels of the neurotransmitter dopamine, and dopamine significantly impacts memory, mood, pleasure, reward, cognition, focus, and attention. Another gene, ADRA2B, plays a critical role in regulating noradrenaline. Noradrenaline — like its closely-related cousin adrenaline — is a neurotransmitter in the brain that acts as a hormone in the body to regulate our response to stress — the famous fight-or-flight response. You can see how too much or too little noradrenaline might make a serious impact on or ability to focus.

These stress- and focus-related genes, like all genes, can occur in the variants we call SNPs, and these variants can entail differing abilities in processing responses. We don't aspire at this stage in medical technology to edit our DNA using CRISPR technology to optimize our focus and stress response, but we do understand much today about the ***expression*** of genes and how that expression can be managed through nutrition, lifestyle, and supplementation.

MAKING A PLEASANT EXPRESSION

Most of us are now aware that throughout much of the industrialized world, we're still eating a SAD diet, that is, the "Standard American Diet", though this moniker may lay too much credit and blame on Americans alone. The SAD is high in processed foods, especially grain-based products containing lots of white flour, sugar, and refined, nutrient-sparse packaged foods. This diet is pro-inflammatory and although acute inflammation is a natural part of the immune system's response to external threats, it is increasingly recognized that chronic inflammation plays a big part in a list of serious diseases long enough to fill this page. Sugar, which we've already met in its role as psychological destabilizer, is highly pro-inflammatory. An abundance of research findings supports these accepted facts: sugar promotes tooth decay, plays a role in joint inflammation and arthritis, causes skin to wrinkle and age prematurely, increases the risk of type 2 diabetes, high blood pressure, heart disease, kidney failure, and erectile dysfunction in men.

As with so much advice out there about what we should and shouldn't eat, and bearing in mind that we aim to keep boosting our mental focus front and center, what should guide us in our daily choices of food? Here is a simple thought that's surprisingly valid scientifically: Eat a rainbow of fruits and vegetables, preferably organic and grown locally.

Red foods, for example, have lots of lycopene, which has been proven to protect the brain against inflammation. Examples are: cherries, grapefruit, cranberries, pomegranate, red grapes, strawberries, watermelon, and most obviously but very importantly, tomatoes.

Orange and yellow foods contain carotenoids, pigments that have already been shown to be protective against several forms of human cancers. Along with bioflavonoids, which are also abundant in these foods, they are the subjects of research as anti-inflammatory agents and protectives against certain eye diseases, cancers and cardiovascular conditions. Meanwhile, these colorful molecules are known to protect brain cells against injury and to promote learning, cognitive function, and focus. Can't think of any except carrots? How about squash, apricots, mangos, papayas, pineapples, yellow peppers, sweet potatoes and yams? Sounds more like a feast than medicine.

Green foods contain lutein, also a carotenoid that accumulates in the brain and is beneficial for cognitive health across all ages due to its potency as an antioxidant. Don't just think leafy greens and broccoli. Think avocados, green apples, kiwis, artichokes, asparagus, and Brussels sprouts.

Blue and purple foods contain anthocyanins, which improve circulation to the brain and protect against neurodegenerative diseases. Think of blueberries, eggplants, Spanish onions, plums, and acaii berries.

I know this seems more a palette than a diet but I hope my message is coloring your thinking: brightly-hued natural foods are almost all great for health in general and often brain health in particular. And, as a general rule, it's not difficult to notice that potatoes and gravy don't seem to fit in this bright array and for that reason they merit a little wariness.

SUPPLEMENTS: MORE OF A GOOD THING

In general we distinguish supplements from medications on the grounds that the ingredients found in supplements are substances often already present in our diet, but ones we may benefit from taking more of. The vitamins are classic examples. In my clinical practice I've had success prescribing supplementation using natural ingredients. When I see patients who have been diagnosed with attention deficit hyperactivity disorder (ADHD) or who simply want to improve their attention and mental focus, I assume from the start that they are not suffering from a deficiency of the drugs Adderall, Ritalin, or Concerta. There are natural alternatives that have been shown in human clinical trials to promote a calm, alert, focused state — without drowsiness. One of these is the amino acid L-theanine, originally identified in green tea. L-theanine has been proven to induce relaxation by increasing alpha brain waves associated with relaxed, yet alert and focused brain activity. I recommend the Suntheanine branded ingredient in particular because it is extracted using a fermentation process that produces the purest L-theanine.

We touched earlier on coffee, which I neither praised nor damned. That's because the coffee picture is a little more complicated than we once thought. First, we need to recognize that the roasted bean lacks many of the natural ingredients useful for focus and attention: they've essentially been roasted out. Green coffee bean extract has enjoyed some popularity as an aid in weight loss, though evidence shows that the weight loss results may be significantly better when the chlorogenic acid in the extract is combined with caffeine. Either way, this extract has nothing to do with improving focus.

A study published in the British Journal of Nutrition examined whole coffee fruit (WCF), the bright red berry that surrounds the common coffee bean, ***Coffea arabica***. The researchers administered a single 100mg dose of WCF extract to a group of volunteers and observed a 143% increase in BDNF in their blood values. WCF contains naturally occurring antioxidants called procyanidins (which are known to protect brain cells) and a profile of polyphenols that may well explain its ability to raise BDNF so dramatically. Another coffee-derived product is whole green coffee powder, the entire raw green coffee bean dried, ground and delivered orally in a capsule. It captures all of the nutrients present in the unroasted green coffee bean and has been shown to improve focus and attention. The caffeine component is buried deep within the cellulose and fiber of the bean and so delivers a slow "time release" of the components — a natural study aid.

MEDITATE ON THIS

When we think of L-theanine and the green tea it's extracted from, we might think of Buddhist monks, who are known to drink a lot of the stuff. Surely the perfect image of calm, focused attention is a Buddhist monk in the middle of a deep meditation. Not only does meditation help keep us cool, calm, and collected, but research has also shown again and again that mindfulness meditation can boost attention span significantly. In one study, 140 volunteers took part in an eight-week course in meditation training. After the eight weeks, all the volunteers showed measurable improvements in attention span and other executive mental functions. But we don't have to spend our days meditating in a monastery to take advantage of this attention-boosting power. Research has shown that just 10 to 20 minutes of meditation a day will do the trick, with improvements in attention span after as little as four days.

Here's a favourite I call the Compassion Training Exercise.

Sit somewhere quiet and begin to focus on your breathing. Think about a time when you felt very kind and caring towards a person or an animal. Don't choose a time when that person or animal was too distressed or injured because the distress will distract you from your kind and compassionate feelings.

Focus on your desire to help the person or animal, and the feelings of kindness that will guide you to help. Remember, it is your intentions that are important, not how the person or animal may respond.

Imagine yourself expanding, as if you were becoming calmer, wiser, stronger, and more responsible, and better able to help him or her.

Pay attention to your body as you remember how it felt to be kind. Spend some time expanding with warmth in your body. Notice the genuine desire for this person to be free of suffering and to flourish.

Spend a minute or two thinking about the tone of your voice and the kinds of things you said, or the kinds of things you did or wanted to do to help.

Spend another minute or two on thinking about how good it felt to be kind to him or her.

Finally, focus only on your desire to be helpful and kind. You feel a deep sense of warmth, expansion, and hear the kind tone of your voice, the wisdom in your voice and in your behavior.

Try this every morning, first thing after waking. When you've finished this five minute exercise, take some notes about how it felt for you. Track whether you feel your focus is improving over the coming weeks.

3

SMARTENING UP

Learn from yesterday, live for today, hope for tomorrow.
The important thing is not to stop questioning.

~ Albert Einstein

Before we get down to work on human intelligence, let's settle an important question in the fairest possible way: a competition.

Who's better? The Boys or the Girls?

The whistle blows. The Boys are first on the field and, yes! They have bigger brains on average! They're between 8% and 13% larger! A full point in the first few seconds of play! One-nothing!

Play resumes and the Boys almost immediately score a cognitive advantage by keeping the ball at the mathematics end of the field. A solid lead! Two-naught, Boys!

There are a lot of women in the bleachers and they've fallen pretty quiet. Now it's a recall play and — wow! — the Girls show enhanced information recall compared to the Boys! Nobody was looking for that and it's a solid goal for the Girls to shrink the lead. We're 2 to 1 in the first half!

The teams are moving into frontal lobes now — that's motor function, ladies and gentlemen, that's problem solving, spontaneity, memory, language, initiation, judgement, impulse control — you name it. That's social and sexual behavior and the Boys have frontal lobes that are a bare 1% larger than the Girls. Will it be enough? What'll they do with them? Score! Alright, that goal just snuck by, ladies and gentlemen, but the Boys retake their commanding two-goal lead. Lotta hoarse and unhappy noises from the stands.

Now play has moved to the amygdala. That's emotions, survival instincts, and memory, fans! Yeah, there's a size comparison study in play and ... and the Boys have a 10% larger amygdala today. Booing from some poor losers in the stands and it's 4-1 for the Boys! Wait! What? The ref's on the field! It's a penalty flag on the play! Seems male brains are larger in general and ... the decision is ... after normalizing for brain size, there's no significant difference in cross-sex amygdala size! Goal discounted! Booing from the stands, friends. It's 3-1 Boys. Let's take a commercial break.

Fans, hope you're enjoying today's game, especially with the stakes so high. I know a lot of you are sitting glued to your screens right now and wondering to yourselves, "What have I done for my brain today?" Folks, a lot of advice is going to come your way over the next few hours, but let me say this: if you do nothing else, don't neglect your Brain Armor, the blend of proven cognitive health supplements backed by world-wide research. Don't enter the field without brain support. Take my advice, suit up with Brain Armor. And now let's get back to the game.

Ladies and gentlemen, we're back! We're back and we've just seen the Girls excel relative to the Boys on incredibly exciting tests that measured recollection. And now ... just moments later, fans, they've taken an advantage on processing speed involving letters, digits and — yes! — rapid-naming tasks. The crowd is out of their seats! Play is moving rapidly to the other end of the field and ... and the Girls have scored! The crowd's going crazy, folks! The girls have scored better on object-location memory ***and*** on verbal memory! Wait! It's unbelievable! The Girls have just performed better at verbal learning! I haven't seen anything like this since Buster Douglas K-Oed Mike Tyson in the 1990 heavyweight championship! The Girls have scored four straight goals while some fans were still looking for their seats! It's over, fans! It's over! Girls 5, Boys 3 in a massive gender upset!

{band plays}

Folks, while things are settling down out on the field, let me just say that studies have shown that exercise increases blood flow to the brain and helps build more connections between neurons, leading to increased concentration, enhanced memory, stimulated creativity, and better-developed problem solving skills. In short, my friends, playing sports — win or lose — helps brains grow and work better in Boys ***and*** Girls. So next time you...

Wait! Wait! There's an announcement! The Boys demand a rematch!

***

We all know what "intelligence" means. We meet people who are more or less intelligent every day. The problem is that, on slightly closer examination, intelligence means something different to everyone. As to the professionals, it's been said that if you ask 100 psychologists for a definition of the word, you'll get 100 different definitions — and many of them long and complex definitions too. Meanwhile, theoreticians have introduced subtle concepts such as fluid intelligence and crystallized intelligence and figurative intelligence and operative intelligence. Yet much remains a mystery. As we saw earlier when we talked about the genetic code, at least a third of the 20,000-odd human genes are expressed in the brain. Yet in a 2009 paper, "Genetic foundations of human intelligence", Deary, Johnson, and Houlihan reported that no finding of a strong single gene effect on IQ has been replicated. Though IQ tests are undoubtedly valuable for measuring parameters of mental ability, the suspicion remains that they're measuring specific abilities while missing others. Certainly we all know what "intelligence" means. We know we're more intelligent than our dog, right? Any of us could find our way two thousand miles back home without a map and without asking for directions, right? Right.

Earlier in the book, we looked at the events of prehistory that contributed to the enormous advances in intelligence that have shaped the ***Homo sapiens*** species. It's rather surprising then to learn that recent studies in the field of evolutionary biology suggest that our brains have begun to shrink since the agricultural revolution of 10,000 years ago — and the grain-heavy diet that was its consequence — made itself felt worldwide. To be sure, we don't yet know whether this shrinkage has been caused by leaving behind our hunter-gatherer behaviors or by the change in diet, but my personal sense is that it's more the latter that insults the brain and limits our ability to think clearly. That's why I recommend we preserve our big, intelligent brains by restricting or eliminating our pro-inflammatory diet of refined grains and carbohydrates. And it looks as though reducing our total daily caloric intake and adding intermittent fasting to our routine may also increase our intelligence. This is not as challenging as it might sound because it doesn't require that we change much about the way we eat. We simply restrict our "feeding window" to eight hours by, for example, not eating after 6 p.m. and delaying breakfast until 10 a.m.

SOME OTHER INTERVENTIONS

Hyperbaric oxygen therapy (HBOT) was originally developed to deal with diving accidents such as the "bends". It involves breathing pure oxygen in a pressurized room or tube and is employed to treat any condition that can benefit from the availability of extra oxygen. In the air you're breathing right now, the oxygen level is around 21% and the atmospheric pressure varies depending on altitude. Sea level is 760 mmHg. In an HBOT chamber, we're breathing 100% oxygen and the pressure is 1.5 to 3 times greater than the 760 mmHg at sea level. The result is a dramatic increase in oxygen flow to the brain. Adequate oxygen flow in the brain is vital for intelligence and low blood oxygen flow to the brain is associated with depression, ADHD, lack of focus, and substance abuse, among other things. Not surprisingly, when our blood is saturated with oxygen to a higher degree than average, our brain benefits. Maybe studying for an upcoming exam or preparing a work presentation is something we should do in an HBOT pod! A typical one-hour HBOT treatment session costs about $60.00.

I've already mentioned pulsed electromagnetic field therapy (pEMF) in the context of brain trauma but its worth bringing it up here again. We know that exposure to pEMF can increase circulation to the head by increasing capillary blood flow and reduce inflammation in the brain. It also appears effective for some persons suffering from depression. Over 2,000 published clinical studies show the benefit of pEMF on brain health from traumatic brain injury to enhanced cognitive function. The FDA and Health Canada have approved pEMF as safe. Because exposure to pEMF can result in a better supply of oxygen to the brain, a better supply of nutrients to the brain, and better disposal of metabolic waste from the brain, it is ideal support for the brain and the intelligence it embodies.

SUPPLEMENTING OUR INTELLIGENCE

Given the physical assaults and chemical insults sustained by our brains, we need every link we can forge in our brain armor. Here are a few that are sturdy in their defence of our intelligence.

◊ *Curcumin* is the bright yellow chemical that is one of the primary components in the spice turmeric. Both curcumin and turmeric have received much favourable attention for years because of their place in Ayurvedic medicine and turmeric's prominent culinary role in Indian curries. On its own, curcumin has some issues of bioavailability and its effectiveness has been disputed despite many studies. However in January 2018 a UCLA research group published the results of a rigorous study in the American Journal of Geriatric Psychiatry. The study strongly supports curcumin's active role in brain health. As Forbes magazine reported on the study, "the memory function of those who'd taken curcumin improved by 28% on average over the 18 months. In contrast, the control group's scores rose slightly (possibly because they got more familiar with the tests) and then declined. The depression scores of those taking curcumin also improved; the control group's didn't change. And interestingly, brain scans revealed significantly less amyloid and tau accumulation in two brain regions of the participants taking curcumin — the amygdala and hypothalamus — which control anxiety, memory, decision-making, and emotion."

Other research suggests that curcumin boosts neurogenesis — the production of new neurons in the hippocampus, essential for learning, memory and mood — and is a potent antioxidant that helps protect the brain from inflammation. Chronic inflammation has been linked to depression and dementia and to a lower IQ.

- *Resveratrol* is the naturally occurring compound famously found in red wine. In recent years it has gained a reputation among neurohackers for controlling brain inflammation, boosting dopamine, helping reverse cognitive decline and fighting brain cell aging.

- *Alpha lipoic acid* is a potent antioxidant with many neurological benefits and can easily cross the blood-brain barrier. Research has demonstrated its powerful protective benefits against cognitive and neurological diseases. It works to protect neurons and boosts the production of acetylcholine, a neurotransmitter involved in memory and intelligence.

- *Tocotrienols* are a sub-group of vitamin E which work to protect the brain from free radicals. Research shows high levels of tocotrienols in blood plasma are associated with a lower risk of mild cognitive impairment. Palm oil is the world's most abundant source of vitamin E tocotrienols. Studies have also shown that having a small amount of tocotrienols in your neurons may help the brain defend itself from stroke damage and may also improve your recovery from stroke. Having tocotrienols circulating in the bloodstream is also associated with improved cognition. Palm-derived tocotrienols can be found in some dietary supplements, such as those labelled "complete E," as well as in red palm oil used for cooking. Look for the ingredient "EVnol Suprabio™" on the label of your supplement bottle. This is a bio-enhanced natural full spectrum form of tocotrienols from sustainable Malaysian red palm fruit oil.

- *Lutein* is the carotenoid pigment found in leafy greens that I mentioned earlier when we were considering nutrients that support mental focus. In supplement form lutein may help with the preservation of so-called crystallized intelligence, the ability to use the skills and knowledge we've acquired over a lifetime.

- ◊ *Molecular hydrogen*
- ◊ *Two hydrogen atoms walk into a bar.*
- ◊ *"Damn!" one atom says. "I've lost an electron!"*
- ◊ *"How d'ya know?" asks the other. "You sure?"*
- ◊ *"I'm positive!" the first atom replies.*

As we saw in our chapter on nerve cell signalling, free radicals are ions — unstable molecules that actually have lost an electron. This makes them reactive and prone to pull electrons from other molecules to regain stability. Free radicals play vital roles in our cellular chemistry but a species of free radical called hydroxyl radicals have the potential to damage not just molecules but the cells they comprise. Antioxidants on the other hand are molecules that can stabilize free radicals and reduce their damage potential. Molecular hydrogen (H_2) — two hydrogen atoms bound together — has potent antioxidant properties that are specific to hydroxyl radicals. Hydrogen is the smallest atom of all and H_2 is a very small neutrally-charged molecule that is able to cross cell membranes and the blood-brain barrier, access the cell's mitochondria and the DNA in the cell core, and there support the cell's anti-oxidant mechanisms.

Research on molecular H_2 is extensive. Scientists have documented positive effects on the brain, on the cellular mitochondria, and energy levels. There is evidence that it may protect against neurodegenerative diseases such as Parkinson's and Alzheimer's, and against the effects of traumatic brain injury — all aspects of the neuroinflammation characteristic of the "damaged brain" conditions. H_2 has no known side effects and an excellent safety profile. It is now available in supplement form as a magnesium hydride tablet that, when dropped into a glass of water, releases H_2 gas into solution, where it forms large bubbles similar to those in carbonated water. These H_2 bubbles remain in solution long enough to drink and achieve the studied systemic effects and brain benefits.

◊ *RiaGev* is a new ingredient technology soon to debut in dietary supplements. RiaGev uniquely combines Bioenergy Ribose and vitamin B_3 to help slow the aging process from the inside out. It supports memory and cognition by boosting cellular ATP and NAD levels, both of which are known to decline with age. It also increases activation of sirtuins, the so-called "longevity enzymes" that help regulate our lifespan in part by promoting DNA repair and playing an essential role in the cellular response to environmental and emotional stress.

◊ *Phenolaeis* is another bioactive palm fruit complex, a new healthy aging ingredient produced by capturing functional nutrients from the water stream that was previously discarded during palm oil production. Palm fruit bioactive complex (PFBc) contains five unique polyphenols plus protein, fiber and carbohydrates. Clinical studies have shown that PFBc might be useful in supporting a healthy antioxidant status in the brain, promote healthy neurons, maintain better mood and clearer thinking, support brain function as we age, and promote cognitive health by supporting a healthy microbiome

◊ *Chewing gum.* Okay, okay. This looks like my little joke, but serious research at Cardiff University and elsewhere suggests that chewing gum improves memory, alertness, mood, and learning as well as reduces anxiety. The exact mechanism is unknown but increased blood flow to the brain is suspected. Studies have suggested that chewing gum for about 20 minutes before taking a test sends blood to the brain equivalent to the effect of mild exercise and measurably improves performance. Cortisol levels fall too, suggesting stress reduction. Choose chewing gum sweetened with xylitol or erythritol and, of course, only walk at the same time if you're comfortable doing so.

THE IQ TEST

Since we have great difficulty defining intelligence, it's no wonder that devising tests to measure it has proved a challenge. The first systematic efforts towards developing a quantitative intelligence test were made towards the end of the nineteenth century with the aim of identifying mental retardation in schoolchildren. Perhaps significantly, Alfred Binet. who was one of the inventors of the 1905 Binet-Simon test to determine a child's "mental age" stressed what he saw as the remarkable diversity of intelligence and the subsequent need to study it using qualitative, as opposed to quantitative, measures. Tests measuring "intelligence quotient" (IQ) — a measure of intelligence adjusted for age — have ever since been devised, revised (to reflect a broader range of aptitudes) but still usually calibrated so that an average score is 100. The Stanford-Binet and the Wechsler Adult intelligence Scale are the most widely used IQ tests today. Brain volume, speed of neural transmission, and working memory capacity have all been correlated to IQ, as have disease, lifespan, parental social status. and parental IQ.

As you can see from the tenor of my comments, I'm not recommending we place huge emphasis on measuring our own intelligence. If it amuses you to do so, do so. But a more worthwhile goal is to enhance and preserve the intelligence we each have.

4

KEEP THIS IN MIND

There is no memory or retentive faculty based on lasting impression. What we designate as memory is but increased responsiveness to repeated stimuli.

~ Nikola Tesla

In the first part of this book, we did a lightning sightseeing tour of the nervous system that culminated in a quick drive-by of the brain itself. We necessarily missed a lot of real attractions but we did linger briefly in the limbic system between the frontal cortex and the brain stem. Not only is the limbic region home to a lot of interesting little parts, but many of these parts are clearly related to memory. And memory — let's admit it, my friends — is of great interest to us all. We may not be overly concerned about whether or not we can solve quadratic equations or juggle four balls, but we're awfully concerned about remembering things.

Let me say at the start that all the processes of memory are far from understood. Science has made remarkable advances through careful study and experimentation. We have some solidly established truths and a great many ingenious categories, classification systems and useful theories. But so complex is our capacity for memory and so dazzling the potential of our 100 trillion (that's a "t") synapses, we must proceed with some humility.

We once believed that memory was a sort of vast filing cabinet packed into our heads. A bit later we refined this to a huge hard drive. Then we realized this was all wrong. Memory is a remarkably subtle process that may involve the whole brain in an ever-changing network, even while specific regions perform specific tasks. Today many neuroscientists believe that memories may be stored primarily in the ***synapses*** rather than the cell bodies of the neurons and that new memories are formed as these synapses are strengthened and weakened. The mapping of that network of connections is the new field of connectomics. To date, these ideas have been difficult to test, but as connectomics matures, scientists may be able to investigate the neural underpinnings of memory storage and retrieval with even greater accuracy.

Back to that tour. You'll remember the hippocampi — the two tiny "seahorses" embedded in the limbic region and now understood to be intimately involved in the creation and processing of memory. As we saw, this is where neurogenesis — the growth of new brain cells — happens, perhaps 700 to 2,000 a day — ***if***, that is, we take good care of our brains.

Clearly the brain can only receive information via the senses. We smell the perfume, see the face, hear the voice, touch the skin. All this sensory input arrives at the brain via separate neural roads. The perceptions are known to be held fleetingly in the senses, then for precious moments in the frontal cortex as short-term memory, where for example a telephone number is held while we dial. Now the powerful little integrator we call the hippocampus melds (or "encodes") these perceptions into a unified experience. Meanwhile more sensory inputs flood in every second. Even if they're successfully integrated with one another, what is the brain to do with this ceaseless stream? Researchers now believe that the hippocampus, in cooperation with the frontal cortex (the big thinker at the front of the cerebrum where among other things we make "deliberate" decisions), determine what will be allowed to dissolve and what will be distributed to other parts of the brain and so retained in long-term memory with its seemingly unlimited capacity and perhaps life-long duration. When called for, these memories will be retrieved, though by a process still rather mysterious to us.

Mysterious, wonderful, but not always accurate. As a product of evolution, the brain might be viewed as a vast improvisation, one that has enabled our species to survive and flourish, though not necessarily through achieved perfection. Remember the family reunion you attended in your twenties? The one at the farm when your cousin Carolyn got stoned? That was great fun, right? Right, but, um, actually you missed it. You were home with the 'flu part of that autumn but so many people have told you about it over the years, it's carved its way into your personal memory cache as if you were there.

We all experience memory failures from time to time, but false memories are unique in that they represent ***distinct*** recollections of things ***that did not happen***. False memories are not about forgetting something or mixing up details of things we experienced. They're about remembering things that we never experienced in the first place. It has been suggested that police line-ups can result in a 50% error rate. The guilty have walked away free and the innocent have been punished on the evidence of well-intentioned witnesses' false memories. It's the consensus of memory researchers that false memories afflict everyone, even those with the best memories of all. But whatever the practical consequences of false memories, they have something to teach us about memory itself.

Some researchers believe that the networks of neurons that constitute a memory are stored adjacent to similar memories and the act of recalling may intertwine one with another to cause new connections and the distortion of the original memory. If there are gaps in a memory as a result of, say, a neurological disease or even the passage of time, the brain may fill in these gaps with related connections. This unconscious "confabulation" may be completely convincing for the person experiencing it. The brain, constructive by nature and inclined to create narratives about our future, may in that process cause related memory distortions about our past. Certainly memory appears to be fragile, malleable and prone to errors for all of us. It might not be difficult to explain this.

Imagine you are in an Indian jungle and you see the grass moving suspiciously a hundred feet away. You panic and run for fear there's a tiger stalking you. However, even if tigers ate computers, a computer in the jungle that spotted the moving grass might calculate that 99% of the time observed grass movements of this kind are caused by wind. Flight would be irrational — and sure enough, if we were persuaded to think like the computer, we'd be eaten only 1% of the times grass moved suspiciously. Our brain however has evolved to make irrational assumptions and make 99 errors out of 100 but the final score is: one disappointed tiger. False memories may be a product of these irrational assumptions, evidence of a memory system that's working well by making rapid inferences.

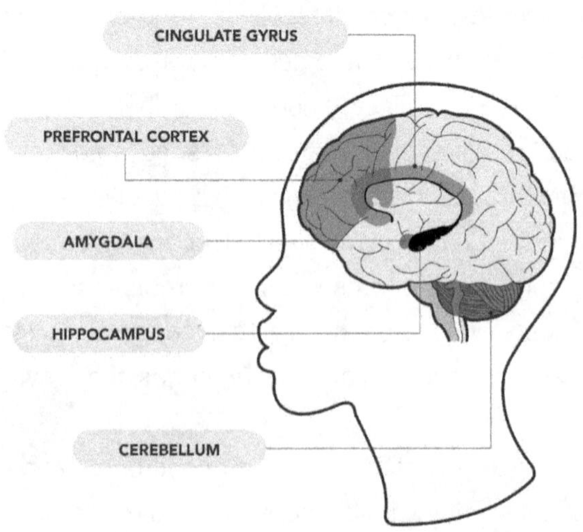

Structures of the limbic system involved in memory formation. The prefrontal cortex in charge of decision making and executive function holds recent events briefly in short-term memory. The hippocampus is responsible for encoding long-term memory. Skill memory of repetitive actions such as tying our shoes or riding a bike are handled by the cerebellum.

Long-term memories are of course more complex than short-term ones, with various long-term systems employed for repetitive procedures, for past life experiences, for language and for other categories of things to be remembered. Memory investigators have for example distinguished between explicit and implicit memory.

Explicit memory is easily recognized. We've almost all gone through that arduous exercise of deliberately remembering (we call it "memorizing") a large volume of material. The night before a final exam is the classic example. Under those stressful conditions, we employ conscious thought to create a type of long-term memory that can be retrieved consciously. Memory champions perform remarkably at explicitly committing large volumes of information into their brains for long periods of time. While the brain of a memory champion is structurally no different than yours or mine, they seem to have cracked the code by using — among other brainspanner techniques — a long-recognized technique called the "Memory Palace". In Part II, I interviewed two world champions: Nelson Dellis and Yanjaa Wintersoul, who gave me some tips and tricks on how ordinary folks can become memory champions.

As opposed to explicit memory, implicit memory, also long-term, does not require conscious thought to create, is both unconscious and unintentional, and cannot be retrieved by conscious effort or verbally articulated. Sound strange? Think about getting back on a bike when you haven't ridden for years. The number of action and perception components to be recalled and assembled to execute this task must be enormous. Yet off you go — and effortlessly too. Afterwards, you can't describe a single thing about those actions that you had to "remember".

Thus does modern brain science slowly untangle the subtle ways of the brain and strives to integrate them with our deepening knowledge of its anatomy. An example is sleep research.

We now know that sleep actively helps our brains consolidate what we learn and store as long-term memory. At brief intervals during non-REM sleep, several types of neural activity — brain waves — sweep through, reinforcing synaptic connections (memories) that the hippocampus/frontal cortex committee determines to be worth remembering, while weakening others. "Neurons that fire together wire together" is the principle and this "re-experiencing" of useful experience during sleep is how it's accomplished. We'll look at it again when we come to our discussion of sleep.

BDNF: A CRITICAL PROTEIN REVISITED

It's time to drop in again on the gene called BDNF, the one that expresses a signalling protein called brain-derived neurotrophic factor (neurotrophin), a member of the growth hormone family. Neurotrophins (from the Greek *trophikós* pertaining to food) promote the survival and general flourishing of specific neurons by preventing them from undergoing the programmed cell death called apoptosis. The neurotrophins accomplish this by stimulating the differentiation of progenitor cells to form new neurons, and by encouraging the sprouting of axons and dendrites that form new synapses between the cells.

The BDNF gene expresses BDNF in the retina, in the central nervous system, in the motor neurons, the kidneys, and the prostate. But we're concerned here with its important work in the cortex, the cerebellum, the basal forebrain, and especially our little friend the hippocampus, because these regions of the brain are vital to learning, memory, and higher level thinking. And since deficiencies of this vital protein have been linked to declines in these mental functions — and even a person's ability to recover from physical and emotional traumas — it makes sense to assure that the brain has an adequate supply.

EATING FOR OUR INNER SEAHORSE

Researchers have shown that BDNF levels are significantly boosted by omega-3 fatty acids, particularly docosahexaenoic acid (DHA). Throughout this book, I cite the omega-3 group. It's the most researched nutrient in the world, with well over 25,000 published papers to date illustrating the positive health benefits of a diet rich in these essential fatty acids. DHA is an omega-3 fatty acid that accounts for approximately 97 percent of the omega-3 fats in the brain. And not surprisingly, dietary omega-3 fatty acid supplements, especially DHA supplements, have been shown to significantly improve brain health and neuronal development, as well as enhance cognitive function. Omega-3s have been convincingly shown to help reduce inflammation, and chronic inflammation is believed to contribute to cognitive decline and memory loss. Centenarians — those people who live to be more than a hundred years old — exhibit high DHA levels compared to the average person.

Salmon is a rich source of omega-3 fatty acids including the brain omega-3, DHA. Our problem is that modern waters often contain mercury, dioxins, furans, PCBs and other potent neurotoxins that can concentrate in the tissues of larger fish. Relying on a diet high in those fish to achieve our omega-3 essential fatty acids is no longer ideal. Fortunately, we are now able to supplement with purified forms of omega-3 that are high in DHA. When you're shopping for a brain-supporting supplement, look for a 2-to-1 ratio of DHA to EPA (another omega-3 essential fatty acid) from an algal source. Omega-3 fatty acids originate within algae, mainly in the form of DHA, and algae are the base of the food chain for fish, whose metabolisms concentrate EPA and DHA omega-3s in their tissues. EPA and DHA from an algal source is every bit as bioavailable as that from a fish source but one kilogram of algal omega-3 ingredient has the potential to replace as much as 12 kilograms of wild fish that won't need to be caught to make fish oil. This makes algal omega 3s a clear environmentally-friendly choice.

Bacopa monnieri is a widespread herb that has long been used in traditional medicine for longevity and cognitive enhancement. A 2014 study published in ***The British Journal of Clinical Pharmacology*** compared the pharmaceutical modafinil (prescribed for the enhancement of attention, executive functions, and learning, as well as sleepiness due to narcolepsy) to ginseng and ***Bacopa monnieri*** and concluded that "these data confirm that neurocognitive enhancement from well characterized nutraceuticals can produce cognition enhancing effects of similar magnitude to those from pharmaceutical interventions." Taking ***Bacopa*** in supplement form has since been shown to improve memory formation in all ages by promoting neuron communication, enhancing the rate at which brain cells communicate by increasing the growth of nerve endings called dendrites. The standard dose for *Bacopa monnieri* is 300mg. When you're shopping for this herb, look for a total bacoside content of at least 55%.

Citicoline is also a potent supplement that can improve memory impairment associated with aging, supply neuroprotective effects, and enhance learning. Published studies show that it can increase dopamine receptor densities and is more effective than the supplement phosphatidylcholine. Dosages range from 500 to 2,000 mg in two divided doses, morning and evening.

In my own clinical practice, many of my patients have reported significant memory improvement when taking a combination of DHA:EPA omega-3 with 300mg Bacopa, and 2000mg citicoline daily.

Déjà Vu

You'll know people who believe the déjà vu experience to be a paranormal phenomenon, perhaps a prophetic one. But modern science regards it as an anomaly of memory, since despite the strong sense of recollection, the time, place, and practical context of the "previous experience" are, er, uncertain. If we travel frequently or watch more movies than the average person, researchers have found that we're more likely to experience déjà vu, and experience it more often when we're under pressure. But just like memory, déjà vu becomes less frequent with age

What's it about? One theory is that experience is "misplaced" from memory centres and contained elsewhere in the brain. Then a similar occurrence might invoke the contained knowledge. This leads to a feeling of repetition because the event being experienced in the present seems already to have been experienced in the past but is not remembered.

Some theorists suggest that memory is a process of reconstruction, rather than the recall of fixed, established events. This reconstruction is assembled from stored components and involves elaborations, distortions, and omissions. Each successive recall of an event is merely a recall of the last reconstruction. A sense of recognition involves achieving a good "match" between the present experience and our stored data. But in the case of déjà vu, the reconstruction may now differ so much from the original event that we "know" we have never experienced it before, even though it seems similar. "I have special powers!" thinks the déjà vu-er.

WORK-OUTS FOR THE BRAIN

There's now plenty of scientific evidence that, in addition to nutrition and supplementation, lifestyle techniques that ***stretch*** our ability to recall — and this will come as no surprise — ***strengthen*** our ability to recall. As an example, try making a list — grocery items, things to do, whatever — and memorize it. An hour or so later, see how many items you can recall. Memory also appears to improve through learning something new such as a recipe, a musical instrument, or a language. Exercise alone has been linked to brain health and memory, but refining hand-eye abilities by learning a new activity that utilizes both mind and body — yoga, golf, or tennis are examples — is just that much more effective.

REPORT CARDS FOR THE BRAIN

Memory can be measured. If you're concerned about your own memory and are considering interventions beyond common-sense brain supplements, you may want to take an online cognitive test, the Montreal Cognitive Assessment, a widely used screening assessment tool for detecting memory impairment. Scores range between 0 and 30 and a score of 26 or higher is considered to be normal. People without diagnosable cognitive impairment typically score between 27 and 30. Those with mild cognitive impairment score on average 22, and those with Alzheimer's disease score around 16 or lower.

Meanwhile, given the intimate link between omega-3s and brain function, you might want to know more about your nutritional status. OmegaQuant, run by Dr. Bill Harris, an internationally recognized expert on omega-3 fatty acids, offers the highest quality analytical services dealing with essential fatty acids. Find the OmegaQuant site at www.TheLivingBrainProject.com

5

IT'S ALL IN OUR HEADS

You, yourself, as much as anybody in the entire universe, deserve your love and affection.

~ Buddha

Mood is a mysterious aspect of human experience, a diffused emotional state that appears as separate from and underlying sharper emotions such as anger, fear or grief, and also separate from and underlying conscious thought. Yet clearly mood interacts with these other aspects of consciousness. We have a hard time saying much about moods except that they're "good" or "bad", "negative" or "positive", yet negative moods are associated with negative thoughts and negative emotions and sometimes negative performance. In their most extreme form, they can constitute mental illness.

In many respects, mood appears to be a proxy for the energy level of the central nervous system. We know that stimulants of the central nervous system such as cocaine and amphetamines (including MDMA, the street drug known as Ecstasy) induce temporarily positive moods and even productivity. When the effect of these chemicals wears off, the depressive effect on the CNS induces a negative mood. And actual chronic depression — perhaps the ultimate bad mood — is characterized by low energy at every level.

Mood is elusive and subtle, yet sometimes appears to control all. What can we do to control *it*?

MOOD STRATEGIES: COGNITION

Research has pointed to ways by which we can harness and control mood and a good example is the role of mood in learning. Someone's estimated that we each have approximately 70,000 thoughts per day, but for many people, 90% of those thoughts are the same thoughts they thought the day before. The same thoughts lead to the same choices, the same choices lead to the same behaviours, the same behaviours create the same experiences, and the same experiences produce the same emotions. The circularity of this surely deserves to be called "unproductive." It smacks of an unconscious process, of someone on "autopilot" and it seems reasonable that the more conscious we become of our states of mind and body, the less likely we are to remain in or revert to "autopilot" states. The mind off of autopilot, almost by definition, is better able to learn and re-learn valuable skills, better able un-learn self-destructive behaviours, and more likely to experience new and better outcomes. This business of becoming conscious of our thinking is called "metacognition." Metacognition is cognition about cognition, thinking about thinking, knowing about knowing, becoming aware of one's awareness. Metacognition is a set of higher-order thinking skills that enable learners to become aware of how they learn, and to evaluate and adapt these skills to increasingly effective learning. Metacognition consists of the ***knowledge of cognition*** but also the ***regulation of cognition.***

Knowledge of cognition has three components. First: knowing the factors that influence one's own performance. Second: knowing general strategies to use in learning. Third: knowing specific strategies to use for a specific learning situation. For example, a student engaged in intensive learning can just blunder ahead by reading and cramming, but it's far more efficient if he or she can become aware of the behaviours that help recall facts, names, and events. Which strategies are most effective for solving problems? What is the student's own style of learning? Visual, tactile, auditory? These are examples of your knowledge of cognition.

Regulation of cognition also has three components. First: setting goals and planning. Second: monitoring and controlling learning. Third: evaluating one's own regulation by assessing results and strategies. As examples, regulation of cognition might include ***developing a plan, monitoring our understanding,*** and ***evaluating our thinking*** after completing a task.

During the ***planning*** phase we may ask ourselves: what am I supposed to learn? What prior knowledge will help me with this task?, What should I do first? What should I look for in this reading? How much time do I have to complete this?

During the ***monitoring*** phase we may ask ourselves: how am I doing? How should I proceed? What information do I need to commit to memory? What should I do next if I do not understand?

During the ***evaluation*** phase we might ask: how well did I do? What specifically did I learn? Did I achieve the results I expected? What could I have done differently? Can I apply this way of thinking to problems in the future? Are there any gaps in my knowledge?

These metacognitive strategies enable us to effectively manage what are in effect mood issues: the anxiety associated with the learning process, the worry related to failure, and the uncertainty we associate with the mastering of new skills. The result is not only that our mood is optimized during the learning process, but the association of a positive mood during learning will help consolidate stronger connections in the brain. It goes without saying that when our mood is predominantly anxious or overly stressed, our brain defaults into fight-or-flight mode and cares only about survival. Retaining new skill sets takes a back seat.

MOOD STRATEGIES: BIO-HACKING

We're bioelectric beings, or more accurately, we're bio-chemical-electric beings. Our brain is the perfect illustration. As we saw when we talked about the nervous system, the billions of brain cells in our head aren't really... well... connected. Chemical neurotransmitters must cross the gaps — the synapses — between those cells and as we've seen, this bio-chemical-electric signalling is what underlays thought. But the behaviour of these neurotransmitters, as we now know, plays a central role in mood and the good news is: we can optimize mood by "bio-hacking" — positively influencing — our brain's inherent flexibility — its neuroplasticity. First, let's review the brain's main neurotransmitters.

GABA functions as the "off" switch in the brain and is the major inhibitory neurotransmitter that improves mood, relieves anxiety, and promotes sleep.

Glycine plays a dual role as a neurotransmitter and as an amino acid that serves as a building block for proteins, improves sleep quality, calms aggression, and acts as an anti-inflammatory agent

Glutamate functions as the "on" switch in the brain and is the major excitatory neurotransmitter that decreases sleep, optimizes learning, memory, and mood, and improves libido.

Histamine plays a dual role in the body as a neurotransmitter and immunomodulator that increases metabolism, promotes wakefulness, and suppresses appetite.

PEA promotes energy, elevates mood, regulates attention and aggression, and serves as a biomarker for attention deficit and hyperactivity disorder (ADHD).

Dopamine, generally regarded as the brain's pleasure and reward molecule, plays a central role in addiction, improves attention, focus and motivation, and modulates movement control. I'll have more to say about dopamine in a moment.

Norepinephrine and ***epinephrine*** function as neurotransmitters and hormones that regulate the "fight or flight" response and elevate blood pressure and heart rate, as well as stimulate wakefulness. We can modify and influence these neurotransmitters through diet, lifestyle, and supplementation.

Serotonin is the neurotransmitter generally regarded as the "happiness molecule". It contributes to the feeling of calm and well-being that eases depression and anxiety, supports sleep, and decreases appetite. So we do understand something of its complex role in regulating mood while modulating cognition, reward, learning, memory, and numerous other neurological processes. But is there anything we can we do to support its work?

"Shinrin-yoku" or "forest therapy" is Japanese. It means "taking in the forest atmosphere" or "forest bathing" and was developed during the 1980s. It has since become a cornerstone of preventive health care and healing in Japanese medicine. Its health benefits don't simply derive from the aesthetic pleasures of forest greenery and floral smells — definitively mood boosters — but can be attributed to the powerful — and long studied — generation of negative ions by the splashing of water and radiance of the sun, the very elements at work in a forest. When we were discussing signalling in the brain and nervous system, we touched on the role of ions — atoms with more electrons (negative ions) or fewer electrons (positive ions) than is usual. But here we're talking about naturally generated negative ions in the environment that have been repeatedly shown to clean the air by neutralizing smoke particles, mould spores, bacteria and other undesirables. Modern pollution has upset the negative/positive ion balance, so those places where negative ions abound are a gift to our systems, including our brains. A review and meta-analysis published in 2013 in the journal ***BMC Psychiatry*** concluded that, for those suffering from seasonal and chronic depression, "negative ionization, overall, was significantly associated with lower depression ratings" and offered as much relief as antidepressants — without the side effects. Other studies have suggested that weather-sensitive subjects who experience negative mood effects with the approach of hot, dry weather systems and associated positive air ions show elevated blood serotonin levels. However, artificially-generated negative air ions induced a return to normal serotonin levels and an improvement in mood in these subjects. Studies such as these and others encourage us to take seriously the claims of forest bathers.

Among the symptoms of chronic dehydration can be depression, anxiety, and irritability. The amino acid tryptophan, famously concentrated in Thanksgiving turkey, is converted to serotonin in the brain but the efficiency of the conversion is limited by the availability of water. If we don't drink enough water, tryptophan can't be effectively transported across the blood-brain barrier and serotonin levels fall.

MOOD THIRST

So yes, there appears to be a hydration-serotonin connection, but dehydration alone can decrease energy production in the body — and the brain. Our cells are fuelled by adenosine triphosphate (ATP), the body's energy currency manufactured by the thousands of mitochondria found in all cells, including the 86 billion neurons in the brain. The mitochondria rely on water as a key ingredient in the recipe for ATP production.

Dehydration can also cause stress, and visa-versa. When our brain perceives stress, our adrenal glands pump out increased cortisol, the stress hormone. Under chronic stress, these glands can become exhausted. And because they also make the hormone aldosterone, which helps regulate the body's fluid and electrolyte levels, as adrenal fatigue progresses, aldosterone production drops, triggering dehydration and low electrolytes. There's a sound basis for drinking plenty of water to maximize brain function. The general rule is to drink half of your body weight in ounces of water daily. For example, if you weigh 180 pounds, you would want to drink about 90 ounces of water. If an average glass is 8 ounces, this would translate to just over 11 glasses daily, depending on your activity level.

You can do a quick check of your hydration status by monitoring the color of your urine. Urine is a very pale straw-yellow when you are properly hydrated. If your urine is dark yellow or tan in color, "urine trouble" as we say.

DOPAMINE AND MOOD

Dopamine — famously the "feel good" brain chemical tied to emotion and pleasure — is one of the most powerful neurotransmitters in the brain. It controls and influences reward, as is evidenced by its release when we eat chocolate, drink coffee or receive a text message from a favourite person.

Recent studies have suggested that low dopamine levels in the brain are associated with cravings and overeating. We're familiar with this endogenous (that is, "from within") mechanism because it sounds so similar to that of the exogenous (that is, "from without") mechanism of the opiate drugs. When we indulge in rich or excessive foods, we may feel good and experience an almost drug-like "high" as a result of the elevated levels of dopamine released in our brains. As the levels fall, we don't feel so good. And if we don't know better, we'll know what to do about it, won't we? More of the same. Right. Eventually over-eating causes a chronic decline of dopamine in the brain and a decrease in the neural receptors in charge of satiety. Ultimately we can crave more and more without ever feeling satisfied. This effect is especially dependant on an individual's variant of the DRD2 gene.

Because the rush of dopamine feels so good, we want more of it. This drives us to repeat the behaviours that create the rush, even when we aren't yet experiencing the end game of success. Because the brain remembers what success feels like, we seek it out again and again and seeking success becomes an even more potent dopamine releaser than the final reward success itself brings. The anticipation of success can be addictive and researchers have concluded that addictive behaviour is in fact rooted in the dopamine reward system.

Besides the biochemical buzz we get from dopamine, it — perhaps unsurprisingly — also boosts our BDNF levels. But the BDNF boost from dopamine only results from healthy activities such as competing in or winning a race, solving a problem, or getting a promotion after years of hard work. Feeling successful — or simply engaging in the act of seeking out success — actually increases neuronal activity, neuroplasticity, and brain health. BDNF levels decline from recreational drug use, alcohol use, work addiction, or gambling.

We can even see this principle at work in the addictive spiking and dropping of dopamine levels that follow behaviors as mundane as your poor food behavior — not ***yours***, of course, but the behaviors of folks who don't realize where they're heading.

1. They make routine late-night trips to the fridge, at least twice a week
2. They regularly eat even when they're physically full.
3. They feel irritable or tired when they try to cut down on their favorite foods.

Many of us are guilty of over-consuming three common dopamine disruptors.

Caffeine: Yes, caffeine can diminish food cravings but many experts believe that it can also rob the brain of dopamine and so induce more cravings. I recommend that we limit our coffee consumption to three cups daily, which deliver about 250mg to 300mg caffeine.

Sugar: It would be hard today to find any medical authority who would not condemn sugar as a nutrient. Repeated blood-sugar spikes can lead to insulin insensitivity and by burning out the dopamine supply, causing cravings — often for more sugar.

Vegetable oil: It has been widely accepted for years that vegetable oils are the heart-healthy alternative to saturated fats. But all may not be as it seems. Vegetable oils — almost universally present in the processed foods we eat — are making us fat by promoting snacking. Research suggests that oils such as canola, corn and soy are not only high in pro-inflammatory omega-6 but are even more likely to increase appetite by inducing a surge of dopamine, which in turn signals the brain to call for more carbohydrates. The ideal replacement for vegetable is olive oil, but not just any type. Extra virgin olive oil (EVOO) is the natural juice cold-pressed (or squeezed) from fresh olives and is the highest grade of olive oil. It displays true olive character with respect to aroma and taste and is free of any defective flavours. It also possesses the superior chemistry that characterise the high quality oils of this grade. The two highest quality EVOOs I've come across (and use personally) are "Cobram Estate" by Boundary Bend and Acropolis Organics.

Snack foods saturated in vegetable oil and sugar just won't polish. At the University of California, researchers found that when animals are given a diet heavy in soybean oil — a diet equivalent to that consumed by a typical American — they gained 25 percent more weight than when on an equivalent coconut-oil diet and 12 percent more than those fed fructose. The soybean oil group also developed larger fat deposits and were more likely to become diabetic. Vegetable oils are arguably among our brain's worst enemies, known to increase the risk of conditions such as Alzheimer's and dementia. On the other hand, foods rich in L-tyrosine — an amino acid that boosts dopamine levels in the brain — tend to diminish cravings. Duck, chicken, ricotta cheese, oatmeal, mustard greens, fava beans, edamame, dark chocolate, seaweed and wheat germ are all high in L-tyrosine. A diet that incorporates as many of these as possible will provide your brain with a firm underpinning of dopamine. And should you run out of recipes that combine duck, chocolate and oatmeal, you can also take L-tyrosine as a supplement, 500 to 1,000 mg on an empty stomach when you wake up in the morning. (If you are on thyroid medication or have Parkinson's disease, speak to your healthcare provider before doing this.) The omega-3 fatty acid DHA works to increase the effectiveness of L-tyrosine and the overall production of dopamine. Try this with supplemental L-tyrosine and DHA for at least six weeks to determine for yourself its effectiveness.

GIVE IT A BREAK

As yet another approach, I recommend a regimen that gives the brain a much-needed break from overstimulation. An individual's variant of the DRD2 gene determines the sensitivity of that brain's main dopamine receptor. Dopamine "fasters" hope to reset this sensitivity from high (more pleasure-yielding) to low (not so productive of pleasure). The ragged effects on our nervous systems that are caused by constant stimulation (think excessive socializing, excessive dinging of text messages) depend on these high sensitivity dopamine receptors. In this regard, you might find interesting the comments about cell phone suppression that memory champion Yanjaa Wintersoul made during an interview I include in Part II. Sleep, meditation, rest and just being quiet may convert dopamine receptors into the low-sensitivity version, which makes us feel calmer. The prescription is for just one day without indulging in food, phones, internet, videos, music, alcohol, drugs, hanging out with friends, talking to people, masturbating or reading books. Instead, you drink water, go for a forest walk, do some light exercise, meditate, and write in an experience journal with pen and paper only. Reset those dopamine receptors and load up on dopamine.

SHOCKING NEWS

Other, more direct approaches to mood therapy are gaining acceptance. As we know, mood is a proxy for brain energy. What if we could, as it were, flip a switch and boost neuronal electricity and so increase the amount of neurotransmitters released, effectively inducing neuroplasticity? Sounds like the product of a Hollywood screenwriter's busy imagination,.but it isn't in fact science fiction. Transcranial direct current stimulation (tDCS) is a non-invasive, painless brain-stimulation treatment that employs two electrodes placed on either side of the head to pass a continual direct current at precise levels (2 to 4 milliamps) to stimulate specific parts of the brain. The tDCS equipment is cheap and easily portable. The therapy is non-invasive, easy to administer, and safe. Multiple studies have demonstrated that it helps treat neuropsychiatric conditions such as anxiety and depression.

"TURNING ON" AND TURNING IN

Scientists have observed for some time that those diagnosed with low mood and depression also exhibit atrophy of neurons in the prefrontal cortex (PFC). Some researchers now believe that the properties of psychedelic drugs such as LSD, MDMA, magic mushrooms, ayahuasca, and particularly ketamine (an anesthetic) can change the structure of nerve cells, causing them to sprout more branches and spines while simultaneously boosting

BDNF. In other words, the psychedelics of the sixties and seventies may be about to make a comeback as enhancers of our ability to induce plasticity in the PFC. This may strike you as unlikely and even disturbing but new evidence points to the possibility that psychedelics — especially perhaps at low dose levels — are capable of making changes in neuronal structures. These changes, as measured by fluorescence microscopy and electrophysiology, appear to be accompanied by increased synapse numbers and functions. The implication is that psychedelics may be capable of repairing the circuits that are malfunctioning in mood and anxiety disorders. With the emergence of this new application of psychedelics, the term "psychoplastogens" has been proposed to describe this class of plasticity-promoting mood-enhancing neuropharmaceuticals. Catch my interview with Chris Kilham in Part II of this book.

Everything old is new again.

A SUNNY DISPOSITION

Meanwhile, exposure to sunlight releases the hormone serotonin associated with boosting mood and helping us feel calm and focused. At night, darkness triggers the brain to make the hormone melatonin, a potent anti-carcinogen and antioxidant responsible for facilitating sleep.

Research has also established that BDNF blood levels are correlated to the number of hours we are exposed to sunlight. And an analysis of 2,851 individuals in the Netherlands found that blood BDNF increased in the spring and summer and decreased in the fall and winter. Scientists have correlated levels of BDNF with diagnoses of depression and with low mood generally.

Supplemental vitamin D may not increase BDNF directly. Elevated BDNF levels may be less about vitamin D (manufactured by the skin in response to sun exposure) and more about the high-energy photons, infrared, ultraviolet B, and ultraviolet A radiation emitted by the sun, with a synergistic impact on the body that ultimately produces BDNF.

THE CLINCHER

A hug is more than just a movement of the arms and a pressing together of two bodies. It's a poignant, powerful gesture of love and support that goes straight to the emotional centers of our brain. A bear hug, a straddle hug, a quick hug, a naughty hug, a London bridge hug, the infamous ass-out hug, the hug accompanied by a pat on the back, and the ever-popular group hug. We hug others when we're excited at the arrivals gate, sad at the departures gate, or trying to comfort the little one who's got a boo-boo. Hugging, it seems, is universally comforting and just makes us feel good. Maybe it should be no surprise that it's now shown to contribute to healthier and happier brains. Hugging research suggests its benefits go beyond that warm feeling you get when you hold someone in your arms.

The neuroscience is quite simple. When someone touches us, they activate pressure receptors within our skin called Pacinian corpuscles. These receptors send signals via our vagus nerve to an area in our brain that plays a vital role in regulating many of the body's key functions such as blood pressure and the "rest and digest" parasympathetic state. As a result, our blood pressure drops, our stress hormone cortisol plummets, calm prevails.

At the same time, hugging deepens our relationship with other persons on a neuro-biochemical level. Besides activating the vagus nerve, it tells the brain to release oxytocin, dopamine, serotonin and other endorphins. These neurotransmitters are collectively responsible for pleasure, reward, safety, general satisfaction, bonding, and pain management.

The effects are immediate. Some experts suggest "hugging it out" for 20 seconds to show you really "mean it". But no matter how long you feel comfortable giving or receiving a hug, research subjects report feeling in a much better mood within nanoseconds.

FINALLY, A WARNING

Researchers at the UCLA brain mapping centre scanned the brains of 32 people as they used social media and observed how reward centres in the brain were activated by FaceBook (and similar) "likes". This is the same area in the brain – the nucleus accumbens – that is activated when we view pictures of a person we love, or when we win money, or – unwisely and illegally – snort cocaine.

Social media appears to create an almost entirely egocentric culture. In conversations with people face-to-face, psychologists observe that we talk about ourselves 30% to 40% of the time. When we use social media platforms, that number jumps to a staggering 80%. The constant stimulation in the form of "likes", "followers", "shares", and "comments" causes dopamine emission and dopamine receptors to become hyper-stimulated. This is the chemistry of addiction.

Addictive behaviour affects neuroplasticity by activating a herd mentality. Instead of learning or re-learning information for ourselves, falling into a herd mentality impedes the continuous processes of remodelling of brain cell connections and brain cell organization that is so pertinent to neuroplasticity. We risk losing our ability to think for ourselves and form our own opinions as we go along with what's most popular or most "liked". Clearly, if we appreciate the potential of our own brain, we don't need to "like" sheep or be like sheep. Critical thinkers stay plastic.

A TEST

A neurotransmitter test can identify and may help correct neurotransmitter imbalances before they become severe enough to cause major symptoms. If you currently struggle with mood imbalance, testing neurotransmitter status can help determine which medication or natural treatments might be most beneficial. I recommend having your health care provider look into the testing service provided by ZRT Labs.

GENES AND MOOD

Among the thousands of genes that are expressed in the human brain, there are unquestionably many that play a role in the regulation of mood. Here are a few, and by the way, don't think it's my error that some of these same genes appear on other lists in this book. The wonder of DNA is that its constituent parts often play multiple roles through their expressed proteins.

The Catechol-O-methyltransferase (COMT) gene produces an enzyme of the same name. COMT is one of several enzymes that degrade the catecholamine family of neurotransmitters including dopamine, epinephrine, and norepinephrine as well as certain prescription drugs. The speed at which the enzyme works in you (to metabolize dopamine, norepinephrine, epinephrine and estrogens) also determines how long you hold onto thoughts and emotions. As we've seen, it is often referred to as the "warrior/worrier" gene

The ADRA2B gene plays a critical role in regulating the neurotransmitter noradrenaline in the brain. There is a strong correlation between individual variants of this gene and personal differences in processing and recalling emotional memory. We can also think of ADRA2B as controlling our predispositions when managing stress or "fight or flight" decisions.

The 5HTTLPR gene encodes protein that affects the brain's efficiency in recycling serotonin.

The MAO-A (Monoamine oxidase A) gene expresses the MAO-A enzyme that breaks down serotonin, dopamine, epinephrine and norepinephrine, a process important to the maintenance of our mood balance and how we handle stress.

The DRD2 gene regulates dopamine levels within the brain, which significantly impacts memory, cognition, mood, pleasure, reward, and plays a significant role in predisposition to addictions.

The PEMT gene encodes the PEMT enzyme, responsible for the conversion of phosphatidylethanolamine into phosphatidylcholine within the liver. Phosphatidylcholine is a key component of all 86 billion neuronal cell membranes in our brain and is a precursor for the neurotransmitter acetylcholine, which plays a role in memory and other brain functions

YOUR PERSONAL GENOME AND THE MARKETPLACE

I realize that many of my patients — and much of the population in general — are still only vaguely aware that it's already possible to analyse their personal DNA — and specific genes within it — to determine what variations of those genes (read about SNPs in Part IV) they may carry, how those variations may predispose them, and what remedial actions can be taken. It's all happened so fast, it still sounds like science fiction. But perhaps most astonishing of all, this technology has already been harnessed by private companies who will increasingly thrive by providing this precious information at affordable prices.

Just by way of illustration, let me quote from some material from The DNA Company, whose CEO, Dr. Mansoor Mohammed, I interview in Part II.

Serotonin and the Gene SLC6A4

An important aspect of your unique emotional response is your ability to stratify and respond appropriately to emotional stimuli based on their urgency.

The neurotransmitter known as serotonin plays an important role in this response mechanism. While on an important phone call, or furiously typing an urgent email, does the ticking of the clock in your room or the knocking of the window blinds compete for your attention, or are you more likely to fade these errant stimuli into the background? Serotonin may be the determining factor. It is often considered the "happy" neurotransmitter for its role in the regulation of mood, circadian rhythm, and eating behaviors. It plays a role in modulating neuroendocrine function by altering hypothalamic and pituitary secretion of hormones. It is also involved in regulating energy intake, body weight, and vascular elasticity. In short, serotonin is one of the most important neurochemicals in the body. Serotonin transport is impacted by a gene known as the SLC6A4 gene. This gene modulates serotonin reuptake in the presynaptic membrane. Stated simply, this gene influences the duration serotonin is available to exert its important role in your brain. A functional polymorphism known as 5-HTTLPR is found within the SLC6A4. This polymorphism exists as either a long version (known as the L allele) or a shortened version (known as the S allele). The S allele results in a significant reduction in transcription of the SLC6A4 gene and reduces the efficiency with which serotonin reuptake occurs in the presynaptic membrane. [Compared to L/L genotypes (who carry two copies of the L allele], S allele carriers (L/S and S/S genotypes) are associated with an increase caloric consumption in response to stress and with an increased risk in developing mood disorders, depressive symptoms, depression, and suicidal feelings.

This, dear readers, is a company — albeit a company of scientists — talking to its potential customers. The future of medicine —the psychological medicine of the brain and the conventional medicine of the body — is already upon us.

6

THE GERMS OF AN IDEA

When we look at 105-year-old people around the world, they carry the diverse gut microbiome of 30-year-old people.

~ Steven Gundry

I'm going to talk in this chapter about native populations, immigration and colonization. I see some of you have already rushed off to get your placards and fire up your social media accounts, but though I regard this as a subject of the greatest interest, our discussion will have nothing to do with politics or human rights. It has however a great deal to do with human health because not only are we born with massive populations of living creatures already settled in and on our bodies, but colonists regularly arrive from outside, most of them living and working as good citizens (and others not).

Research biologists have been tackling the question of cell numbers for a while now. The latest — ridiculously rounded — number of human cells in the human body is thought to be 40 trillion, tops, or 35 trillion more likely. A big number, to be sure, but just as sobering are the estimates of the number of ***non***-human cells in the human body, numbers that easily exceed the total number of human cells. We are, it seems, as much non-human as human. Welcome to our microbiome.

Bacteria make up the vast bulk of these non-human organisms living on and in us in almost every nook and cranny: the skin, mammary glands, placenta, seminal fluid, uterus, ovarian follicles, lung, saliva, oral mucosa, conjunctiva, biliary tract, and gastrointestinal tract are popular locations for settlement. These bacteria are really too small to count as micro-animals so we don't need to think of them as parasites, though in fact the harmful ones ***are*** classed as parasites. The rest are very often relatively benign fellow travellers or just as often have a "mutualistic" or a "symbiotic" relationship with us, their hosts — not surprising, since bacteria evolved with us, were here long before us, and will be around when we're gone. By taking them aboard with their various useful molecular tricks, we more complex beings saved ourselves having to evolve some of these now indispensable metabolic engines.

But how do we reconcile these facts with the rise in modern antimicrobial treatments, powerful disinfectants and harsh cleaning products marketed as necessary for good human health? Clearly we've needed to understand our germs better and in 2007 the United States National Institutes of Health established the Human Microbiome Project to analyse this unique relationship and determine its role in human health and disease. The project's work since 2007 has enormously advanced our knowledge of the human microbiome, which some scientists now label a 'superorganism'.

Some nice crumbs of trivia from this important initiative are that some 10,000 microbial species occupy the human ecosystem, with a combined genome of ten million genes — 150 times larger than the human genome. Having said that, and though it may be unfair to those trillions of bacteria living elsewhere in our bodies, I really want to talk about those living in our gastrointestinal tract. I know, this is a book about the brain, but bear with me: It's a gut feeling I have.

Let me begin with a caveat about bacteria. There's no use whitewashing them as a group; some of them aren't good for us at all and some are catastrophically bad. Our gut microbiome has evolved a sort of balancing act by which the trillions of benign bacteria keep the harmful ones in check. When for whatever reason that balance is upset, we call it "dysbiosis" — and preventing and healing dysbiosis is what this chapter is actually about.

Back to the brain. Of course we now know that there's an intimate relationship between the brain and the gut, connected as they are by the vagus nerve. The vagus nerve (from the Latin for "wandering") is actually a pair of complex branching nerves that comprises the main component of the parasympathetic nervous system and mediates a vast array of bodily functions, including control of mood, immune response, digestion, and heart rate.

As an aside, and speaking of gut and brain, the term "hypochondriac" (from ***hypo***, meaning "under" and ***chondria***, meaning "rib cage") was used in the past to refer to people who suffered from "depression and melancholy without cause". Physicians then had no scientific knowledge of the brain-gut connection, but doesn't "hypochondria" suggest an intuitive sense of that connection? Certainly it must have been evident to the ancients that when the ancient mind entertained thoughts of extreme fear or disgust or excitement, the thoughts were vividly experienced in the gut of that ancient.

Whatever, we've understood for a while that the vagus nerve is the direct "hotline" between the brain and the gut, such that when one is upset the other is upset too. Much more recently, however, has been the discovery of another rich channel of communication between the two, a channel using signals we hardly imagined a few decades ago. And it's the bacteria in our gut that act as its medium.

Key players in this chain of signalling are the "enteroendocrine" cells embedded in the lining of our digestive tract. (The root "entero" refers to the digestive system and "endocrine" to the hormonal system.) We know that these enteroendocrine cells react to various stimuli in the gut in several ways including the production of neuropeptides, hormonal molecules that enter the bloodstream and influence the enteric nervous system. The enteric nervous system consists of about 500 million neurons — five times more than in the human spinal cord — and is the only autonomous neural system outside the central nervous system. The enteric nervous system may be its own boss in certain situations but it also sends signals up to the brain. Gut bacteria connect to this chain of signalling. What could they be saying?

Well, for example, the bacterial population varies from stage to stage along the digestive tract and the many sub-types of enteroendocrine cells vary too, providing a subtle feedback flow of data to the enteric nervous system and the brain. They are responsible for the release of different products, particularly gastrointestinal hormones that have effects on appetite control, gastric acid secretion, insulin modulation, intestinal motility and contractions, and appetite regulation. Recent studies have shown that "good" bacteria ferment nutrients in our diet and release short-chain fatty acids that help optimize our use and storage of nutrients. Pathogenic "bad" bacteria do the opposite: They consume fatty acids, impeding healthful metabolism. This is the sort of information that could be useful to a brain — and a body.

Or how about this? Gut bacteria play a clear role in the metabolism of tryptophan, which is the precursor to the production of the "feel good" neurotransmitter serotonin, most of which is produced in the gut. And many species of ***Lactobacillus*** and ***Bifidobacterium*** — significant players in a healthy microbiome — produce GABA, the main relaxing neurotransmitter in the brain.

Gut-associated lymphoid tissue (GALT) is found at strategic locations in the lining of the gut and plays an important and independent role in the body's immunity to disease. Its job is to initiate immune responses to specific antigens and so defend against harmful microbes. The GALT's defender and supporter is the microbiome, and these two remain in constant cross-talk with one another.

So dysbiosis — an imbalance between good and bad bacteria — is going to have its consequences. Researchers are demonstrating that one of these consequences can be intestinal hyperpermeability, the weakening or loosening of the gut lining I spoke about earlier. That lining, if it's functioning properly, modulates the traffic through the gut lining into the blood stream and prevents dangerous organisms and molecules from crossing over into our bloodstream and leaking into, for example, our brain. In our earlier discussion of toxins and lectins and zonulin, we referred to this breakdown as "leaky gut syndrome". Many health practitioners are increasingly aware of its invidious effects. Studies have shown that depressed patients and persons suffering from chronic fatigue syndrome often have excessive gut-derived Gram-negative bacteria in their blood and lymph systems. These elevated levels are strongly related to inflammatory, oxidative, nitrosative, and autoimmune processes in the body — and none of these are good. My point is that when the gut is leaky, so is the brain, and when the brain is leaky we can feel foggy, lack focus, and can't find the car keys.

BADMOUTH

And by the way, just as the gut is host to a plethora of bacteria, so is the mouth, which is of course part of the digestive system. Most of our oral microbes are benign contributors to our mouth's bacterial population and their presence there confers health benefits. Some unfortunately are downright bad and known for releasing toxins that make their way to the brain. This often comes as a surprise to people but it shouldn't. The mouth and the brain are very close neighbors in the head. When our teeth feel slimy and need brushing, it's a sign this population of bacteria are gaining in strength. If we neglect our oral hygiene, the result can be chronic low-grade inflammation of the gums. The seal between the gums and our blood circulation eventually breaks down and the bacteria proceed to enter places in our bodies where they don't belong. The parallel with leaky gut syndrome is obvious. ***Porphyromonas gingivalis***, a bacterium notorious for its role in periodontal disease, is on our immune system's most wanted list. Like an evil influencer, it can turn good bacteria into bad bacteria and release toxins into our circulation and sneak across our blood-brain barrier. It can cause pneumonia, rheumatoid arthritis, heart disease, hepatitis, and — as some studies are suggesting — contribute to cancer. I personally find it most disturbing that clusters of ***Porphyromonas gingivalis (PG)*** have been found inside the brains of deceased Alzheimer's patients. Brush your teeth, dear friends. Brush them well.

Flossing to dislodge food bits that collect bacteria and contribute to inflammation and infection on the gums, and brushing our teeth for a full two minutes twice a day, are together ideal regimens for managing our oral microbiome. Proper brushing massages the gums with a downward stroke that disorganizes the biofilm that harbours *PG* and prevents acid attacks brought on by other, cavity-causing bacteria lurking in patches on the enamel. And while we're at it, we skip the fluoride toothpaste. There's plenty of evidence that fluoride is neurotoxic and we're already overexposed to it in our environment. Finally, go easy on the mouthwash. It may be effective perfume for the breath but it *is* antibacterial and that means *all* bacteria. Overuse can disrupt the oral microbiome by inhibiting proper growth of good bacteria. Instead, rinse with water after each meal, especially after high-carb meals and snacks. And here's a final tip unfamiliar to many people: chew some probiotics. BlisK12 is an oral probiotic strain that attaches to cells in your mouth and works to crowd out 'bad' bacteria in a process known as bacterial interference. This innovation diminishes *PG* and other bad guys and has been proven to fight cavities, bad breath, and even cure sore throats.

THE CARE AND FEEDING OF MAN'S BEST GERMS

If nothing ever went wrong, maybe our microbiome would always remain in perfect balance. But it's not a perfect world and my experience — and that of many clinicians — is that an optimal gut microbiome requires a little care and feeding.

When you're in the grocery store and see those labels of yogurt containers that talk about cultures, they're talking about bacteria, the kind of bacteria with which we have a "mutualistic" relationship or at least a "commensal" relationship to our advantage. Yogurts, of course, are fermented milks and many cultures — the human kind — have long appreciated the value of fermented foods, even without direct knowledge of bacteria and the human microbiome. Today, with our greater consciousness of food and nutrition, we recognize that it's wise to have at least one serving of fermented food every day. Yogurt is a good example, but only those varieties labelled as containing live or active cultures. Sauerkraut is another familiar ferment, but choose only homemade sauerkraut or that found in the refrigerated section since processing destroys the bacteria. Some other fermented foods, though perhaps less well known, are miso, kefir, kombucha, tempeh, kimchi, and fermented cheeses such as Pecorino. Some may be acquired tastes but there are people everywhere who love them, they're increasingly popular and available, and they're relatively easy to incorporate into our diets. Again, purchase these products in the refrigerated section because any type of canning or pasteurizing kills the bacteria that convey the health benefits.

When we go over to the supplement aisle, we should keep in mind that there's no such thing as the best probiotic. Specific strains and species have been studied with respect to the health benefits they convey. For example, we've got strong evidence that the ***Lactobacillus acidophilus*** strain CL1285 offers protection against and treatment for antibiotic-associated diarrhea. On the other hand, there's no evidence this strain of probiotic would do anything for brain health. The combination of ***Lactobacillus helveticus*** R0052 and ***Bifidobacterium longum*** R0175 however was specifically developed with brain health in mind. They support the gut-brain connection and research has shown that their use can reduce anxiety and depression.

A diet high in fiber — particularly soluble fiber — is gratefully received by our gut bacteria. Soluble fiber dissolves in water and forms a thick gel in our digestive tract that regulates gut transit time and helps us to feel fuller for longer. The gel also acts as a sponge during digestion, attracting fluid and softening stools to allow waste to move through the bowel more easily. Soluble fiber is found in some vegetables and fruit, oats, lentils, legumes, nuts and seeds. Some foods and supplemental fibers can cause gas and bloating, though, so look for a tasteless, odorless soluble fiber made from the guar bean plant that you can add to a shake or mix into water. Look for the ingredient SunFiber on the label. Your microbiome will love you for it.

OUR MICROBIOME BY NUMBERS

So for those of us who care — really care — about our microbiome, how do we get the information we need to proceed?

There are many hundreds of probiotic products on the market. Which is right for our inner self? Have we tried the right kind? Fortunately accurate testing is now available that can tell us what we're missing or what isn't growing properly. A simple stool sample sent through your health care provider to a functional medicine laboratory can shed light on what strains and species are right for you. Genova diagnostics laboratory, for example, offers a test called GI Effects. Doctors Data is another laboratory offering a test they call the Comprehensive Stool Analysis. Commercially available tests are popping up all over the place. See also Viome, DayTwo, UBiome, and Thryve. And we can now test for and diagnose leaky gut, with the lactulose-mannitol urine test as well as zonulin. Both can serve as biomarkers using no more than a "finger stick" of blood or a simple urine sample. We have every reason — and many ways — to optimize our microbiome and more and more informed people are doing this because what's good for our gut is good for our brain.

When you can't get your hands on this level of laboratory analysis, take a look at this clinical guide to evidence-based indications for select probiotic products: **http://www.probioticchart.ca**

7

BRAINSTORMS
(AND CALM)

The truth is that there is no actual stress or anxiety in the world; it's your thoughts that create these false beliefs. You can't package stress, touch it, or see it. There are only people engaged in stressful thinking.

~ *Wayne Dyer*

Brain health affects and is affected by our daily life. It's a no-brainer but some of these connections may not be obvious at first. I'm going to start with one familiar to us all.

Biologists refer to changes in our environment as "stressors" and our responses to those changes as "stress." From this it follows that stress in unavoidable since change is unavoidable, and the key factors are the nature, duration and intensity of the stressors and the nature and intensity of our responses. Research has determined that for different individuals under different circumstances and at different stages in life, stress can result in our acquiring hardy resistance to its negative effects or, sadly, in our suffering negative or fatal consequences. There's evidence that in North America stress is our number one silent killer, contributing to heart disease, diabetes, and cognitive decline.

Knowing that individual responses to stressors vary so widely, what can we do for ourselves?

In Part IV, when we look briefly at brain anatomy, we'll visit a deep region of the brain where the hypothalamus and pituitary gland form part of the "border" or "limbic" system between the cortex and the brainstem. The body's stress response is primarily governed by an interaction between the hypothalamus and pituitary gland on one hand and the adrenal glands that sit on top of the kidneys. Together they comprise the so-called hypothalamus-pituitary-adrenal (HPA) axis, a "neuroendocrine" system that, as its name implies, interfaces between the brain and the hormonal system. When it's activated, the HPA axis integrates the many physical and psychosocial stressors and sets off a cascade of signals that leads to the release of hormones and neurotransmitters such as cortisol, norepinephrine and epinephrine that regulate the metabolic system, cardiovascular system, immune system, reproductive system, central nervous system and others. Our understanding is that the HPA axis evolved early to allow organisms to adapt to their environment, use resources, and optimize their chances of survival. Since the axis is clearly a long-term evolutionary survivor, we know it's still mighty useful. The problem arises when a complex human environment presents too many stressors and the HPA interaction calls forth an excess of hormonal responses that the body does not or cannot use. Researchers have established links between HPA excess and anxiety disorder, bipolar disorder, insomnia, posttraumatic stress disorder, borderline personality disorder, ADHD, major depressive disorder, burnout, chronic fatigue syndrome, fibromyalgia, irritable bowel syndrome, alcoholism, attention deficits, schizophrenia, and metabolic syndrome associated with many diseases including diabetes and coronary heart disease.

I had a lengthy and revealing conversation about managing the HPA axis with Dr. Andrew Weil, the guru of integrative medicine and the mind-body connection. You can find his excellent advice in Part II.

The Little Bit that Goes a Long Way

Sometimes an agent is damaging to an individual organism at higher doses but induces a beneficial response at lower doses. This phenomenon is called hormesis and the agents that bring about hormesis are called hormetins. Moderate or intermittent stress is such an agent.

Hormetins have been broadly classified into physical, psychological, biological, and nutritional. Physical factors such as moderate exercise, irradiation, thermal shock, and cold stress are grouped as physical hormetins. Factors which lead to social and mental well-being of an individual are classified as psychological hormetins. These include mental engagement such as intense brain activity and focused attention such as meditation.

The evidence is clear that some stress – just the right amount of stress – can be good for us. We call those stressors the "Goldilocks hormetins". I don't recommend that you go out and expose yourself to various forms of radiation but I want to emphasize that intense exercise, intermittent fasting, and thermal shock – the kind you survive – can be great for your brain.

HAVING A HEART

Today we recognize that the reduction of stress's detrimental effects are vital for the preservation of our mental and physical health. But this book is about ***brain*** health so you may wonder why I'm now talking about the heart. And you may be surprised to learn — I was — that the heart sends more signals to the brain than the brain sends to the heart. In fact the heart hosts so significant a cluster of nerve tissue, it qualifies as a mini-brain that can learn, remember, and make functional decisions independent of the brain's cerebral cortex. Experimenters have demonstrated that the signals that the heart continuously sends to the brain influence the function of "higher" brain centers involved in perception, cognition, and emotional processing. To this extensive neural network linking the heart with the brain and body, the heart adds the body's most powerful and most extensive rhythmic electromagnetic field, which can communicate information throughout the body via electromagnetic field interactions. We think back to those ancient Greek philosophers and wonder if the heart may not be the true seat of emotion after all. When we experience the stress of negative emotions, our heart rhythm may be erratic, disordered. Our positive emotions and a state of relaxation are often associated with a smooth, ordered heart rhythm. The implications are clear when we consider how so many biological systems function as feedback loops: by optimizing our heart rhythm, we can positively influence our state of mind.

One of the most powerful implications of this information is that by optimizing your heart rhythm, you can positively influence your state of mind. One of the most effective ways to do this is a proven breathing technique.

Touch the tip of your tongue to the roof of your mouth. Keep it there while you exhale completely through your mouth, making a loud whoosh sound. Close your mouth and inhale quietly through your nose to a mental count of 4. Hold your breath for a count of 7. Exhale completely through your mouth, making a whoosh sound to a count of 8. Do that for two minutes and your heart will tell your brain that "everything is just fine in the world".

I've found effective the tools and techniques developed by the HeartMath Institute, based on their 25 years of research on the psychophysiology of stress, emotions, and the interactions between the heart and brain. Over 300 peer-reviewed or independent studies have utilized HeartMath's techniques and technologies to achieve beneficial outcomes. While researching this book, I had a chance to interview Rollin McCraty of HeartMath and you'll find the interview in Part II.

THE BRAIN AND THE NOSE

If the heart sends signals to the brain, why would the nose not, being so much closer? The smell of a pine tree brings you back to your family's holidays at the cottage. The smell of fresh sheets hung outdoors on a spring day reminds you of your mother tucking you into bed as a child. Folding open the first pages of a new book brings you back to a beach-side vacation. Memories flood in with a fresh pot of coffee on a Sunday morning. Why are these memories so effortlessly recalled by smell? Back to the brain, of course, where rich neuronal connections link the sensory receptors in our brain's olfactory bulb to the limbic system, where they influence emotions and memories, instinct and mood. This "neurocircuitry of olfaction" — a nerve cell's interpretation of a molecule in inhaled air — is the basis of our sense of smell. The olfactory bulb has about 400 unique types of receptors but by responding simultaneously to a variety of molecules these 400 can register countless distinct scents. Through eons of development our olfactory sense has enabled the detection of hazards, of the edibility of food (and in association with our sense of taste, the flavour of foods), and even of the pheromones that we don't consciously register but play an important role in sexual attraction. From the limbic region, signals may loop on to the "higher" brain centers where they can modify conscious thought. We may recount to our kids the events of our long-ago holiday or perhaps lay plans for a future one.

Folk wisdom has long recognized that certain plants have unique scents with unique effects. For thousands of years, people have known how to capture the natural essences of these plants and preserve them as "essential oils" — the basis of what we know today as aromatherapy. Despite its intuitive appeal, aromatherapy's potential to reduce stress might have seemed doubtful until we understood the brain's circuitry as we now do. The calming sense induced by certain smells may in fact be the absence of stress.

The claim for lavender is its ability to lull us to sleep and as a calming and able aid in depression, anger and irritability. Like lavender, bergamot is believed to relieve anxiety, agitation, mild depression and stress.

Peppermint is a potent brain booster, acting as an energizer that can be used to stimulate the mind and calm nerves at the same time. Like peppermint, rosemary oil has a reputation as uplifting and able to stimulate the mind, improve cognitive performance, and enhance mood.

Lemon oil is one of the best studied and most effective oils and research shows it can improve memory. Ylang Ylang is often combined with lemon oil to boost brain activity.

I use and recommend the Saje line of essential oils. They utilize 100% natural ingredients (most are vegan), not tested on animals, made without synthetics, and sourced from sustainable farms all over the world and from certified organic sources wherever possible.

Maybe, just maybe, common sense can be enhanced by common scents.

THE BRAIN AND THE PRESENT

By now most of us have encountered the practice of "mindful meditation" (or "mindfulness meditation"), an ancient stress-reduction technique rooted in such traditions as Zen Buddhism. In essence, mindful meditation is about centering the mind on the present without drifting into concerns about the past or future. This is usually accomplished by adopting a comfortable sitting posture and focusing on our breathing. This type of meditation has gained wide currency and attracted scientific interest, though the design of meditation studies that meet scientific standards faces challenges in selecting control groups and unbiased subjects. But a research team at Johns Hopkins University in Baltimore surveyed 19,000 meditation studies and found 47 to be well-designed and worthy of review. Their findings, published in ***JAMA Internal Medicine*** in 2014, made the case that mindful meditation can reduce psychological stresses such as anxiety, depression, and pain.

Over the next few years, the number of randomized, controlled trials involving mindful meditation had jumped from almost none in the 90s to over 200. The most promising findings were in the areas of depression, chronic pain, and anxiety, where, according to the ***Harvard Gazette***, "well-designed, well-run studies showed benefits for patients engaging in a mindfulness meditation program, with effects similar to other existing treatments." It was at Harvard, in fact, that researchers using fMRI machines established that there are persistent changes in amygdala activity in meditators — even when not meditating. And as evidence that the effects of meditation go beyond relaxation, another team of researchers reported in ***Frontiers in Psychology*** in 2015 that "hippocampal dimensions were enlarged both in male and in female meditators when compared to sex- and age-matched controls." Specifically, eight weeks of mindfulness-based stress reduction increased cortical thickness in the hippocampus, which governs learning and memory.

AN EXERCISE

We can combine breathing, olfaction, and mindfulness into a technique I find potently brain-calming.

Choose an essential oil known for its calming effects. Lavender's claim to fame is its ability to sooth depression, anger and irritability. Like lavender, bergamot is reputed to relieve anxiety, agitation, mild depression and stress. Take a few deep sniffs of the oil or add it to your diffuser. Next, touch the tip of your tongue to the roof of your mouth. Keep it there and exhale completely through your mouth, making a loud whoosh sound. Close your mouth and inhale quietly through your nose to a mental count of 4. Hold your breath for a count of 7. Exhale completely through your mouth, making a whoosh sound to a count of 8. Close your mouth and inhale quietly through your nose to a mental count of 4. Repeat this for two minutes.

For the next ten minutes, return to a relaxed breath and focus on the sensations of air flowing into your nostrils and out of your mouth, with your belly rising and falling as you inhale and exhale. Once you've narrowed your concentration in this way, begin to widen your focus to become aware of sounds, sensations, and ideas. Embrace and consider each thought or sensation without judging it as good or bad. If your mind starts to race, return your focus to your breathing, then expand your awareness again.

8

WHERE DO YOU GET THE ENERGY?

You are responsible for the energy that you create for yourself, and you're responsible for the energy that you bring to others.

~ Oprah Winfrey

The subject of energy often comes up at dinner parties and everybody has an opinion. Sometimes it's power plants, sometimes solar panels, sometimes electricity bills. We use too much energy, right? Or sometimes it's energy drinks. Good or bad? Sometimes it's energy levels. Whew. Don't seem to have enough these days. Dragging our butts before lunch.

But rarely is there mention of a staggeringly important energy consumer that dominates our lives: the kilo and a half of jelly inside our skulls that consumes 25% of our body's energy, as much energy as burning a ten-watt light bulb, and consumes it twenty-four hours a day, even when we're sleeping. In fact, the brain consumes roughly as much energy at night as it does during the day. While we rest, our neurons are still busy communicating, updating each other on what's happening, soaking up energy.

Research a decade ago established that maybe a quarter to a third of this energy goes to keeping the brain cells ticking; all the rest is consumed in signalling — sending and receiving ionic messages across the synapses. The brain needs to be supplied with this huge allocation of available power on a continuous basis — cut off the flow for only a matter of minutes and its neurons and glial cells begins to wink out — because storing the energy on board (the way muscles do) would drastically cut processing efficiency. If the brain contained cells that stored backup power, those cells would expand the distance between neurons and increase the travel time for signals. This would require yet more energy and more time. Our brain's actual set-up makes us vulnerable to injury but offers a huge gain in efficiency. The result: a lean, mean but hungry thinking machine.

The obvious corollary to all this is that shortfalls in the supply of brain fuel — whether or not our lives are in imminent danger — must wear the brain down just as food shortages wear the body. We now know such shortfalls mean slowed mental function, memory deficits, mood disorders, vulnerability to Parkinson's, Alzheimer's and dementia, and poor recovery from trauma. By contrast, readily available brain fuel means a high-performance, focused brain.

What then do we really mean when we talk about brain fuel?

MEET YOUR MITOCHONDRIA

We've already made the brief acquaintance of ATP when we talked about mood and dehydration but we're not quite done with it yet.

Our 86 billion neurons and (by the latest count) 85 billion glial cells are necessarily small indeed. But as with so much else in this universe, there are wheels within wheels. Inside many cell types, along with the nucleus and its DNA, are numbers of much smaller structures called "organelles." And of primary importance among the organelles are the mitochondria. These "little organs" are usually depicted in diagrams as tiny dirigible-shaped capsules but in reality mitochondria are constantly dividing and fusing in ever-changing networks as they perform a dazzling array of critical tasks on behalf of their cells. Mitochondria even contain their own DNA, quite separate from the DNA housed in the cell nucleus. For our purposes, though, let's review just one crucial mitochondrial function: the generation of energy within the cell.

Scientists now have a pretty clear understanding of the complex reactions by which the mitochondria convert the chemical energy ultimately derived from the food we eat into energy the cell can use. Within the mitochondria's membrane-within-a-membrane structure, these reactions use lipids and glucose to create a molecule called adenosine triphosphate, which for obvious reasons we'll now refer to as ATP. The ATP molecule has many roles throughout the body but it is often characterized as the cell's "energy currency" because it's a convenient way to transfer and store energy. This it can do because the adenosine part of the molecule has three phosphate groups attached to it in a chain (thus the name) and the bond between the second and third phosphate group is unstable. When energy is needed for a certain task within the cell, the phosphate bond is broken and energy is released and transferred to the cell via enzymes specific to that task. The "spent" ATP is now adenosine diphosphate (ADP), which is usually immediately recycled in the mitochondria to become again ATP. At any given moment, each one of the trillions of cells in the human body contains a billion ATP molecules. In the words of author James Trefil, "hooking and unhooking that last phosphate [on ATP] is what keeps the whole world operating."

The complex processes involving ATP within a cell's mitochondria respond to the special needs of that cell. The grey matter of the brain consists of the neuron cell bodies and requires far more mitochondrial output than the white matter that consists of bundles of signalling axon extensions and myelin, the fatty sheaths that insulate them.

Energy usage and mitochondrial activities also depend on the area and function of the brain that is active. The brain circuits responsible for auditory processing for example require more energy than the olfactory system devoted to smell. Our very survival may depend on fast and precise processing of the sound of danger. Relatively slower processes such as smell don't have the same intense energy needs.

BRAIN ENERGY AND MITOCHONDRIA

When the mitochondria in our brain cells are dysfunctional due, say, to a poor diet causing excess inflammation, or to dehydration or toxins or a leaky gut, they can't make ATP efficiently and we can't think clearly or function optimally. For example, we know that Parkinson's is a mitochondrial disease that can result from insults to the brain in the form of toxins, infections, inflammation, or poor diet. We know too that malfunctioning mitochondria accumulate in the Alzheimer's brain. In clinical practice, I support the mitochondria of patients with these conditions and they feel better, function better, and regularly show significantly improved outcomes.

Some of the threats to our mitochondria do not originate in our lifestyle choices but were with us from conception. When this happens we have a special challenge to offset these handicaps to lengthen our brainspan and sustain our quality of life. Here's an example.

Free radicals are compounds containing highly reactive oxygen ions (charged atoms, as you may recall) that we touched on earlier. Superoxides are a specific and common type of free radical produced in the body as a by-product of oxygen metabolism and, in excess, capable of causing many types of cell damage. Mitochondria are especially vulnerable to free radicals, which are toxic to several of these vital organelles' energy pathways, so the enzyme superoxide dismutase (SOD) — a so-called "antioxidant" — degrades superoxide compounds and in this role is a potent protector of mitochondria.

Our discussion of genetics in Part IV will trot out a gaggle of brain-related genes. SOD2 is one of these, the gene that encodes for the expression of SOD.

Unfortunately our DNA sometimes contains variations called SNPs within particular genes and these variations are sometimes undesirable. Such a variation on the SOD2 gene can cause the expression of imperfect versions of the SOD antioxidant enzyme, variations that can hinder its ability to protect us against free radicals and oxidative stress. When SOD2 isn't optimal, increased free radical activity causes excess cell damage, especially to the cell's mitochondria. The result can be an increase in the risk of developing neurodegenerative and other brain-debilitating disorders. What can we do to counter this?

Research has shown that SOD's antioxidant effectiveness is dependent on the trace minerals manganese and magnesium. Both of these are found in nuts — particularly brazil nuts — and seeds, wheat germ, wheat bran, greens, and pineapple, among other foods. Whether or not an investigation of our personal genome reveals a detrimental SOD2 SNP, it makes sense to do whatever we can to support this enzyme that supports the mitochondria that fuels our brain.

PUSH-UPS FOR THE BRAIN

Meanwhile, other research has proven that exercise — and in particular so-called high-intensity interval training (HIIT) — causes cells to make more proteins for energy-producing mitochondria. HIIT has been shown to reverse the brain-dulling effects of obesity, has anti-inflammatory and cardiovascular benefits, and appears to prevent age-related cognitive decline. HIIT involves alternating short periods of intense anaerobic exercise with less intense recovery periods, until the exerciser is too exhausted to continue. Even people who are new to working out can engage in a HIIT-related regimen. Details of this Brainspanner workout appear in an interview in Part II with Brent Bishop, celebrity trainer and author of *Think Fitness*.

THE FAST TRACK

And while we're on the subject of lifestyle activities that boost our mitochondrial function and brain energy, again, I strongly recommend intermittent fasting at least a few days a week. We can't do without food, it's true, but eating regularly — even the appropriate calories — comes at a price: the processing and combustion of food within our bodies release radical oxygen ions that wear on our tissues and stress our mitochondria. As we've seen, the science points toward a strategy to condense our eating window on select days from the typical 12- to16-hour all-day graze routine to 8 hours — simply by eating breakfast later and dinner earlier.

BRAIN ENERGY SUPPLEMENTS

Diet and lifestyle are such sensible ways to boost and maintain the cellular energy generated by our mitochondria, I've put them in first place. But there is another and powerful way to support this critical part of our brain's activity. Three ingredients play important roles in mitochondrial function and I recommend supplementing with them.

Ubiquinol (also known as ***reduced co-enzyme Q10***) is a co-enzyme — that is, a helper molecule that works with an enzyme to enhance the function of the enzyme. The body produces CoQ10 to protect mitochondrial DNA against free radical assaults, but levels decline rapidly with age and regular CoQ10 is not well absorbed as a supplement. Research has shown that ubiquinol does not suffer from this limitation.

Pyrroloquinoline quinone (PQQ) demonstrates antioxidant and B-vitamin-like activity, with a wide range of benefits for the brain and body. It promotes cognitive health and memory by combatting mitochondrial dysfunction and protecting neurons from oxidative damage. It thus supports energy metabolism and healthy aging and creates new mitochondria in the process.

Nicotinamide Riboside (NR) is a form of vitamin B_3 that helps to boost the energy output of mitochondria. It is the direct precursor to nicotinamide adenine dinucleotide (NAD) which is essential to all cells, since cells depend on NAD to convert food into the energy they need to perform their tasks. But this is especially true of those cells hosting mitochondria, such as the neurons.

***

An optimal brainspan requires taking good care of our mitochondria to ensure we're getting the best ATP output performance from our cells' energy engines. In clinical practice, I've tested many hundreds of patients with suspect mitochondrial dysfunction. The most comprehensive test that I can recommend is called the "NutrEval" by Genova diagnostics. If you happen to be a fan of biochemistry, I'll pass on that this test uses a blood and urine sample to look at citric acid, cys-aconitic acid and iso-citric acid levels as measures of mitochondrial energy output. It looks at B-butyric acid levels to measure ATP energy molecule production. It looks at suberic acid, adipic acid, pyruvate and magnesium levels to determine the rate of catalyzed lactic acid build-up, which can impede mitochondrial ATP production. And it looks at many vitamin B metabolites. Technical, yes, but a surprisingly uncomplicated, non-invasive way to examine and measure the efficiency of your mitochondrial energy system's status. All you need is a clinician who is willing to run it.

9

PERCHANCE TO DREAM

There will be plenty of time to sleep once you are dead.

~ Benjamin Franklin

Many healthcare professionals — more than half in fact — report not having enough time during regular office visits to discuss insomnia and other sleep problems. This is unfortunate because when it comes to brain health, more important than any supplement, super food, exercise, trick, tactic, or hack, is a deep restful sleep. This is what repairs, resets, and optimizes our brain. Sleep is what, as Shakespeare famously said, "knits up the ravelled sleeve of care."

I believe strongly that, all other factors being equal, healthy sleep patterns are what establish and maintain an optimal brainspan, and in these pages we'll explore the wonderful and in some ways still mysterious mechanisms of sleep, so intimately connected with the brain.

THE TIMEKEEPER

Deep inside our brain lies a cluster of about 20,000 brain cells dubbed the suprachiasmatic nucleus. It's part of our old friend the hypothalamus and sits just above the optic chiasm, the place where many of the axons of the optic nerves cross over to the other side. that go from your eyes to the back of your head. The suprachiasmatic nucleus communicates with the nearby optic nerves to control our cycles of sleeping and waking. When light hits our eyes — whether the lids are shut or not — the suprachiasmatic nucleus signals the production of serotonin, the day-cycle hormone. At night, the lack of light triggers a shutdown of serotonin production and initiates the production of melatonin, which lulls us to sleep. This delicate balance we call the "circadian rhythm" defines our sleep-wake cycles and when the circadian rhythm is imbalanced we don't sleep well. Annoying, of course, but far more serious are its consequences. If we don't get enough sleep, for example, our levels of leptin, an appetite-regulating hormone, fall and we experience a significantly increased appetite-promoted weight gain. Lack of sleep also contributes to digestive disorders, irritable bowel issues, constipation, cardiovascular disease, memory failure, and — significantly — brain shrinkage.

HUMANS: THE ANIMALS WHO MURDER SLEEP

Veterinarians are rarely called upon to deal with cases of insomnia because we are the only mammal that willingly delays sleep or at least engages in activities we know to be inimical to sleep. Why should this be?

Clearly our modern urban and industrial environment is remote from the world our species evolved in. Our days and nights surround us with noise and sights that simply didn't exist in our ancestral past. Some of these aren't conducive to sleep.

We've talked about stress in other chapters and we are all familiar with how the agitation of worry can disrupt the process of falling to sleep. It's unlikely that earlier humans were free from stress but things haven't improved in this regard: work, finances, family life, death or illness of a family member or friend — they still take their toll.

Illness and pain can make sleep a longed-for but elusive condition. Gastroesophageal reflux, prostate enlargement, Parkinson's disease, Alzheimer's disease, stroke, and other medical conditions including mental health conditions such as depression and anxiety: these can all be enemies of sleep. As though these torments weren't enough, there are even conditions such as apnea and restless leg syndrome that are specific to sleep itself.

Too much noise, light or heat are obvious problems but these can be more subtle and unrecognized and still rob us of sleep.

Substances ingested can work directly on our nervous systems to make sleep difficult. It doesn't matter whether these are illegal recreational drugs, prescribed medications, or social drugs such as nicotine, caffeine, and alcohol. Your nervous system doesn't react on the basis of where you got your chemicals. We're the only animals who consume large amounts of caffeine, a central nervous system stimulant. We know that caffeine in excess contributes to sleep interruption and yet caffeine is the most popular drug in the world. All over the globe people consume it on a daily basis in the form of coffee, tea, cocoa, chocolate, soft drinks, many over-the-counter medications and some prescription drugs.

Finally, there are lifestyle choices that militate against sleep: vigorous exercise before going to bed, and (conversely) inactivity during the day, poor sleep habits, the introduction of artificial daylight by watching TV or other screens late at night. And a significant number of us are shift workers whose working hours are intermittently out of whack with their circadian rhythm, putting them at increased risk of desynchronosis — a chronic upset of that rhythm.

THE LAG THAT SUCKS

Nobody is immune to jet lag. In animal research, subjects exposed to chronic jet lag created new neurons at about half the rate of normal stay-at-home members of their species and showed significant memory and learning deficits.

Our circadian rhythm is the tight schedule of regular sleep-wake cycles and body functions that our brain establishes. When the suprachiasmatic nucleus decides it's time to get some sleep, the natural time-keeping system releases the hormone melatonin. But the body also likes regularity — especially as it relates to hormonal balance — so this natural clock is accustomed to going off at the same time every night. When we cross time zones we force drastic and sudden resets. The problem is at its worst when we fly eastward, say from Toronto or New York to Paris. When it's nighttime at our destination, our body still thinks it's late afternoon and we wind up lying sleepless in our hotel bed all night, finally dozing off when it's time to get up.

Jet lag sleeplessness disrupts just about every biological function in the body by causing the release of stress hormones that make us feel anxious and grumpy. It drives up our blood pressure, and sends inflammation-stimulating chemical markers flooding through our arteries. Poor sleep rhythms disrupt the release of appetite-regulating hormones. Complicating matters further, clinical evidence shows the average human circadian rhythm to be slightly longer than 24 hours, so that most of us have a natural tendency to drift slightly later each day. That may be why the body adjusts better flying east to west.

Light isn't the only thing that influences sleep. Our brains manage body temperature, which also fluctuates during sleep, reaching its minimum temperature about three hours before we typically rise. Some scientists theorize that this temperature shift is necessary for the glymphatic system (you'll recall how it's responsible for toxin elimination from the brain during sleep — but more on that below) to work at peak performance. Jet lag symptoms tend to be the worst when we're forced to awaken while we're still at a normal temperature.

If you're traveling abroad, I recommend using a time-release melatonin. Here's how to take it:

- **Dose:** 1mg/~50lbs body weight (preferably a slow release form)
- **Timing:** 1 hour prior to desired sleep time in new time zone
- **Duration:** one night for every two time zones you've crossed
- **Repeat** once you've arrived back to original time zone

THE NATURE OF SLEEP

We know from studies of sleep that there are two basic types: rapid eye movement (REM) sleep and non-REM sleep, which has four stages, each linked to specific patterns of electrical activity in the brain – brain waves. The average person needs to cycle through all five stages at least four or five times a night for optimal brain function during the day and each cycle takes approximately 60 to 90 minutes. That's how scientists arrived at the notion of seven to nine hours of sleep and why we so often hear "get your 8 hours". However, it's not about simply clocking those hours on your pillow. The quality of sleep is a major factor.

Stage 1 non-REM sleep is the transition from wakefulness to sleep. During this short, relatively light sleep, our heartbeat, breathing, and eye movements slow, and our muscles relax with occasional twitches.

Stage 2 non-REM sleep is a period of light sleep before we enter deeper sleep. Our heartbeat and breathing slow further, and muscles relax further. Our body temperature drops and eye movements stop. Brain wave activity slows but is marked by brief bursts of electrical activity, of which more below.

Stage 3 and 4 non-REM sleep is the period of deep sleep that we need to feel refreshed in the morning. It occurs in longer periods during the first half of the night. Our heartbeat and breathing slow to their lowest levels during sleep. Our muscles are relaxed and it may be difficult to awaken us. Brain waves become even slower. These stages are the most important type of sleep for optimal brain health.

REM sleep first occurs about 90 minutes after falling asleep. Our eyes move rapidly from side to side behind closed eyelids. Brain waves are similar to when we're awake. Our breathing becomes faster and irregular, and our heart rate and blood pressure increase to near waking levels. We are now in the zone of dreaming. Our arm and leg muscles become temporarily paralyzed, which prevents us from acting out our dreams. As we age, we spend less time in REM sleep.

Why do we sleep? In many respects this remains one of science's mysteries, though modern brain research is beginning to throw real light on the role of sleep. It's apparent that sleep is a sort of compromise state since, however necessary it may be and for whatever reasons, deep sleep in a world of predators and prey must expose the sleeper to the risk of waking up as someone else's meal. Sleep has evolved as a balancing act, since there must be evolved reasons for sleeping that offset the survival risk.

It's becoming increasingly clear, for example, that one reason we sleep is to facilitate the repair of our DNA, a complex and necessary process. It's also been long understood by brain scientists that sleep in closely tied to the reinforcing or "consolidation" of memories. More recent research in several centers has brought us closer to understanding how sleep accomplishes this. Particularly interesting is the observed correlation between two types of brain wave patterns occurring in non-REM sleep — rapid "sleep spindles" and slow oscillations — and the ability to retain learning, that is, "declarative memory". The research drills down further, demonstrating in the process how scientists are increasingly able to link mental processes to brain structure. In this case, wave patterns such as sleep spindles and slow oscillations have been traced to activity within specific brain regions (such as our old friend the hippocampus) and — drilling still deeper — to the branching dendrites of neurons there, where the spindles seem to be evidence of new signalling pathways being formed or strengthened. This may be the actual mechanism of memory consolidation during sleep — not something we want to short-change ourselves on.

But now a factor has appeared that may be the most important of all.

Our "glymphatic system" which is in charge of detoxifying the brain functions almost exclusively when we're in deep non-REM sleep. That's when the spaces between the brain's cells enlarge and the accumulated detritus and waste that arises naturally in the course of brain metabolism is flushed away by a convective surge of cerebrospinal fluid and drained into the lymphatic system. It makes sense by analogy that this can no more happen during waking hours that a railway crew can repair tracks when the trains are running.

So what's being flushed away? This question brings us to investigations that bear directly on the concerns of this book. The glymphatic flow, along with its other roles, sweeps away β–amyloids, which are small protein molecules called peptides. To quote a 2010 paper, "Alzheimer's disease pathogenesis is widely believed to be driven by the production and deposition of the β-amyloid peptide." Indeed, "all prevalent neurodegenerative diseases are characterized by accumulation of aggregated proteins."

So sleep allows the glymphatic system to clear away β–amyloids – and β–amyloids, which accumulate as "plaques" in the brain, are clearly associated with Alzheimer's Disease.

Further, and unfortunately for all mammals, glymphatic flow declines with age and is a striking feature of traumatic brain injury. It's no coincidence, then, that Alzheimer's strongly correlates with both aging and brain trauma. All these dramatic findings have come too recently to allow for "magic bullet" interventions yet it's impossible to miss the central role of sleep in protecting the brain. So for the balance of this chapter, let's chase that sometimes elusive quarry.

KNITTING THE RAVELLED SLEEVE

Since this "activity" consumes much of our lives and has an obvious bearing on our waking hours, what can we do to help it do its job?

In general, though some individuals can function without sleepiness or drowsiness after as little as six hours of sleep and others can't perform at their peak unless they've slept ten hours, most healthy adults need seven to nine hours of sleep a night. Sadly, some people have DNA variations that make it difficult to sleep in the first place. Such a variation is in the "serotonin transporter gene-linked polymorphic region" or "5-HTTLPR" of our DNA.

This gene is in charge of manufacturing a protein critical to the regulation of serotonin function in the brain. It terminates the action of serotonin at the synapses by re-uptaking the neurotransmitter when its job is done. Because a serotonin-melatonin balance is so crucial to a healthy circadian rhythm, those people with the "low-expressive short version" of this gene may experience sleep interruption. Researchers have now found that such people may benefit from supplemental 5-hydroxy-tryptophan (5-HTP) prior to bedtime.

I briefly mentioned "sleep habits" earlier when listing some causes of sleep problems. "Sleep hygiene" is a conscious regimen to help us get our optimal quality of sleep for good health. It many respects it's no different than daily washing, exercise or brushing our teeth, except that its purpose is to regularize our circadian rhythm. It usually entails stopping all caffeine by 11:00 in the morning, going to bed at the same time every night to achieve about seven to nine hours of sleep, and strategies such as setting the phone alarm an hour prior to bedtime to remind us to turn it off (with all other electronic disturbers), keeping the lights on low to prepare our brain for a surge of melatonin, and setting the bedroom thermostat to about 68 degrees. Change your pillow regularly and your mattress every ten years: it's hard to sleep if you're uncomfortable. And if you're easily awakened, invest in an inexpensive white noise generator to drown out random sounds. Don't forget to close your blinds, but also don't forget to take in that burst of natural sunlight first thing on waking.

Some people feel they benefit from a daytime nap. If you do nap, don't risk upsetting your rhythm. The best time is in the mid-afternoon, but not for longer than 20 minutes – the "trucker's nap". After 20 minutes, you quickly enter a deep phase of sleep, and to wake up abruptly from that descent may make you groggy and rob you of a proper sleep at night.

In general, exercising regularly makes it easier to fall asleep and contributes to sounder sleep. However, exercising sporadically or right before going to bed will make falling asleep more difficult. This is because exercise elevates body temperature and your brain and body desires to be cooler for an optimal sleep. Time your exercise to the first few hours after waking.

Sleeping supplements need not mean powerful drugs. A number of supplements can help with getting to sleep and staying asleep.

Magnesium is one of my favorites for calming the mind and body. Look for the L-threonate form and try 100mg before bed. I also like passion flower and hops extract.

I've already mentioned melatonin in the context of jet lag. As a supplement sleep aid, it helps many people establish or maintain that natural circadian rhythm. Research has shown that the use of melatonin can shorten the time it takes to fall asleep and reduce the number of awakenings. As a bonus, it's a potent brain-healthy antioxidant.

California poppy is a little-known supplement that sounds as though it may be related to opium but It isn't. It's non-addictive. There's good evidence though that extracts of this flower can both help with the low back pain that can interrupt sleep and act as a potent sedative.

In addition to these strategies, there are endless numbers of free apps that may help ease you into sleep. Others monitor audible snoring or read heart and respiration rates as well as night movement.

NOT IGNORING SNORING

Hemoglobin is an element in the blood that binds with oxygen to carry it through the bloodstream to the organs, tissues, and cells of the body. Normal oxygen saturation is usually between 96 and 98 percent. Anything less than 95% is damaging to the brain, which requires approximately 3.3 ml of oxygen per 100 g of brain tissue per minute. If oxygen gets low, the body responds by redirecting blood to the brain to increase cerebral blood flow. But if oxygen saturation in the brain isn't corrected because blood flow can't be increased or if doubled blood flow does not correct the problem, symptoms of cerebral hypoxia will begin to appear.

If you do snore, your brain is very likely not getting the level of oxygen it requires. Optimal blood levels of oxygen while you sleep is something you can test yourself for. A simple technology called pulse oximetry can measure your blood oxygen levels overnight. You can purchase a unit for less than $30 online. If you find your levels are below 88 percent for longer than five minutes during a night, a condition called hypoxemia may be happening. This is dangerous for your brain and many people experience it without knowing. Snoring is the primary cause of sleep disruption for approximately 90 million North American adults. It's often a sign of sleep apnea — potentially dangerous interruptions in breathing caused (usually) by nighttime restriction of the airway.

Sleep apnea's pauses in breathing or shallow breaths during sleep can cause a significant reduction in oxygen saturation. People with sleep apnea often stop breathing for ten seconds and up to a minute or more. Symptoms of hypoxia caused by snoring can include difficulties in learning tasks and reductions in short-term memory. If oxygen deprivation continues, cognitive disturbances and decreased motor control can result. It only gets worse from there, and over time the brain's grey matter starts to diminish.

The good news is that if you snore (and therefore likely have sleep apnea), you can increase the volume of grey matter in your brain by using a technology known as continuous positive airway pressure therapy (CPAP). Research using magnetic resonance imaging shows that CPAP significantly increases grey matter volume in the hippocampus and frontal areas of the brain after only three months and this increase in grey matter volume in these regions is specifically correlated with the improvement of executive functioning and short-term memory.

Overnight oximetry alone is not adequate to diagnose sleep apnea and cannot be used for insurance purposes to qualify for treatment such as a mask that delivers continuous positive airway pressure. If you are snoring, ask your family physician for a referral to a sleep specialist who can order a nocturnal polysomnography which monitors heart, lung and brain activity, breathing patterns, arm and leg movements, and blood oxygen levels while you sleep. And by the way, CPAP isn't the only known solution. Sometimes a customized dental appliance, or surgeries called uvulopalatopharyngoplasty and lingual tonsillectomy may also work.

PART II

TALKING TO THE THINKERS

INTERVIEWS WITH THE WORLD THOUGHT LEADERS

It is the mark of an educated mind to be able to entertain a thought without accepting it.

~ ***Aristotle***

During my years as a clinician, it's been my privilege and pleasure to make the acquaintance of many researchers and physicians who have devoted themselves to their practices, their studies, and often their convictions. In writing this book I realized how many among them had made contributions to brain science or had relevant opinions on the subject, and to these I can add persons with whom I'm newly acquainted or who may not be practitioners in a formal and professional sense, but with unique insight to offer. I felt there could no better way to round out my thoughts on the brain than to add the thoughts of people whose combined experience outweighed any of my own. And who better to voice those thoughts than the people themselves?

10

THOUGHTS ON THE BRAIN

From an interview with Dr. Andrew Weil

I think all of the brain is concerned with the mind, but not all of the mind is in the brain.

~ Andrew Weil

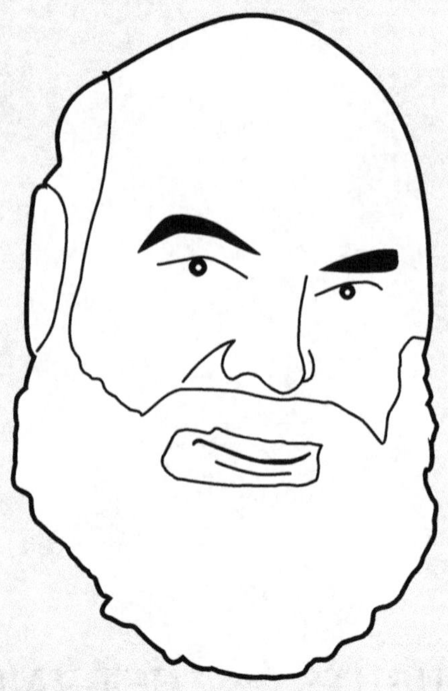

DR. ADREW **WEIL**

Dr. Andrew Weil is a world-renowned leader and pioneer in the field of integrative medicine. He takes a healing-oriented approach to health care which encompasses body, mind, and spirit. Dr. Weil is an internationally recognized expert for his views on leading a healthy lifestyle, his philosophy of healthy aging, and his critique of the future of medicine and health care. Combining a Harvard education and a lifetime of practicing natural and preventive medicine, Dr. Weil is the founder and director of the Andrew Weil Center for Integrative Medicine at the University of Arizona, where he also holds the Lovell-Jones Endowed Chair in Integrative Rheumatology, and is Clinical Professor of Medicine and Professor of Public Health.

Wylde: About eight months ago, my own mother was diagnosed with Alzheimer's. As a result, I've decided to write a book focusing on solutions that help those with everything from TBI to CTE to Alzheimer's. We've all been focusing so long on the heart and exercise and losing weight to prevent diabetes, I think we've lost focus — in fact I've never had one — on the brain. So I'd like to supplement my own years of clinical experience by calling on some of the world's most recognized brain health researchers and practitioners, including yourself. Can I start, then, by asking what you, Dr. Andrew Weil, have done for your brain today?

Weil: You mean this very day? Well, let's see, I got a good night's sleep. I didn't have a cigarette because I've never smoked. I've taken my dogs for a long walk and got my cardio-respiratory function up. I'll go for a swim later. I had some salmon for breakfast for my omega 3s and after some desk work I've done my breathing exercises.

Wylde: That's probably a lot more than the average person will do in an entire day.

Weil: I've also I've also taken a supplement of turmeric and of various mixed mushroom supplements that include lion's mane. Oh, and I had a bowl of matcha green tea.

Wylde: You start this on on a daily basis, don't you? Most people aren't taking the right matcha. Where can we get the "right stuff"?

Weil: The problem is it is very finely powdered so it has a huge surface area, and if it's exposed to air and light and heat, it oxidizes quickly and loses its bright green color, its flavor and aroma and probably some of its health properties. Most matcha I see in North America has not been properly stored. It's sometimes yellow or brownish green and often tastes bitter. I think many people here have never tasted really good matcha, so I started a company, www.matcha.com, and I made arrangements with a major producer near Kyoto, which is the best tea-producing region.

Wylde: I had the opportunity to drink that very stuff in Japan while I was studying with some Buddhist monks on the base of Mount Shigisan. So anyway, I have a question for you, appreciating your history and your deep interest in the mind/brain connection. This is maybe partly scientific, partly philosophical. Do you think the mind and the brain are one and the same?

Weil: Hm. How shall I put this? I think all of the brain is concerned with the mind, but not all of the mind is in the brain.

Wylde: I'm sure you'd agree that stress is North America's number one killer, contributing to heart disease, diabetes, cancer, etc.. But what impact is chronic stress having on our brain, particularly on our overall mental well-being?

Weil: Here's one very sobering fact. Cortisol, the main stress hormone is directly toxic to neurons.

Wylde: So what would we do on a daily basis to manage that cortisol level?

Weil: There are many possibilities. Whatever suits you. My personal favorite is a breathing technique, especially a four, seven, eight breath count that I teach because it's so time- and cost-efficient and uses no equipment. If you practice it, it literally takes two minutes a day. And I think the effects are very dramatic.

The 4-7-8 Breathing Exercise

The 4-7-8 Breathing Exercise is utterly simple, takes almost no time, requires no equipment and can be done anywhere. Although you can do the exercise in any position, sit with your back straight while learning the exercise. Place the tip of your tongue against the ridge of tissue just behind your upper front teeth, and keep it there through the entire exercise. You will be exhaling through your mouth around your tongue; try pursing your lips slightly if this seems awkward.

Exhale completely through your mouth, making a whoosh sound.

Close your mouth and inhale quietly through your nose to a mental count of four.

Hold your breath for a count of seven.

Exhale completely through your mouth, making a whoosh sound to a count of eight. This is one breath.

Now inhale again and repeat the cycle three more times for a total of four breaths.

Note that you always inhale quietly through your nose and exhale audibly through your mouth. The tip of your tongue stays in position the whole time. Exhalation takes twice as long as inhalation. The absolute time you spend on each phase is not important; the ratio of 4:7:8 is important. If you have trouble holding your breath, speed the exercise up but keep to the ratio of 4:7:8 for the three phases. With practice you can slow it all down and get used to inhaling and exhaling more and more deeply.

Wylde: You're known as the guru of alternative medicine, but how can we help people understand that this sort of advice is not anti-medicine, but more integrative and evidence-based?

Weil: I like the word integrative because it suggests inclusivity ... and it works. The aim is to expand the paradigm with conventional medicine and make it more effective and cost effective by focusing on prevention and on health promotion, especially with attention to lifestyle issues. It works by looking at the whole person, not just the physical body, and then by making use of all therapies that are not going to cause harm and show reasonable evidence of efficacy no matter where they come from.

Wylde: When you say harm, is the biomedical model of managing mental health becoming obsolete?

Weil: I think it's extremely limited in its effectiveness and it depends entirely on medication and sees all disturbances of mind and emotion as simply the effects of disturbances of brain biochemistry. I think that's a very limiting paradigm.

Wylde: Are there some useful drugs?

Weil: I think that drugs are sometimes necessary for the management of bipolar disorder but I think the antidepressants are much less effective than their manufacturers would have us believe; the anti-anxiety drugs are a disaster and I see almost no reason to take them. Their efficacy is greatly exaggerated and their dangers are greatly downplayed. They're being far too widely prescribed.

Wylde: From what you know, what are we observing in terms of the nations that have the lowest incidence of depression, or bipolar or schizophrenia?

Weil: Well, Iceland has the lowest rate of depression. I think that correlates with high blood levels of omega-3 fatty acids. I think that in countries that are often rated high on the happiness scale — such as the Scandinavian countries — a lot of that has to do with community and social networks taking care of people. I think we're ***not*** in great shape here. And one of the things that most alarms me is the rate of giving psychiatric drugs to kids. We have no idea what the long term effects are on the developing brain. it's a vast experiment with our nation's kids.

Wylde: It's worrisome.

Weil: Here's something about Alzheimer's. A few years ago I was in the in the Republic of Pulau, a group of islands in the far western Pacific. Alzheimer's is almost non-existent there and nobody has any idea why that is. The islanders' health has deteriorated dramatically in a relatively short space of time. After World War II, we Americans introduced all our worst foods and there's epidemic obesity, hypertension, type-2 diabetes. Their general health has really suffered. But interestingly, there's almost no Alzheimer's disease and people live long lives. They chew betel – maybe that's protective. I don't know about that, but someone should study it.

Wylde: The Scandinavians eat a lot of fish, but they also do sauna. We know the heat increases BDNF – brain derived neurotrophic factor. Maybe the people of Pulau do things other than chewing betel nut that heat the brain.

Weil: They live in a hot climate. That's interesting.

Wylde: Does the evidence support that we can actually evolve a healthier brain by what we eat or supplement?

Weil: I would say definitely. And just looking at one issue, I think that a lot of the neurodegenerative processes in the brain begins as inflammation. Controlling inflammation is certainly one strategy. And there's accumulating evidence of environmental causation of things like Parkinson's and A.L.S. and possibly there's an element of that in Alzheimer's as well. But I would bet money that Parkinson's and A.L.S. will turn out to be due to toxic injury, so protecting ourselves from environmental toxins is crucial.

Wylde: If there was a favorite brain-healthy food for you, what would that be?

Weil: There's an old saying that fish is brain food., and I think that's true, especially oily fish that are sources of EPA and DHA

Wylde: How much would you recommend on a weekly basis?

Weil: I would say something like three to five servings a week

Wylde: What about healthy spices?

Weil: Most certainly turmeric and ginger for their anti-inflammatory effects and cinnamon for its blood-sugar-lowering effects. Many of these spices and herbs have unique, vital protective compounds in them so I think the bottom line is, we should be eating a variety of herbs and spices, just as we should be eating a variety of vegetables and fruits.

Wylde: What are your thoughts on this burgeoning area of nootropics — supplements that may or may not be cognitive enhancers and provide benefit to mental focus, concentration, alertness, or energy?

Weil: We can get some of these active agents from natural sources such as green tea and matcha, but others such as turmeric and lion's mane mushroom, for which there's good evidence of efficacy, are better taken as a supplement if you want a therapeutic dose.

Wylde: Lastly, if there was one brain-healthy exercise that you wished you'd put into place long before you discovered it, what would that have been?

Weil: I guess learning another language, especially young in life, is very useful. And even ***attempting*** to learn another language, I think is a great brain exercise at any age. You don't have to master it — it's just the act of trying to learn it.

11

ENDING THE SLOSH EFFECT

from an interview with Dr. Julian Bailes

I've been most interested for several years in the use of omega-3 fatty acids, which are the main structural fat of the brain

~ ***Dr. Julian Bailes***

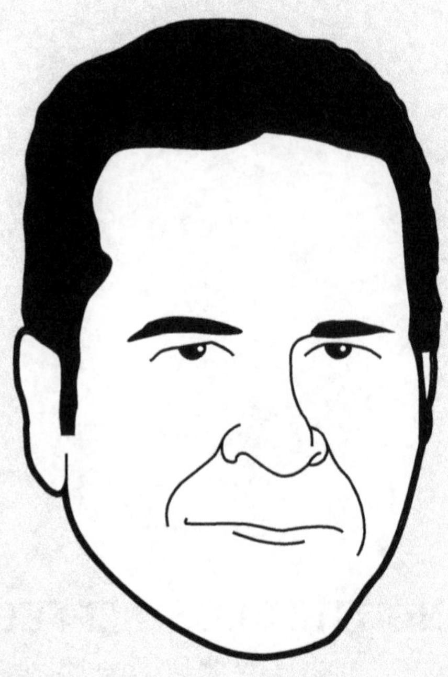

DR. JULIAN **BAILES**

Dr. Julian Bailes is a neurosurgeon and the former team physician of the Pittsburgh Steelers and has been a team physician in either the NFL or NCAA Division I for 25 years. He may be best known for being featured in the movie Concussion (played by Alec Baldwin) for the work he conducted with Dr. Bennet Omalu (played by Will Smith) to identify the first clinical evidence of chronic traumatic encephalopathy (CTE). He is a founding member of the Brain Injury Research Institute, Co-Director at the NorthShore Neurological Institute and Clinical Professor of Neurosurgery at the University of Chicago Pritzker School of Medicine. Dr. Bailes is a recognized leader in the field of neurosurgery and both the short and long-term impact of brain injury on cognitive function.

Wylde: We've been talking about the intricacy of the brain, which you as a neurosurgeon confront every day. But what about that brain when it's damaged, even lightly but repeatedly?

Bailes: On the question of repetitive head impacts, concussion, and CTE, these are an issue in a lot of sports: American football, lacrosse, rugby, the fighting arts such as boxing, and many others. All players in these sports risk brain injury because of the speed involved and the style of play that exposes players to hitting their heads. In football and ice hockey, of course, they wear helmets, but in soccer, the world's most popular sport, there's no head protection. In the vast majority of instances, impacts cause no apparent harm, but ***repetitive*** hits to the head — particularly in American football, where the helmets may give players a false sense of security — are a concern. The problem is that the human brain is floating inside the skull and the presence of the helmet doesn't stop the brain from moving or twisting or stretching or tearing fibers. It's possible that these repetitive head impacts can cause some concussion, and when they happen hundreds or thousands of times, we're concerned about accruing injury to axons or neurons or astrocyte cells that would lead in time to brain degeneration.

Wylde: Helmets are certainly protective, but do they protect against concussions specifically?

Bailes: No. They're designed to prevent skull fractures and scalp lacerations and facial and dental injuries. But they weren't really designed to prevent concussion and they don't. In fact, there's no concussion-proof helmet because, again, the brain is freely mobile inside the skull and there's no way to stop it when the helmet suddenly strikes another surface. Some people call that brain slosh.

Wylde: Is there anything coming down the pipe as it pertains to contact sports — some technology that you could wear that would perhaps reduce the incidence of trauma and concussion?

Bailes: We've done a lot of work here at a lot of work here at the NorthShore

Neurosurgery Department with a technology that is worn around the neck. It appears in multiple studies to limit the brain's ability to move or twist or tear— the slosh phenomenon. It seems to be beneficial and is the only technology I'm aware of that provides protection from ***inside*** the head. It is moving through FDA approval at the moment, so that's as much as I can discuss. But I can tell you that it's development is referred to as "biologically inspired discovery". How can a woodpecker sustain what is believed to be 83 plus million head impacts — pecks — in its lifetime without getting concussion? Far as we know — because they keep pecking — they don't even get a headache. But it seems woodpeckers have a special adaptation of their tongue, which has divided in two so that one half goes out one nostril and wraps around the cranium like a kind of strap and makes their brain less freely movable inside the skull. Bighorn sheep have their own complicated adaption by which a hollow pneumatic horn core increases vascular pressure in the cranium. These examples observed in nature are the so-called "bubble wrap" effect. Now some researchers have noticed that football players at higher altitudes are less prone to concussion, maybe because the lower air pressure increases the volume of blood in the cranium just like the bighorn ram — and our helmet.

Wylde: So this is a technology that may prevent head injury. What about technologies that help to recover from these injuries?

Bailes: Unfortunately there's no pharmaceutical solution for severe brain trauma, no drug that can repair the brain in the case of major trauma or mild trauma or concussion. But I've been most interested for several years in the use of omega-3 fatty acids, which are the main structural fat of the brain. And there's been a lot of work in multiple labs around the world showing the benefits of a omega-3, particularly DHA, as applied to improvements or healing or reducing injury after concussion. In some instances, it may even be prophylactic if someone's already taking it. If so, it would be a cheap and affordable and accessible solution and should be available worldwide for traumatic brain injury, especially in light of the fact that there's no effective pharmaceutical solution.

12

THE LAND OF OZ

From an interview with Dr. Mehmet Oz

My mom's genetics is the highest risk for Alzheimer's disease as you know, because you did my testing as well

~ Dr. Mehmet Oz

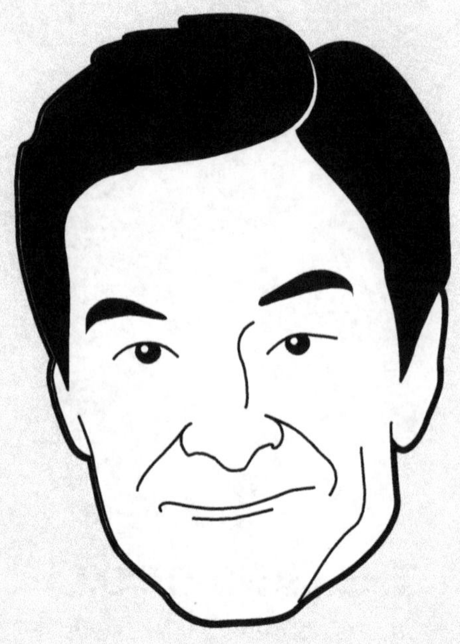

DR. MEHMET **OZ**

Dr. Mehmet Oz is an Emmy Award-winning host of the The Dr. Oz Show and Vice-Chair and Professor of Surgery at Columbia University. He directs the Cardiovascular Institute and Complementary Medicine Program at New York Presbyterian Hospital. His research interests include heart replacement surgery, minimally invasive cardiac surgery, complementary medicine and health care policy. He has authored over 400 original publications, book chapters and medical books, has received several patents, and performs more than 100 heart surgeries per year.

Wylde: What have you, Dr. Mehmet Oz, done for your brain today?

Oz: I'm having oatmeal with flaxseed oil right now, so that's a little bit of help. You and I talked this morning and I did 10 minutes of yoga. Then I woke my brain by doing a TV interview.

Wylde: Most people hear your name and they think of America's doctor or the doctor on TV. But first and foremost, you're a leading cardiothoracic surgeon, one of the most papered. You still hold hospital privileges. You operate routinely. So tell us a bit about that side of your career.

Oz: My calling has always been medicine. Since I was a little boy, I wanted to be a doctor. Cardiac surgery is the perfect field for me because you have to make quick decisions, sometimes fail and yet get up and go back again. That was always what my life has been like, my personality. I also like the fact that when I went into heart surgery, it was at the dawn of a massive improvement in what we could do. And so I thought, hey, I'm in a major field that is on the cutting edge. I didn't want to go into a field where I thought the best advances were in the past or so far in the future.

Wylde: And has it served you?

Oz: Very well, I mean, I got to invent a device we use to fix heart valves. Been involved in a lot of endeavors that shape innovation in the field. I've hosted the biggest conference for innovation, the first week into every year for a decade. The medical societies that I joined have grown dramatically because it was the right place, the right time. It would be like joining the Internet in 2000. There was a lot of stuff that was going to happen. You could tell it

Wylde: Your mom and her recent diagnosis of Alzheimer's, which you opened up about and how the initial signs eluded you as a physician. Tell us about that.

Oz: My mom, she's a very stubborn woman but she began to get even more stubborn than usual. As one of her children, it was hard to figure out because you can't figure out whether they're being obstinate because they don't feel well or that you you're having trouble communicating or maybe you're the problem. I wrote it off as that for a long time, probably a year, as she got more more difficult to deal with on simple issues. She'd been away from us for a while and a problem arose I had to deal with her on. I realized that she was not being rational about it. I knew this was not right. So we had to re-evaluate neurologically -- just a simple series of questions and the results indicated that she was borderline Alzheimer's, not quite there, but borderline. We didn't want to admit it at that point. My father denied it. One of my sisters wouldn't acknowledge it. But after six months finally we all agreed earlier this year that she had Alzheimer's.

Wylde: How did you deal with that when you finally came to realize that that was the diagnosis?

Oz: Well, the first thing was to get everyone in the family on board. Your family is the biggest obstacle. They don't want to admit it's true. If you don't want to call out the truth, you won't get very far. I got my one sister on board and we could begin with some simple things, like make sure that she didn't give away everything she owned without realizing it. She would walk down the hall — she did this this year — and start giving jewellery away to strangers. Of course, people very ethically would give it back. But she could get lost. She could take advantage of you. But she still recognized me. If I sat down with her, for the first five minutes I wouldn't be sure what was going on. And then you start thinking, "Now wait here..."

Wylde: As an intelligent woman, I'm sure she was intellectualizing a lot of these symptoms early on or somehow evading detection.

Oz: She was. My dad enabled her. People do this. They cover up for each other. They finish your sentences. "You're talking about those things from last year. I'll help you." And then, next thing you know, you've got a whole conversation going where they don't actually say anything because they don't know what to say.

Wylde: All right, so then the family's on board and everyone's banding together, which is the right thing to do. But then it must become a time when you think about your risk, your family history is a risk factor. You also played football, so there are head trauma factors into the risk. Is this something that's now weighing heavy on your mind as it relates to prevention of this disease for yourself

Oz: I've worked on it. I met with some top notch neurologists exactly along the lines that you described to get genetic testing. My mom is ApoE4 twice and the fact that she didn't have Alzheimer's until she's in her 80s is itself stunning and my risk is actually a little bit below average because other genes are protective, which I learned from Dr. Tansey, who's a superb neurologist at Mass General.

Wylde: So this leads to the next obvious question. What program have you ultimately established? Now that you've had your risk evaluated and tests done for yourself to keep a healthy brain?

Oz: Well, there are a couple of supplements that I need to deal with. One is, because of my genes, I'm especially dependent on omega-3 fats. And I need to take folic acid more studiously, so I've started. That's not for everybody but for me it's an important contributor. I don't really have a lot I can change. I don't smoke. I'm not overweight. However sleep is something I put a lot of emphasis on over the last year. Actually, the last couple of years, I'm doubling down on that. That's really important for mental health. You just have to be attuned to the fact that you're not the same as everybody else. My cholesterol numbers are good enough that I wouldn't need to do anything about them in respect to my heart, but with regards to my brain, they're not quite where we want them to be. So I pretty much gave up meat. I'll eat meat if I'm at an event and there's no other food. If they serve me the big filet mignon, I may return it and get fish or vegetable. At home, we don't eat meat anymore.

Wylde: Would you say pescatarian, maybe even ovo-pescatarian — eggs and fish with a variety of fruits and veggies? Would you suggest that's probably the healthiest diet?

Oz: The healthiest diet is the vegan diet but I don't want to do that right now. It's too much of a hassle. I can't spend my whole day trying to figure out what to eat. People who bring me food at the show know not to bring me meat. I eat primarily vegetables, but I'll have fish now and again just for diversity's sake. I cut back the amount of eggs I eat. We had chickens so I used to eat a lot of eggs but now I eat no more than 5 a week, usually none on weekdays

Wylde: There's the vegan trap, of course. A lot of people are going vegan. It's a trend. It's not necessarily healthy unless you know how to manage your diet. You often refer to Alzheimer's, for example, as Type 3 diabetes. So help us understand the connection between brain health and sugar, because that is the vegan trap: overeating refined carbohydrates.

Oz: Many vegetarian and vegans are carbarians. They just eat carbs. Potato chips are vegan. Off you go. You can pervert any diet. However, at its very core, avoiding inflammatory substances in your body is valuable. The most important inflammatory substances to avoid are the unhealthy fats the transfats and the simple sugars, which our insulin tries to catch up with. And then right behind these are the saturated fats, though the saturated fats aren't as bad as the sugars. Probably the keto or paleo diets — fats instead of carbs and sugars — are good options for many people. I think I can do both. I think I can have complex carbs, which I'm eating right now, with a little less of the sugars — I just avoid adding sugar to food — and then I don't have to have saturated fats. My fats are primarily healthy vegetable fats and things like that.

Wylde: On your show, you often talk about knowing your numbers. What numbers should we know for our brain? And that includes any screens or tests we might take at home or with family physician to help evaluate our brain health today.

Oz: Most important is your waist size. You can do it right now. Get a measuring tape — put it over your hips, your belly button and suck in. See how much fat you have in your belly. Remember that waist size needs to be one half your height or less. I'm six foot — seventy two inches — and half of that is 36 inches. If my waist size is below 36 inches, the risk of inflammatory conditions caused by belly fat — high cholesterol, high blood sugar, high blood glucose — are diminishingly small. Above that number, the risk rapidly increases. And that's probably the best tactic for people to use. In addition, when you go to a doctor, your LDL, cholesterol, blood sugar numbers should be in two digits — under 100, ideally less than 95. A third of the population is pre-diabetic. So their numbers are 100, 200. That's not acceptable.

Wylde: As a heart specialist, what can you tell us about the brain-heart connection, perhaps even specifically as it relates to stress because they're both so deeply affected by this number one silent killer, as you often emphasize?

Oz: It's how you cope with stress that matters. If you cope with stress in a thoughtful, intelligent way, then you can go to it. When you play sports, it's very stressful. You put your body under stress. You have mental stress trying to win. And I think people don't appreciate there's a benefit to that. That's what we try to highlight.

Wylde: Well, how do you do it?

Oz: How do I manage stress? Meditation, which I do, usually in the evenings. But I dare say, I'm not a very anxious person. I never have been. One of my genetic tests showed I have a gene mutation where I tend to have more oxytocin. I'm not alone. Probably 50% of the general population is like me, but things that should stress me don't bother me as much. And maybe I'm a heart surgeon because, you know, when someone's about to die — I mean, I obviously care about it — but it doesn't bother me the way that it affects some others. And that's a good thing in my case because of my profession, though maybe bad in other settings, if you can't empathize with people and connect with them. You play the cards you're dealt. But for me anxiety and stress aren't the big issues.

13

ENDING COGNITIVE DECLINE

From an interview with Dr. Dale Bredesen

There is accumulating evidence Alzheimer's comes from multiple sources... number one, the microbiomes of patients with Alzheimer's are indeed different

~ Dr. Dale Bredesen

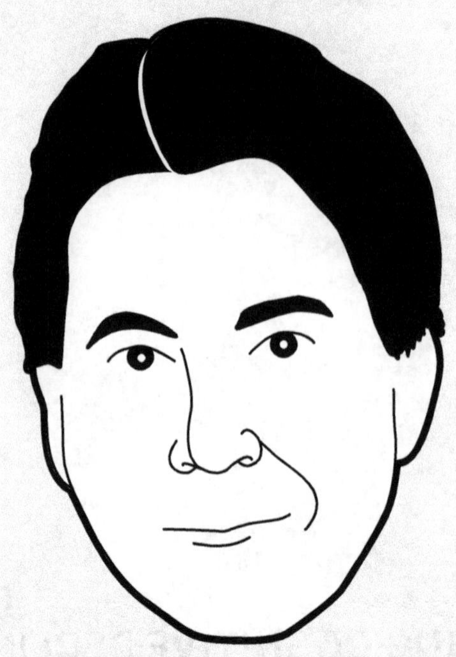

DR. DALE **BREDESEN**

Dr. Dale Bredesen is the professor of neurology at UCLA and best-selling author of "The End of Alzheimer's". He is internationally recognized as an expert in the mechanisms of neurodegenerative diseases such as Alzheimer's disease. He graduated from Caltech, then earned his MD from Duke University Medical Center in Durham, NC. He served as Chief Resident in Neurology at the University of California, San Francisco (UCSF) before joining Nobel laureate Stanley Prusiner's laboratory at UCSF as an NIH Postdoctoral Fellow. He held faculty positions at UCSF, UCLA and the University of California, San Diego. Dr. Bredesen directed the Program on Aging at the Burnham Institute before coming to the Buck Institute in 1998 as its founding President and CEO.

Wylde: My first question is, what have you, Dr. Dale Bredesen, done for your brain today?

Bredesen: First and foremost, I'm getting eight hours of sleep at night and making sure that I don't have any issues with sleep apnea, snoring, that sort of thing. I often sleep on my side for that reason, which I know a lot of guys, aging as I am, have resorted to that. The second thing is to try to keep this stress to a minimum. The third thing is to get exercise each and every day. I was just trying to get a little in before you called here. And then the fourth thing, of course, is diet.

We always think about diet, exercise, sleep and stress reduction as being the four pillars and try to eat more a plant rich diet that is good with high fat things like good fat, things like avocado, things like unsaturated oils, things like olive oil. So all of those. And things like brain exercise. And it's typically just either working on the book last night or looking at new patient material, things like that just to keep active. And then I do take a set of supplements and I don't take all of them all every day. But I do take some magnesium when I look at the fact that most of us are deficient in magnesium. Most of us are deficient in iodine, most are deficient in zinc, and most of us are deficient in potassium. Those are sort of the big four. So I try to deal with that. Of course, there's more and more on ancestral diets. And so we've tried to recognize that the failures we have in terms of our eating habits. I try to stay away completely from processed food. We do sometimes have some popcorn and stuff like that but in general, try to stay away from any sort of processed food and eat a largely plant based diet. We do have some meat. It's a condiment, basically. So all those are the kind of things that I actually found out I was low in the hormone pregnenolone and low in thyroid hormone. So I take some of both of those hormones in small amounts. I also take some products to heal my gut. I take some short-chain fatty acids and then also some probiotics and prebiotics and then I also take a multivitamin. And then some omega-3. I try to get my omega-3 ratio appropriate. And those are the main ones. I do have some vitamin D and I do take some mixed tocopherols and tocotrienols. And, again, not every single day. I basically try to balance the fact that many of us are deficient in these things or at the very least we are suboptimal in them. But I do think that the difference between true deficiency and being suboptimal is not well enough understood. Some are told by their doctor "you're not really that low, your B12 is 350 so fine because it shows in the normal range." But we know this is not fine. So I do take some B12 and methylfolate as well.

Wylde: I always start my day with exercise. I can't get by without it because my genome shows that I have an unfavourable BDNF variant. But I've recently just had to start looking into and trying an oral appliance because I started to snore a bit. I understand that even active snoring, whether you're apneic or not, is ultimately brain toxic. As you point out in your work, even having a two percent difference in O_2 saturation can make an impact on your brain and may be harmful.

Bredesen: Right. We've spent 30 years in the lab looking at the molecular drivers of the degenerative process. If you trace backwards from a cell committing suicide, committing programmed cell death and you ask what triggered that? — this is basically what we did for all those years and then asked how can we now translate that into a clinical approach to different people? Then a couple of things emerge. Number one, we're just doing something very simple, which is asking of each person: what are the things that cause your decline and then let's go after each of those. So if you have a great B12 level, that's probably not contributing to your decline, you won't worry about that. Dozens and dozens of things that are contributory. And so it's a little different for each person. No surprise. And so all we are trying to do is look at what are the things that drive the process. We typically find 10 to 25 sub-optimal values. And these things do seem to contribute to your lack of neuroplasticity, and to your decline. I mentioned I found out I was very low in pregnenolone. Okay. So I take pregnenolone. And what's beautiful about it is that you can actually trace the molecular paths, for example, from testosterone or estradiol and NFKB and inflammation directly through ATP itself and why the ATP would be cleaved in the alternative approach, which is the one that gives you the amyloid. So you can you can literally trace the molecular pathways and see why it is that you get this disease we call Alzheimer's, which is ultimately actually a protective response to these different insults. It's a scorched earth retreat.

Wylde: In your book, ***The End of Alzheimer's***, you discuss at great length the idea that there's more than one form of Alzheimer's. Tell us about that.

Bredesen: Right. First of all, you realize that you have to have a larger data set. This old idea that we're just going to give you a predetermined treatment, which only has a single mechanism of action is really, I think, very biologically naive. You're going after something that's a complex problem with a simple solution that will not work. And so therefore, when we now start looking, we say Let's look at someone's status with respect to their inflammation. Let's look at their status with respect to their trophic factors. In fact, there are several different metabolic syndromes are called Alzheimer's disease. I won't get into the details, but here is how we classify them:

> **Type 1:** Inflammatory ("Hot")
> **Type2:** Atrophic ("Cold")
> **(Type1.5:** Glycotoxic ("Sweet"combines 1 and 2))
> **Type3:** Toxic ("Vile") – a fundamentally different problem.
> **Type 4:** Vascular ("Pale")
> **Type 5:** Traumatic ("Dazed")

There are about twenty-five contributing factors to type1 and about a third of all Alzheimer's cases have a non-amnestic presentation.

Wylde: I'd like to talk about the idea and this concept that most of us it's been driven by our primary health care provider and even through society in the media to think about heart health, keeping a healthy weight or liver health, but we don't often think of the brain until it's too late. So my question is, ultimately, how early should people start to think about looking at their brain health and considering these various types that maybe they are predestined to in a meaningful way? In other words, what may be a good time to start running tests to determine a baseline for brain health? I think you refer to this as cognoscopy. [https://www.bcna.ca/2018/02/have-you-had-a-cognoscopy/]

Bredesen: Right. So we recommend that everybody get a cogonoscopy at the age of 45. And if you pass 45 and you haven't had one yet, still go, go by and get one because in fact, as you indicated, you have about a 20-year run up from the beginning of the pathophysiology. The best data so far in terms of looking at early changes in cerebrospinal fluid and early changes in PET scan, it suggests that this is about 20 years between the beginning of the pathophysiology and a diagnosis of Alzheimer's. During that time, you can certainly have some subjective cognitive impairment and mild cognitive impairment. So certainly you may have some symptoms, but we want to recommend that everybody get a cognoscopy at 45. Now the only exceptions are the rare cases, less than 5 percent, where you actually have a familial Alzheimer's who get symptomatic in their 30s. And so in those rare cases, of course, you should have one and you should come in. We are dealing with one guy whose family gets Alzheimer's in their 20s. He's 42 and asymptomatic. We want to keep it that way. So the goal is get on prevention and don't worry if you've started to have mild symptoms. These are very treatable. And we see it again and again and again. The problem is when people wait and they say, well, I'm not that bad yet. This is one thing that sneaks up on you, as you probably saw just a week ago. Dr. Oz reported that he had missed the signs and symptoms of Alzheimer's in his own mother. This happened right in front of his eyes and he missed it. It can sneak up on you. As I said, it is a stealthy reaper. Again, the old idea is backwards: I'm going to wait as long as as long as I can, because there's nothing that can be done. No, it's just the opposite. Come in as soon as possible because there's more to done early on than there is later on.

Wylde: Absolutely. I like to refer patients that are concerned about this early on and want to maybe check why they're losing a name or forgetting why they're standing at a fridge, I want to refer them to the Montreal mini mental test. Do you have a favorite or best online assay that folks can do at home?

Bredesen: There are a number of things that we recommend. I like the Montreal cognitive assessment, but as you know, it is not terribly sensitive to the early changes. And so we think of it in terms of what is the dynamic range for each thing. MoCA (Montreal Cognitive Assessment) has a good dynamic range for late MCI (mild cognitive impairment) and early Alzheimer's. For later Alzheimer's, we want the MMSE (Mini Mental State Examination) which is very insensitive but good for late-stage Alzheimer's. The MoCA is in between, but then the things that you really want are the ones upfront that are the most sensitive to early changes and we use CNS vital signs.

[ed. note: MoCA and MMSE are similar but different. Both the MMSE and the MoCA are routine cognitive screening tests rated on a 30-point scale. They are both brief, though the MMSE is a little shorter, taking about 7 to 8 minutes to administer. The MoCA takes approximately 10 to 12 minutes.]

But other people use Cogstate. There are a number of things. There's a Cambridge product that people use, but I like CNS vital signs. Again, there are multiple things that are very sensitive. And of course, there's the standard 4 hour neuro or quantitative assessment. The concerns I have about that, if you've actually got any sort of changes, that is a very stressful four hours and stress certainly can damage your brain. You don't want to stress people out too much while testing.

Wylde: Right. I'll refer my readers to your book ***The End of Alzheimer's***. Meanwhile, I'd like to talk about leaky gut. You've experienced that yourself. You've fixed it or are always in the process of fixing and preventing it. What can you tell us about the relationship between leaky gut and ultimately leaky brain?

Bredesen: Yes, it's a very good point and I think that at this point, there's probably a little more data on leaky gut — and a change in microbiome — and its relationship to Parkinson's, because that's been done nicely with animal models. With Alzheimer's, though, there is accumulating evidence from multiple sources that, when you put it all together, it's very suggestive. Number one, the microbiomes of patients with Alzheimer's are indeed different than the microbiomes of people without Alzheimer's. Number two, in animal models where you actually do alter the microbiome, you can make an impact on an animal model of Alzheimer's, which we call mouseheimer's. So it argues that there is a direct effect between the microbiome and you're likelihood of developing Alzheimer's disease. Third, a lot is published on diet and its relationship to Alzheimer's and diet obviously has multiple impacts. The fourth thing is, of course, that leaky gut is associated with systemic inflammation and everything that's been published. Anything that is associated with systemic inflammation — and I include things like metabolic syndrome, cardiovascular disease, people with high hs-CRPs (high sensitivity c-reactive protein which is a blood-borne inflammatory marker) — all of the above are associated with increased risk of cognitive decline. Metabolic syndrome is in fact a multiple-fold increased risk for Alzheimer's disease — and of course type 2 diabetes as well. So all of those things add up to a strong suggestion that in fact, leaky gut and altered microbiome, they're very important in your likelihood of developing cognitive decline, which is why we want to — and we talk about it in the book — heal the gut and then provide pro-biotics and pre-biotics to create an optimal microbiome. You're probably aware there's been some interesting recent A.L.S research on a specific organism ***Akkermansia muciniphila.*** I think over the years you're going to see more and more use of specific parts of the microbiome to be part of the treatment, part of the overall treatments for various degenerative conditions

Wylde: So interesting! And as the saying has gone for some years now in the world of functional medicine, when it comes to metabolic syndrome at least and a shift the microbiome: the larger the belly, the smaller the brain. That sounds like a pretty straightforward accurate statement.

Bredesen: Yes, I think that is a very accurate statement.

Wylde: Are there any other genetics beyond the APOE variants that you're paying close attention to as it pertains to a predisposition to, not just Alzheimer's but cognitive decline at large.

Bredesen: That's a very good point. It used to be thought that your genetics are your fate. Now it's your tendency, but not necessarily your fate. Epigenetics and its effects have been a big part of functional medicine. So again, we recommend that everyone evaluate their genome or at least the critical drivers for cognitive decline. And I think as whole genomes become less and less expensive, this will be something for everybody to be doing. Yes, the APOE4 genetic variant is the big one, its the common one. About two thirds of people with Alzheimer's have it. And as you know, if you've got zero copies of APOE4, you've got about a 9 percent chance of developing Alzheimer's during your lifetime. If you've got a single copy, it's about 30 percent, but if you've got two copies, it's well over 50 percent. So it makes a big difference. We've studied this for years in the lab to look at the underlying mechanisms and found, in fact, APOE4 has a big impact on the overall inflammatory response of cells. Stephen Gundry sent me a paper that just appeared this morning showing that in the iPS cells (Induced Pluripotent Stem Cells), the APEO4 was associated with a decreased phagocytosis and decreased mobilisation of microglia. That went pretty well with what we described genetically. We published a large genetic study looking at the genes affected by APOE4 and we discovered something really interesting. APOE4 actually enters your nucleus and binds to the promoters of seventeen hundred different genes — literally changing the programing of your cells. So what we always thought of as our butcher — APOE4 — carrying around the fat, the lipid, turns out also to be our senator making the laws of the land, literally changing the programming in our cells. And interestingly, in the cells there is a mutual antagonism between NFkB and a SERT1. So literally you can set yourself up in different modes. And this is almost like thinking about it as sleeping or awake. In one mode, of course, you are directing the resources of yourself away from inflammation and toward protection. You're doing the very thing that you need to do to repel invaders. On the other hand, you can direct your cell to shut that down and focus resources on building, on structure. It's no different than a country would do in wartime versus peacetime. So SERT1 is your peacetime approach. You're building new things, you're making new synapses. And APOE4 actually alters that balance towards NFkB, towards fighting inflammation, fighting infection. So in fact, no surprise, if you are APOE4 positive, you do better in a third world setting where you have a lot of parasites, you're eating raw meat, you're in squalid conditions. You actually live longer and better. When these same challenges aren't around, and you now want longevity and you don't want to use so much of your resources on protection, you actually do better with an APOE3 or APOE2 genetic variant. So those are less protective, but support longevity.

Now, there are actually several dozen other SNPs that are associated with increased risks of Alzheimer's disease. It's been less clear how to impact these, although as you can imagine, they tend to fall into just a couple of groups. Genes like TREM2 have to do with inflammation, and they have to do with the innate immune system, which turns out to be absolutely critical. The innate immune system such as CR1 (compliment receptor 1), such as NLRP1 — those are critical. They are involved with the innate immune system and they are part of the overall response and they are part of the risk for Alzheimer's. Vitamin D receptor (VDR) another one that was more on the atrophic-type side of things. Of course, vitamin D is associated with your inflammatory response, and when you are low, you have an increased risk for Alzheimer's disease. Then there are also things such as ABCA1 that are lipometabolism-related. There are multiple dozens of SNPs associated with Alzheimer's. It's become more and more clear what to do if you're APOE4 positive. There's a whole website (APOE4.info) where many thousands of people who are doing this sort of protocol and are looking at increasing their own Alzheimer's prevention plans and I think in the long run they're going to have a decreased likelihood of developing Alzheimer's given their APOE4 status because they have addressed it and they've addressed it early on. And that is the way of the future. And I think we'll be seeing the same sorts of things with all of these different SNPs as people begin to look at these earlier on in life.

Wylde: On the APOE variants, what you were just describing reminds me to remind readers that APOE4 is, in fact a favorable variant as it pertains to our evolution. But what I'd love you to describe is how that explains why blockbuster drugs have failed so miserably.

Bredesen: It's a great point. Let's look at what a drug is. A drug is a way to allow an underlying disease process to go on while trying to circumvent the root cause of this problem. But imagine that you have something where you've got 36 holes in your roof — different types of holes, but they're all letting in water. And now you're going to take a really great patch, an excellent patch, for one hole. You're not going to get much of the change. You get a little change but typically not significant. And that's exactly what's happened. When you have people with APOE4, we know that their Alzheimer's disease is driven by several different things but a large part of what's driving their disease is multi-factoral. When we grouped those seventeen hundred genes I mentioned where APOE4 bound to their promoters, we found you couldn't tell a better story for Alzheimer's. They absolutely impact your inflammatory state. They absolutely impact NFkB. They impact your tumor necrosis factor (TNF-a) but they also impact your glucose homeostasis. They also impact things like microtubules, disassembly and pulling back on your neurites. They impact your trophic support. So what's happening when you're giving a drug, you're not impacting those things that are actually driving the process — especially you're not impacting the inflammation — and in fact, you can be harming the person because once you understand that amyloid beta is actually an anti-microbial peptide — and this was discovered by Robert Moyer and Rudi Tanzi at Harvard a number of years ago — you start to realize this is a protective response. You're now impacting your own protective response, so it's a little bit like firing the CFO of your company. You might allow people to spend a little more for a short time, but ultimately you're going to hurt yourself more. And so when you give these drugs, number one, they're not hitting the root cause. Number two, they may actually be impacting what is a protective response, especially in the case of APOE4 where you've got more inflammation, you may not do very well. The observation has been that people with APOE4 do more poorly on the drugs and often have more side effects. Interestingly, it's just the opposite when you take a root cause approach, such as we published. The APOE4 positive patients tend to respond even better than the APOE4 negative patients.

Wylde: You talked about the cost of sleep. Tell us a little bit about sleep in context of what we're learning about glymphatics, particularly in context of brain clearance and let's call it detoxification and maybe in context of mitophagy. Why do we need to sleep? Why should we pay attention to brain health at night?

Bredesen: Yes, sleep is one of the most critical pieces. And in fact, sleep reduction affects you in multiple ways. But let me do a quick preamble here, because, in fact, there's something that's come up relatively recently and it's turning out to be very important. In evaluating patients, you have to include nocturnal oximetry and preferably also some daytime oximetry, because many of our subjects are dropping their oxygen saturations at night. One physician who trained in this protocol reports that he's getting the best and most rapid responses in people who have this reduced nocturnal oximetry. He's followed the desaturation evidence and typically addressed it with a continuous positive airway pressure (CPAP) device at night. During the day, you can address it with

EWOT, which stands for exercise with oxygen therapy to improve oxygenation. And that's one of the reasons exercise has been so good for so many people and for everybody who has any cognitive decline. Please get your oxymetry checked at night and address this and optimize. And we should all be in 96 to 98 percent saturation while we're sleeping. We're finding people dropping not only into the 80s, which is horrible, into the 70s and even low 70s, which is actually scary. Now, as you indicated, a number of other really critical things happen during sleep. With the glymphatic system, you literally have a change in the micro-anatomy of your brain during sleep that allows you essentially to wash out, as it were, some of the waste products that naturally accumulate during the day. In addition, of course, sleep is a critical time for fasting. And after about 12 hours of fasting, you are beginning some autophagy, decreasing your damaged components and destroying and essentially recycling damaged proteins, damaged lipids, damaged carbohydrates and other cellular components. Interestingly, if you just stop the autophagy of mitochondria, you get a Parkinsonian-type of phenotype. So it's very clear you need to get rid of the bad batteries and replace them with good batteries. You need mito-genesis and you need mitophagy. You need autophagy for these damaged proteins. Imagine that you don't go through this. You're going to now increase the presence of these damaged components in your body and especially in your brain. So sleep is absolutely critical. And it's critical that you while you're sleeping, you are able to give it appropriate oxygenation. You've got to have the appropriate energy to carry out these processes. And by the way, your body makes less amyloid while sleeping. And it now is removing more, whereas when you're awake, you're actually making more of the amyloid. So for many reasons, many different molecular mechanisms. Sleep is an absolutely crucial part of preventing and reversing cognitive decline.

14

DO THE HEART MATH

From an interview with Dr. Rollin McCraty

The heart has a causal role of modulating perceptions and brain function.

~ Dr. Rollin McCraty

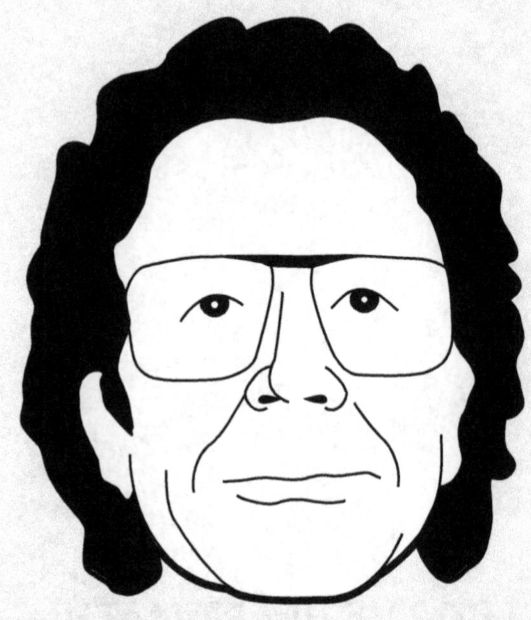

DR. ROLLIN **McCRATY**

Dr. Rollin McCraty Ph.D. is the director of research at HeartMath Institute Research Center. McCraty, a professor at Florida Atlantic University, is a psychophysiologist whose interests include the physiology of emotion. One of his primary areas of focus is the mechanisms by which emotions influence cognitive processes, behavior, health and the global interconnectivity between people and Earth's energetic systems. He has served as principal investigator in numerous research studies examining the effects of emotions on heart-brain interactions and on autonomic, cardiovascular, hormonal and immune-system function. The members of his research team regularly participate in collaborative studies with scientific, medical and educational institutions in the United States and around the world.

Wylde: Rollin McCraty, what have you done for your ***brain*** today?

McCraty: I started the day with about a ten-minute heart lock-in meditation. My practice is to try and start every morning with a five to ten-minute period of really prepping for the day by stabilizing my system and aligning with my own deeper heart and setting my intention to have a more caring, appreciative day. To be kind to people and not be so emotionally reactive if something comes up, to be able to really maintain compassionate latitude for people and others. And so I just sit in that coherent state for five to ten minutes. This morning I actually got about ten minutes. That has a carryover effect – I won't say all day because life happens and then you have to reset. But at least that's what I do to prepare my brain for the day.

Wylde: Just for readers to understand the difference generally between the heart lock-in and the routine form of meditation, whichever form they may be practicing that's great for the brain.

McCraty: Let me preface by saying that most of the HeartMath techniques, with the one exception of the heart lock-in, are really techniques that are intended to be used in the moment when something stressful or uncomfortable comes up. I call those moments the traffic jams of life, literally and figuratively. We aim to self-regulate in those moments, to really bring the emotions back into a deeper alignment. The heart lock-in is more of a meditation technique, but it's a heart-focused meditation where basically you really focus on the heart and really activate genuine feelings of appreciation, compassion, care, rather than the more dissociative state of some meditation techniques, and then you radiate those feelings to yourself, to your body, and then out to the world, to others, into the field environment.

Wylde: What is the mission of HeartMath?

McCraty: Our simple mission statement is "activating the heart of humanity".

Wylde: And from a bio-physiologic perspective, what exactly is heart rate variability and coherence?

McCraty: Everybody knows about heart rate is, simply how many times the heart beats in a minute. But in reality, especially in a healthy or resilient person, our heart rate is changing with each and every heartbeat. To measure heart rate variability, called HRV, we have to accurately measure the time between each pair of heartbeats. And that's really what heartbeat variability is. It's that beat-to-beat variation in every pair of heartbeats. Or you can spend an entire career trying to understand it and all that it's reflecting about the inner workings of the brain and body. It's simple but complex at the same time. In a healthy person, as I've already said, we have a lot of this beat-to-beat variability, this natural, intrinsic variability, and we have more of it when we're young and it gets less as we age. In fact, there's a rather linear relationship between the amount of HRV we have and our biological age. We can tell fairly close to how old somebody is, if they're on a healthy trajectory in life, by measuring their heart rate variability and determining how much of it they have. Heart rate variability, of course, has become huge, has actually crossed out of the medical and clinical worlds now into the market in a lot of ways, because we know that if you have lower heart rate variability than you should have for your age, that is a an independent and strong risk factor for future serious health problems. In fact, low HRV correlates with all-cause mortality rates in several studies. So it's a great measure of the overall functional status of our whole neural axis — the brain, the heart, the nervous system. It's pretty clear now that one of the main reasons that people tend to have low HRV is chronic long-term stress. We live in a very stressful world these days so we see a lot of people with relatively lower HRV because of the accumulation of long-term stress. Of course, disease processes can also lower HRV, especially inflammatory type processes. We know that lower HRV will occur in many people several years before the onset of symptoms. It's a great early warning indicator. Then there's coherence, independent of how much HRV we have, and coherence — the pattern of the HRV — reflects a deeper process. So when we plot the actual heart rhythm, we can see that it's reflecting many things, but for sure a person's emotional state. So when for example, someone's impatient or frustrated, anxious, or feeling overwhelmed — these types of stressful emotions — they're reflected in the heart rate variability pattern as what we call an incoherent heart rhythm. This is where a picture is worth a thousand words and it reflects activity in our brain and nervous system that is out of sync. Ultimately, it's the higher brain systems, the frontal cortex, the subcortical and inputs down into the brainstem and how those higher brain activities are reflected into the nervous system and the body. So we have, I think, a fairly clear understanding of why people who are frustrated a lot or tend to get angry or experience these types of unmanaged emotions over the long term also experience negative impacts on health and well-being. I love the analogy of a car here where you're driving with one foot on the accelerator and riding the brake with the other. That's a great analogy because it's pretty easy to see in the car context that you're going to put more stress on the brakes and the drive train and wear those parts out faster and you're going to use a lot more gas. It's not energy efficient. It's the same thing in our body. It's one of the questions I tend to ask when I do presentations and things to audiences. How many of you would like more energy than you currently have at the end of the day? Of course, everybody raises their hand. But let me digress for a moment. It's our emotions that really drive physiology much more than our thoughts. Of course, thoughts are important to manage, too, but once you feel something, that's when you really see activation in the nervous system and the hormonal systems. So back to those folks raising their hands, if we're going through the day getting triggered by all these little under-the-radar impatiences and frustrations, that's all activating the system and mobilizing energy, which at the end of the day depletes our energy reserves. So we tend to be exhausted. And that's one of these neat things that's reflected in heart rate variability.

Wylde: So what about coherence?.

McCraty: This goes back to our research in the early 90s when we were one of the first groups to look at positive emotions, not just the stressful and negative stuff. This was many years before the positive psychology movement. I think maybe there were only three or four papers in the medical literature at that time on anything positive. Anyway, we were looking at things like appreciation and compassion and gratitude — these types of emotions — and what we found there was not only that the heart rhythm was the most reflective of emotional states in general, but especially positive emotions. When you really feel appreciation or compassion, love — these kinds of emotions — the system naturally shifts into a different functional state, which we call coherence, and that's reflected in the heart rhythms again in this beautiful, sine-wave, smooth-looking heart rhythm pattern. That was a neat discovery back then, but following that rabbit down the hole, as you might say, led to many other discoveries and understandings about how the heart and brain communicate with each other. We saw that when the heart was in a coherent state, the brain was the big winner in many ways. The heart sends far more neural information to the brain through the afferent or ascending pathways of our nervous system — both the vagus nerve and the spinal column — than the brain sends to the body. A conservative estimate is 80 percent of the fibers in the vagus or afferent or ascending nerves — more people say 90 percent — carry information from the heart. The majority of signals are coming from the heart and cardiovascular system, far more than any other system in the body. So the heart and brain are intimately interconnected. We now know that the signals on these afferent pathways, once they get up to the medulla, can follow direct neural pathways to almost every major brain center. In the very late 60s, early 70s, researchers were starting to observe that the activity of the heart was having profound effects on the brain, including perception and emotional experience and cognitive function. I introduced two terms back then — cortical facilitation and cortical inhibition — to describe the effects that the heart was having on the brain. What wasn't known at that time was how this all worked. It was just observed that this was happening and it took a lot of years and many different groups around the world to really sort out the mechanisms, which are pretty well understood now. Most in the field of psycho-physiology would agree with one of the most famous hypotheses in the field, which was introduced back then, that the heart has a causal role and modulating perceptions and brain function. The history is fascinating. If you look back at the older literature, they were talking about how the heart was acting as though it had a mind of its own. It was believed that the autonomic nervous system was this dumb system, just a bunch of wires, and that the brain controlled the body and the body danced to its tune. People had this perception back then that the body and the nervous system were there just to support the brain and theoretically, if you cut the head off and give it a blood supply, everything would be just fine. We now know that's kind of absurd, but it was really these observations of the heart back then that started the paradigm shift. For example, you might observe a sympathetic arousal and the heart rate should in theory be increasing. But the heart rate would decrease instead of increasing — and vice versa. These were the early observations that really started that paradigm shift back in the understanding that the body and the information being sent from the body to the brain is very fundamental and has to be there for proper cognitive function and emotional experience and a textured life.

Wylde: I'm very interested in the phenomenon of centenarians. You mentioned that, as we age, we lose HRV. Do we know if anyone's looked at centenarians and their HRV?

McCraty: That would be a great study to do from my own observations over the years. In fact, a lot of my mentors in life — the Karl Pribram or Joseph Chilton Pearce and a bunch of other folks like that — who we've done HRV analysis on just because they were here and hanging out with us a lot — these were people who were in their late eighties and nineties — in fact, almost all of them lived well into their nineties — and were very active. Retirement was not something that was even in their world view. They had amazingly high HRV. I would say every one of them we looked at, these older people who really had that passion for life and were on a mission in their research careers, they were outside the box: their HRV was double or three times what it typically would be for someone their age. I can't generalize from that because there were maybe ten of them. But we certainly saw a pattern there.

Wylde: Ultimately, you can't practice yourself into a better HRV. Frankly, you don't even need the technology. But whether it's the emWave® or the Inner Balance, you can pass it along to a friend because at a certain point, through biofeedback, you understand what it takes to quickly get into coherence and optimal heart rate variability..

McCraty: We developed the emWave® and Inner Balance technologies to facilitate people learning the skills to shift into a coherent state and better self regulate in the moment. This is highly relevant to the brain because one of the neural pathways from the heart goes directly to the amygdala. In fact, the core nucleus of both amygdalas are synchronized to the cardiac cycle, to the heartbeat. So every time the heart beats, you have a firing of the cells in the amygdala. Whatever the heart rhythm pattern is — coherent or incoherent and everything in between, with different patterns reflecting different emotions, with anxiety looking different from frustration and frustration looking different from anger — the amygdala sees those heart signals and rhythm patterns right in its core nucleus. One of the things I learned from Dr. Karl Pribram who was a regular here for a week or two every year and most of what I know about the brain, I learned from him — one of the things I learned is the role of the amygdala. It's actually kind of embarrassing to say that he tried to explain this to me over a few years and it took a while for the penny to finally drop. From Karl's perspective, a lot of people have it wrong about the amygdala. In his model, the amygdala actually determines what is familiar and what is not familiar — both from the external sensory systems — what we see, hear, smell and so on — but also from the internal body systems, what we tend to call interception. The amygdala determines what's familiar, what's safe, what's comfortable or what's not comfortable — all those types of feelings and emotions that are generated from this process. To do that, the amygdala has to have a reference state that it can compare the current input to. That's what we call the familiar baseline reference. And it's an adaptive process. Everything we perceive goes through this process and filter. But say somebody is starting a new business or going through a divorce with a lot of stress over a sustained period — then that becomes the new familiar. And once that's set as the baseline the brain wants a pattern match — a maladapted familiar pattern. So that let's say anxiety becomes our new familiar. That's what the brain is going to seek to feel comfortable. For any type of sustained behavior or attitude, for any sustained emotional or world change, you can't accomplish it without shifting the familiar baseline references, especially if it's in the maladapted state. Now, here's the part that took me a while to grasp. Karl actually proved this in his work when he went back to Stanford: the only way to establish an internal reference pattern is to change the inputs from the body to the brain, especially the heart's inputs. That's such a fundamental and important understanding that psychology doesn't get yet. As you said, you can't think yourself into a new reference pattern, or a new internal baseline. If you're going to establish a new baseline, it's common sense to establish a coherent one. That's where our technology is so important. That's where heart lock-in is so important. But anytime we become more self aware and interrupt the old familiar patterns — such as getting pissed off in traffic jams or at that same person in meetings — and choose to take a different approach, use a technique and self-regulate, we're starting to interrupt the old baseline pattern and starting the process of establishing a new one. And if we do that long enough, this new pattern is going to become a coherent and self-regulating state and so become the new familiar. That's when this kind of work really becomes transformational in people's lives. It becomes the new automatic. You don't have to think about it or work on it so hard. So that's when you can pass on the technology, as you were saying.

Wylde: Let's talk a little bit about "heart intelligence". Because just as the brain thinks, we now know the heart is essentially a thinking organ.

McCraty: Let me just read you a quote, if that's okay. It's from the Founder, Chairman and Co-CEO of HeartMath, Doc Childre. "Picture heart intelligence as the flow of awareness, understanding and intuitive guidance we experience when the mind and emotions are brought into coherent alignment with the heart. This intelligence steps down the power of love from universal source into our life's interactions in practical, approachable ways which inform us of a straighter path to our fulfilment.." During our research back in the late 90s, so many people were testifying that after they learned the Heartmath skills, that their intuition was on steroids. There was a noticeable shift in their inner voice, their inner guidance. And they would usually say that the synchronicities in their lives were noticeably different. And of course, that made sense to us based on how that definition of heart intelligence. We started looking into the electrophysiology of intuition to see if we could actually measure this stuff. Our findings surprised us. What we found was that the heart was the first organ in the body to get intuitive signals about an unknown future event. The heart would send a measurably different neural signal to the brain. Then you had a brain response in the pre-stimulus period and then you triggered a conscious body response — the gut feeling or the hair on the back of the neck — a conscious feeling as long as you were paying attention to those body changes. So the gut tends to get the credit, but it's really the heart first, then the brain, and then the body makes a conscious response. That particular research has been replicated now and the heart's always the big player in these pre-stimulus experiments. I think it confirms what you were talking about a minute ago. We have all these sayings in our language. "Listen to your heart, it'll never fail you" or "play from your heart". They go on and on. But this intuition research is some of the best I know of and actually confirms that what the poets and great religions of the world talk about — the heart is the window to the soul, the source of courage and wisdom — has been right all along. That's really what we're suggesting here at Heartmath: we have the physical heart and what we call the energetic heart and the energetic heart is not a metaphor. It's a real thing with real structure. It's the transformation point or transceiver to that larger part of ourselves, our energetic self, who we really are.

Wylde: I'd like now to talk about the Global Coherence Initiative, about some of the work you people have done, about getting everyone engaged in feeding the field and, putting together these global monitoring sites. Could you explain this project and what the intention is in feeding the global field?

McCraty: The Global Coherence Initiative is twelve years old now. One of our four main hypotheses is that our cognitive functions, our behaviors and so on are affected and impacted by the background magnetic fields we live in — the field line references and Schumann resonances, magnetic fields from other people, and so on. That's not really a hypothesis; that's well established. We know that when there are solar flares and the Earth's magnetic fields goes into a disturbed state, there are significantly increased hospital admissions for heart disease and strokes, but also incidents of mental and emotional disorders, depressions and suicides go up. That's well established. One of our other hypotheses is that all living systems are connected to the Earth's magnetic field so that our thoughts and especially our emotions are actually literally feeding that field, radiating externally to the field. And just as a side note here, we've looked under the hood of that and there's a surprising amount of evidence that we may not be that crazy here. Ask any mother if she knows when her kids are in harm's way or doing something they shouldn't be doing. There's a non-local connection here. They could be on the other side of the planet but I don't know a mother who hasn't told me that had that experience and there has to be a mechanism for that and our hypothesis is actually a plausible mechanism. So we're all feeding the field – the global information field, as I call it – so my call to action here: throughout the day, pause, and take an inner weather check. Ask yourself, what am I feeding the field? How much of it is impatience and frustration or anxiety versus how much of it is feeding the field feelings of kindness and appreciation and compassionate attitude for people in these types of feelings? I believe that all counts. The second part of the Global Coherence Initiative is really bringing people together to shift their baseline of what we're feeding the field into large enough groups that we put a more coherent signal into the field environment, a more stable, consistent, coherent signal, that really helps others wake up and become more aligned and discover their own heart and heart intelligence.

In my view, that's the best thing people could do for humanity and the planet. At the personal level, it's very similar. What am I feeding my personal field environment? The heart generates a measurable magnetic field, the strongest magnetic field in the body by far, that permeates every cell in our body and radiates externally. So, our emotions are affecting us energetically, not only us, but also those around us. So, one of the best things we can do for our personal health and well-being is to really become more aware of our emotional diet and learn how to align with the heart that has the power to finally manage the mind and emotions to bring more coherence into our daily lives.

Wylde: One thing that really strikes me is that, as you suggest, it's not just the brain listening to the gut. It's probably the heart driving the brain driving the gut.

McCraty: If you look at the neural anatomy, the gut of course has afference – all the glands and organs do – but it has very few relative to the heart and the heart has the rhythmic ongoing complexity of the afference to the brain. The biome is important but in terms of the nervous system, the gut has very little afference to the brain. It's mostly an effector organ where we feel stuff rather than sending information back to the brain. And then there's infections. Have you seen the recent work on gingivitis and potentially a new understanding of what's called Alzheimer's?

Wylde: Yes. And a group in New Zealand may potentially have partial solutions. We talk a lot about the gut microbiome; now we're learning more about the oral microbiome. I'm not sure if you're familiar with these two strains — Bliss K12 and M18 — but these species of bacteria, may keep *P. gingivalis* at bay. Of course, what we've seen in the cadavers of Alzheimer's sufferers is that their brains are often riddled with *P. gingivalis* among other things. As we know, there's not one magic pill for the disease. I've learned from Dr. Dale Bredesen that it's a complex immunological dysfunction of which there's probably four or five subtypes, one of which is immunological and another pro-inflammatory, another toxicologic, etc. But as for *P. gingivalis*, when there's a pro-inflammatory immunological dysfunction, that sucker is just going to take advantage of that person. But once again, I really appreciate everything you do in helping individuals to learn about how to manage their number one silent killer and predisposer to whatever their genes or otherwise environment dictate, and that is stress.

McCraty: I agree. And I think it's becoming more and more clear that that stress and inflammation are strongly linked.

15

BRIGHT MINDS

From an interview with Dr. Daniel Amen

If you want to keep your brain healthy, if you want a long brain-span, you need to be working in multiple areas and get away from the idea that one pill is going to fix you.

~ ***Daniel Amen***

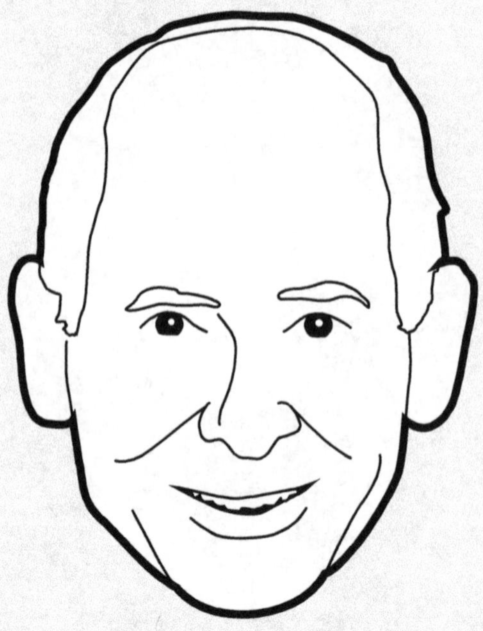

DR. DANIEL **AMEN**

Dr. Daniel Amen is one of America's leading psychiatrists and brain health experts. He has helped millions of patients change their brains and lives through his health clinics, best-selling books, products and public television programs and has the world's largest database of functional brain scans relating to behavior, totaling over 150,000 scans on patients from 120 countries.

He has authored or coauthored 80 professional articles and more than 40 books, including New York Times mega-bestseller Change Your Brain, Change Your Life. The Washington Post wrote: "By almost any measure, Dr. Amen is the most popular psychiatrist in America." He has appeared on numerous television shows including Dr. Phil, Larry King, Dr. Oz, The Doctors, and The View.

Wylde: Dr. Amen, we've been talking about brain injury. But Alzheimer's disease reminds us that "mental" illness is brain illness — and another kind of injury. What, based on your experience, should we do to keep our brain healthy?

Amen: You want to keep your brain healthy or rescue it if it's headed to the dark place. You'll have to prevent or treat the eleven major risk factors that steal your mind. In 2004, I wrote a book called Preventing Alzheimer's with the same idea: go after all the risk factors. We created a mnemonic: BRIGHT MINDS.

B is for blood flow. Slow blood flow is the number one brain imaging predictor of Alzheimer's disease. You need to care about your blood vessels because anything that damages your heart or your vasculature damages your brain. Your brain uses 20 percent of the blood flow in your body. That means you have to take care of things like hypertension and any form of heart disease. You need to get your cholesterol optimal. We have it backwards in this country where we're trying to get cholesterol as low as possible — except that makes all your hormones tank. It's not a good idea to have a cholesterol of 130.

R is for retirement and aging.

I is for inflammation. That's where your gut work is so important to your brain.
G is for genetics.
H is for head trauma. It's an epidemic here in North America, but nobody knows about it because nobody's looking at the brain.
T is for toxins.
M is for mental health.
I is for immunity and infections.
N is for neuro-hormones.
D is for diabetes.
S is for sleep.

If you want to keep your brain healthy, if you want a long brain span, you need to be working in multiple areas and get away from the idea that one pill is going to fix you. That's dumb. That hasn't worked.

Wylde: But what would be a brain-smart program for somebody who's already playing soccer? What do they do? Do they just stop cold? Are there ways to protect their brain?

Amen: I have active NFL players. One of them has just signed an $80 million contract and he's ***not*** going to stop playing. So if you are in a brain damaging sport, own that truth and don't do anything else to hurt your brain. NFL player Tom Brady is a great example. He's 40 years old and he's still probably the best quarterback in the game today. How did that happen? Well, he's doing everything else right. He gets nine hours of sleep. He takes supplements. He thinks sugary cereal is the devil. But this sort of lifestyle doesn't just apply to contact sports. My football players aren't heroes; they're entertainers. Firefighters are heroes. Police officers are heroes. They are in brain-damaging professions. Firefighters have to deal with toxic smoke debris, with the emotional trauma they experience on a regular basis, with head trauma from falls and things falling on them. It doesn't mean we're not going to have firefighters. It means we should own that this is a brain-damaging profession and we should be rehabilitating them all the time. But all of us should be on a rehabilitation program because ageing sucks for your brain. I published a study on how the brain ages based on sixty two thousand four hundred and fifty four scans. The news is not good. The things that accelerated aging? Marijuana was one of the worst. Not a surprise. Alcohol. Not a surprise. Having untreated mental health conditions like bipolar disorder or ADHD. Those are problematic for the brain.

Wylde: Of course some of us have it worse off than others by virtue of our genetic susceptibility. What's your impression of the relationship between neuroplasticity and the BDNF gene that expresses the brain-derived neurotrophic factor? Can we do anything about that gene if we don't happen to have the optimal variant?

Amen: You absolutely can. If you know your weakness, you want to strengthen it. I think it was Rocky Marciano, the boxer, who early in his career had weak shoulders. So he started swimming and he just swam and swam for months to strengthen his shoulders and he became one of history's best boxers. Know your vulnerabilities and then do things to change your situation.

Wylde: Speaking of vulnerabilities, I'm intrigued by your work with convicted felons. You say that people who do bad things also have damaged brains. What are you seeing within this cohort that's different from the average person in society who has no convictions?

Amen: I published a study on our work with murder. We found that young murderers had reductions in their prefrontal cortex — the most human, thoughtful part of us, often called the executive brain, involved in things like forethought, judgment, impulse control. Older murderers had global brain damage — the whole brain was less active. But clearly, in almost every case, their brains are not healthy. Dostoevsky said you can tell about the soul of a society not by how it treats its outstanding members, but by how it treats its criminals. And our soul is stained because it's easy to call someone bad — that's easy to do. Think of Adam Lanza, who committed the Sandy Hook atrocity. After that happened, President Obama said we need more money for mental health. That upset me because virtually all of the school shooters had seen mental health providers. Most of them had taken psychiatric medication. If we do more of what we're doing, we're going to get more of what we have: an international nightmare. We need to change the paradigm. These things aren't "mental". They're brains. If we don't understand that and don't pursue a revolution in brain health, we'll continue with this escalation of suicide. It's gone up 33 percent since 1999, while cancer has declined 27 percent. Why? We have the wrong paradigm. We need to go after this integrative medicine approach to the brain. We need to look at the brain, because if you don't look, how the hell do you know? Is it traumatic? Is it toxic? Does it work too hard or not hard enough? How do we know? My colleagues call me crazy, but I'm right. We need to stop lying about it. I'm just completely unhappy with my profession. I mean, how in good conscience can we be the only medical specialty that never looks at the organ we treat? "Oh, there's not enough research," they say. Come on. Go to med.gov today and type in brain. You'll get 14,415 abstracts. Don't tell me there's not enough science. Maybe they haven't read it?

Wylde: So your *patients*. How do you explain to *them* the difference between mind and brain if they think something is perhaps wrong with their mind? Do you help them refocus on how this is just as much their brain being "off" or "mismanaged" as their "mind"

Amen: I think of it as circles: hardware, software and network connections. The hardware is the physical functioning of your brain. The software is how you've been programmed and how you think day in and day out. You can optimize both of them. The network connections are your relationships. You become like the people you hang out with. And ultimately there is a "why?" Why should you care? Why are you on the planet? All of these circles work together to create who we are. Damage the brain — damage the mind.

16

THE BRAIN ON STEROIDS

From an interview with Dr. Mark Gordon

My turning point was 2004, when I realized all roads led back to hormone deficiency and when I realized most physical traumas in life — accidents, falls, etc — are obscure in memory. The first phase is trauma, the second phase is all of the biochemical aberrations precipitated by the trauma.

~ *Dr. Mark Gordon*

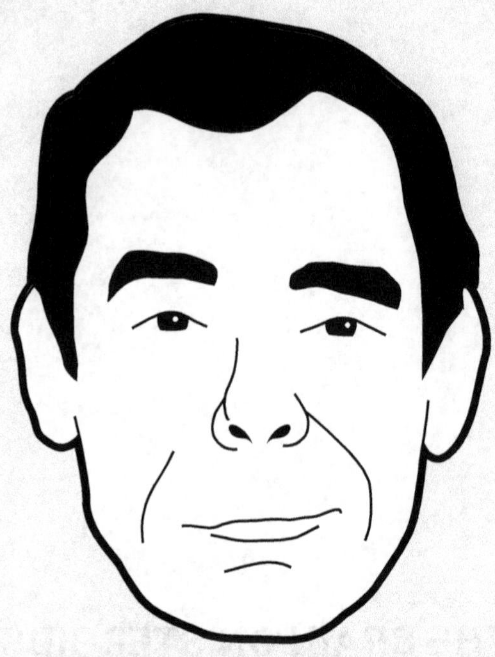

DR. MARK **GORDON**

Dr. Mark Gordon is a strong advocate of Integrative and Functional Medicine and the promotion of wellness medicine through the correction of underlying hormonal deficiencies. He is instrumental in promoting the recognition of Traumatic Brain Injury as a cause of hormonal deficiency. His book, The Clinical Application of Interventional Medicine, is recognized by his peers as a primer for the standards of care and assessment for Interventional Endocrinology. He holds the position as Voluntary Associate Clinical Professor at the Keck School of Medicine and Medical Director of CBS Studios, and has also participated on projects with HBO, ESPN, CNN, FOX, Good Morning America, and a number of international news programs.

Wylde: Dr. Mark Gordon, what have you done for your ***brain*** today?

Gordon: I monitor my neuroactive steroids and replenish them to a healthy youthful level of 25 to 35 years of age. In addition to this, there are a number of ingredients in the literature that can be helpful, products such as quercetin, NAC, and resveratrol. The list is long. These help with hormonal (that is, neurosteroidal) replenishment – especially in liposomal form – and they also help with inflammation that accumulates in the brain. I used to supplement with injectable testosterone for years but after doing a three-year veteran study that used clomiphene citrate to help stimulate the body to make its own testosterone, I switched over to that protocol. So now I take a tablet every other day. I also exercise. I have a daughter who is in naturopathic medicine who works with me. She monitors my nutrition and monitors my levels of inflammation. But I'll tell you right now, I can't go vegan. That's for sure. So, what I do is a composite of hormones, good nutrition, exercise and a cleaner lifestyle.

Wylde: Can you elaborate on the mechanisms that underlie these choices?

Gordon: A group of hormones called neurosteroids regulate all the functions in our brain that trickle down into all the functionalities of our body including a good contraction of the heart, a deep enough breath, a regulation of the cells of the pancreas that produce insulin, the control of muscle contractions that you might do for bicycling or weight lifting. I start off with assessing the presence in the brain of neurosteriods and neuroactive steroids that come from below the neck but also influence functionality in the brain. We've got a misconception of neurosteroids or hormones. They have a pleiotropic effect, not just in respect to sexuality but also work to keep the youthfulness of our brain. Dr. Caleb Finch at USC wrote about this in his book ***The Biology Of Human Longevity*** and in the thesis, ***Neuroendocrine Theory of Aging***, he covers the hormones that help to preserve the functionality of the brain. Living 100 years is meaningless if you're living a life with any sort of dementia such as Alzheimer's disease or Parkinson's or ALS or MS, or even depression, anxiety or psychiatric disease, which are all related to deficiencies of hormones.

Wylde: Let's unbox this further. What percentage of your clinical practice do you feel is neurosteroidally deficient or imbalanced?

Gordon: Out of the 350 veterans and active military, 100%. Out of the 2,800 civilians — also100%! And the average clinical practitioner doesn't know that their patient is hormonally deficient unless they conduct an appropriate laboratory assessment. The conventional ones most typical clinicians run — if they run anything at all — are too limited to recognize that a hormonal deficiency exists. A key hormone is pregnenelone. Pregnenelone becomes progesterone and progesterone becomes allopregnanolone. These three hormones regulate all of the hormones in our brain and they are responsible for neuroregeneration, synaptogenesis (the communication between neurons), free radical scavenging, and they upregulate the production of GABA. So, when supplementing pregnenelone, one tends to sleep better, regenerate the brain, and wake up better in the morning. If you look at the literature just on pregnenelone there are some 9,000 articles referring to pregnenelone deficiency linked to social anxiety, anxiety, panic attack, depression and in April of this year a new medication came out called brexanolone for $34,000 USD a year for treating postpartum depression, depression, and anxiety.

TESTING

We all benefit from being properly and comprehensively tested. I'm medical director of education for **Access Medical Lab** over the last nine years, where I have helped build proprietary testing panels that are only available to physicians who have gone through appropriate training. There is a significant difference between how clinicians typically interpret test results and how we interpret them. We employ optimal individualized parameters. Most physicians aren't aware of the differences between RIA (radioimmunoassay), chemiluminescence, ELISA, or liquid chromatography mass spectrometry with two or three channels. We educate clinicians on this technology because if they are not testing comprehensively and they are using antiquated technology, they're going to get poor results.

Wylde: You said, "I could never be vegan!" Why?

Gordon: I'm in the habit of individualizing my patient and comprehensively testing them to determine whether they should be on a particular diet, whether it be low glycemic, gluten free, or whatever type of diet. But I'm a great believer in "the middle of the road" where you don't do excessive anything. You'll have some people who are adamant about being vegan but they don't know they have an intolerance to tomatoes. I should bring up the "ketogenic diet" and the fad that it has become, including for those with traumatic brain injury. Theoretically when you significantly lower carbohydrate intake and increase fat intake in the diet, free radical damage to the brain drops. But what we know is that the brain runs on carbohydrates and you can switch over to fats so that it runs on fats such as hydroxybutyrate. But what we are finding is that if we starve glial cells, because they need glucose they can't do their job. They can't detoxify the neural environment because their glial mitochondria become damaged and begin spitting out more reactive oxygen species which leads to apoptosis (cell death). So, if folks are interested in the ketogenic diet, I highly recommend the modified version which doesn't go down to 20g of carbs daily. You still need to feed the brain.

Wylde: We are on the same page. People often exercise ***and*** diet. But when you exercise — especially intensely — you need glycogen stores. Glycogen is only stored if you consume carbohydrates. It's all about personalization. To switch things up here, do you think the majority of the population have been mildly to moderately concussed at least once in their lives?

Gordon: I think that we have all had traumatic brain injury and likely don't remember. I was talking with Lance Armstrong about his bicycle accidents and I had a flashback about an incident when I was twelve years old that I had totally forgotten. The thing about injury is that amnesia or retrograde amnesia can occur. The problem with the terminology that we use is that it's so fixed. We need to move away from "recovery from traumatic brain injury" (TBI) to "neuroregenerative". When we say TBI, we think loss of consciousness. The analogy I use is monetary. You could have a dollar which could be either a single bill or ten dimes. A dollar represents one major event where ten dimes represents ten events over time that culminate into one event. I have so many patients that say they have never had a TBI nor have been officially concussed but when I run the labs and tally the numbers, boom... there it is! Our labs will show in four different directions where a patient has had central trauma to the brain that ends up disrupting hormonal function. As we age, hormones that manage all of this downregulate and drop below healthy age-matched levels.

Most clinicians aren't used to looking at findings as a group — they are used to line-by-line assessment (ie. low, normal, high). But it turns out we need to properly understand the interactions of each line item. We must consider multi-tiered cross correlational assessment of our labs, which is the foundation of a new piece of software I've been writing the algorithms for over the last three years. My daughter Alison has been working on this for about eighteen months, learning what I do. But the software package can do this in about fifteen minutes. Clinicians still need to take a minimum four-hour course to be able to understand how to interpret the labs. My last book ***Traumatic Brain Injury*** outlines this general approach.

I think labels such as "chronic traumatic encephalopathy" (CTE) are a distraction. The military with "PTSD" is a great example of how the description of traumatic brain injury is so restrictive. All these labels — TBI (mild, moderate, severe), concussion, post-concussion syndrome, Alzheimer's, Parkinsons, depression, bipolar, obsessive compulsive, MS, ALS — all refer to the same thing! Fortunately the literature supports the fact that all these labeled psychiatric /psychophysiological / neurodegenerative conditions are all due to inflammation. Recent research shows that all patients diagnosed with Alzheimer's have had physical traumas in their past. My turning point was 2004, when I realized all roads led back to hormone deficiency and when I realized most physical traumas in life – accidents, falls, etc – are obscure in memory. The first phase is trauma, the second phase is all of the biochemical aberrations precipitated by the trauma.

Wylde: How much of all of this resides in genomics?

Gordon: it's a great question but very difficult to answer. Scientist are trying to unravel the APOE gene and its relationship for example to the risk of Alzheimer's disease. But it turns out that no matter what your genetic variant, it is epigenetics that matter most. It is inflammation that turns on beta-amyloid. So much of what causes Alzheimers is the pathway our brain chooses to convert the Alzheimer's precursor protein (APP) into beta-amyloid. But there is another pathway – one of which is to ***alpha***-amyloid. There are three enzymes responsible for conversion of this APP to either beta-amyloid or alpha-amyloid – three enzymes called secretases: secretase alpha, beta, and gamma. If you have secretase beta or gamma cleaving the APP you end up with amyloid-beta – the precursor to Alzheimer's. But if you have the alpha secretase and gamma secretase cleaving the APP, it becomes the ***inert*** form of alpha-amyloid. So the question is: why is it that we are not preferencing alpha- and beta- secretase? It comes down to one mineral! Alpha-secretase is zinc dependent, so if you have a zinc deficiency (which is common), you have a predisposition to beta-amyloid preference. Inflammation in the brain causes a loss of zinc-SOD (zinc bound to superoxide dismutase). When you lose zinc, you lose magnesium – it gets tied up in the inflammatory process. I have discovered that we need to supplement extra zinc citrate to manage this inflammation. Zinc citrate is responsible for over 300 known biochemical processes in the body. One important thing it does is to downregulate NFKB [ed. note: nuclear factor kappa-light-chain-enhancer of activated B cells. NFKB is technically a transcription regulator that is activated by various intra- and extra-cellular stimuli such as cytokines, oxidant-free radicals, ultraviolet irradiation, and bacterial or viral products.}

If you look at the studies from the NFL, if a player has even a single concussion on the field they are 19 times more likely to develop Alzheimer's disease between the ages of thirty and forty-nine years of age. So, what happens? The inflammation destroys the zinc-SOD, allowing for beta- and gamma-secretase to produce beta-amyloid. Now, we can naturally get rid of beta-amyloid — there is a membrane transporter called neprilysin which helps to remove the beta-amyloid from the cell. But unfortunately as we age, Alzheimer's may set in because what helps to upregulate neprilysin is testosterone, estradiol, progesterone, pregnenelone, DHEAS. All these hormones help to boost neprilysin. As we get older, we become deficient in all of these hormones. As we get older, these hormone levels drop and some authorities say its normal. It might be common, but it's not healthy. In other words, it's a normal finding but it's an abnormal condition. We know this from studies. As one example, look at DHEAS — the activated form of DHEA. In cardiovascular studies over 600 articles that look at the role DHEA plays in protecting the heart from ischemic heart disease.

Wylde: How important is sleep in recovery?

Gordon: It turns out that if you have inflammation in the brain, you develop insomnia. If you look at the meta-analyses of TBI you see it is associated with widespread objective and subjective sleep deficits. If patient suffers from sleep disruption due to TBI, I work to increase GABA naturally along with a small dose of melatonin and add a small amount of pregnenelone. This approach effectively drops inflammation and stimulates growth hormone production. I personally only sleep five hours at night. I use a device that monitors theta, delta, and alpha waves and see that I achieve three to four full cycles every night. I go to sleep by midnight and wake up by five a.m. and feel great. So, what I've learned by studying my sleep architecture is that I go into deep sleep very quickly. Some people take longer to move through their sleep cycles, thereby requiring they spend a longer time in their bed.

Wylde: What supplement products do you think anyone could take daily to improve brain health?

Gordon: I use and recommend a product called "Brain Care 2" that uses liposomal technology. It has taken me fifteen years to create. I personally formulated it. I introduced it to one of the military bases in Kentucky where all participants are medics – medically trained – and have all been downrange out of country in the theatre of war and have sustained injury and in 90 days they report feeling 50% to 60% better using this all natural product called Brain Care 2 that contains gamma tocopherol vitamin E, DHA omega-3, quercetin, NAC, ascorbyl palmitate vitamin C, EGCG from green tea. We have also started 200 patients in house on this product.

Wylde: What else are you up to?

Gordon: Soon, I'll be coming out with a product that focuses on mitochondrial optimization using, among other things, PQQ (Pyrroloquinoline quinone)

Wylde: Awesome. We know that mitochondrial support is key for brain energy.

17

WORKING MIRACLES

From an interview with JJ Virgin

On the other hand, if you live in Iceland, where they eat four times more fish than in any other country — and it's also one of the happiest and healthiest countries in the world — then you probably don't need to supplement.

~ JJ Virgin

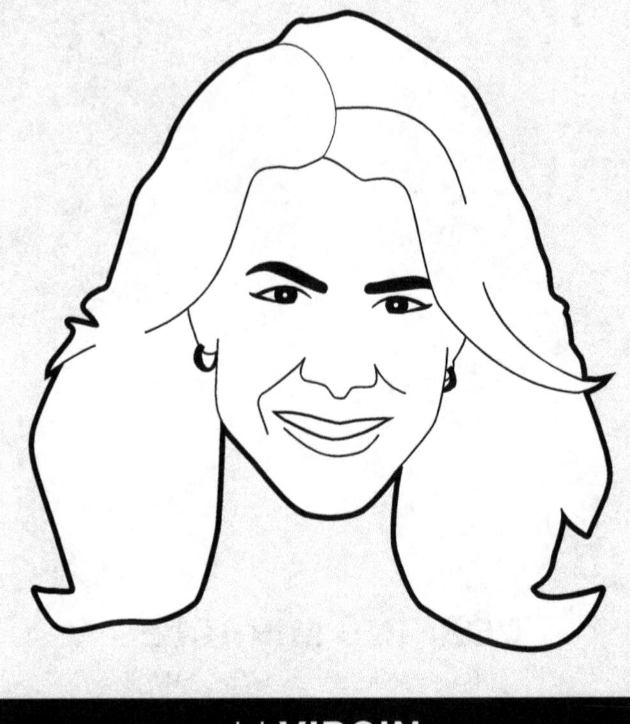

JJ **VIRGIN**

Wylde: What has JJ Virgin done for her brain today?

Virgin: What I do almost every morning is get up, pull out a really good, inspirational, motivational book — right now I'm reading Wayne Dyer — and then I write in my journal.

Wylde: Wayne Dyer. Poor guy. Wish we hadn't lost that genius.

Virgin: Oh, my God, the most amazing human.

Wylde: What do you think those morning practices are doing for your overall health and more particularly, your brain health?

Virgin: Well, as we know, thought creates, and what you focus on expands and you expand what you focus on. That was this morning's learnings. I think that the single most important thing you can do is continue to grow your mindset and you have to guard it, with all the negativity out there in the world. Twenty-six years ago, I had a mentor — my business mentor I thought, but she was actually my mindset mentor. The first thing she taught me to do was tightly control my environment. Be careful what you listen to. Don't listen to the news. Read the people you hang out with and just stay elevated. So that's why I always start that way. And I also have a process such that if I start getting in a pissy mood throughout the day. I can interrupt it and change my state.

Wylde: As a nutrition health expert, do you have a particular favorite brain food or for that matter, brain exercise, that you eat or do every day?

Virgin: My favorite brain food is coffee. In Iceland, I was so excited when people said, we love coffee. I thought to myself, I need to move here. Because for years I felt like I was the only person out there saying coffee is healthy for you. Besides the antioxidants in it helps me to focus. So I always start the day with coffee. And then if you want to pick one thing for your brain — and I think David Perlmutter says it best when he talks about the best thing for your neurons — one thing that if it was a drug, would be the most prescribed drug: I'm talking about exercise. Exercise is the single most important thing you can possibly do for your brain. That's something I work on every day, but I do a variety of things, everything from some long distance walking with my dog to hit training, resistance training. And I finally have put yoga into the mess, which took me years and years and years. The final thing was incorporating yoga, my missing piece. But I do think the best thing you can do for your brain is exercise.

Wylde: I have to agree with everything you just said, in particular, the exercise component. I feel that if we could encapsulate exercise into a pill, it would probably heal 80 percent of what ails us. I'm a huge fan of coffee as well, the coffee first thing in the morning to perhaps enhance a fasting regime. But is there anything that you believe we should all avoid that perhaps most significantly depletes our brain health? I'm reminded of that question because we've come to learn about microtoxins as important things to avoid. Are there other things that you believe we shouldn't expose yourself to — things other than negativity? I mean ingredients or supplements or artificial sweeteners?

Virgin: Artificial sweeteners. I mean, I know how they actually got out on the market, but they should never have been allowed. They're the worst chemistry experiment ever done to us and it's gone wrong. They're clearly neurotoxic and bad for so many different things. The other thing to manage is stress. You can't avoid stress so it's really knowing how to tolerate it, work with it.

Wylde: So how do we manage that?

Virgin: That's the big joke. What are you going to do? Can't really fire your family, right? You can't fire your boss either. So it's whatever practices help you tolerate stress. When you look at truly successful people, it isn't that their life is easier, it's that they got stronger, they got better. They learned how to tolerate higher and higher levels of stress. I think one of the things out of its many benefits that high-intensity interval training does best is retrain your sympathetic nervous system to be able to get stressed out and recover. We need to learn how to say, okay, I've got stress coming up. How do I recover from this? What do I need to do? What works for me? It might be tapping my deep breathing. What other things might help me? For me, my dogs are my stress reducers.

Wylde: I think you hit the nail on the head. I think we all have to realize there's no such thing as "no stress". It's about tolerating and managing it better. I believe one of the most stressful times of your own life was when your son was hit by a car and left for dead on the side of the road.

Virgin: Yeah, that is an understatement. But here's what was good before that happened. I'd gone through a lot of stressful situations. Prior to that, I'd had a family member commit suicide. I'd had a father die of cancer and basically wither away in front of me, and I'd just gone through a brutal divorce. I'd gone through highly stressful situations and trained my mind and body to handle them so that when this happened, I didn't just crumble. In fact, when it happened, I went into overdrive to be able to *perform* in this situation. If you look at a Navy SEAL, what are they learning how to do? They're learning how to tolerate ridiculous, stressful situations. My first processing when this happened was like I was watching the movie. I think your brain goes, "No, this is not happening!" because it could not be real. "Protect yourself!" But then I went into, "Okay, now what do I need to do?" Ultimately what was going to happen was going to happen, but I knew I had to do everything possible in my power to help my son recover and be 110 percent. But I knew the only way to do that was that I had to be playing full out, to be at the top of my game, and I had to take care of myself first in order to do everything to save his life.

Wylde: Let's take a step back. I appreciate you've told this story a million times before, but if you don't mind sharing with us what happened, how bad was it? What did you end up doing about it?

Virgin: I had two boys at the time. They were 15 and 16. Grant and Bryce. Grant had bipolar disorder and he'd had a lot of different struggles when in school but was finally on track. Everything was going great. He went out to walk to a friend's house at dusk. He didn't have anything on him — no I.D., no nothing. He was crossing the street in a 40-mile-an-hour zone. A neighbor driving nearby saw a woman get out of a white car, gasp, get back in the car and drive off. The neighbor pulled around to the side, protected my son from oncoming traffic and called 9-1-1. The paramedics came. They had Grant airlifted to the local hospital in Palm Springs and then my ex-husband and my son Bryce went out to look for Grant because they didn't know where he'd gone. They see this big accident. They asked the policeman what was going on and they looked at Bryce and said a boy was hit, a boy who looked just like Bryce. We raced to the hospital. He was a John Doe. No I.D. We get there and the doctors usher us into a conference room. Now, here's the big challenge. We were in Palm Springs, where the average age of a person coming into the trauma center in Palm Springs is about 70-plus years old. There's a trauma doc. There's a neurosurgeon. The trauma doc walks in and tells us that my son's type of injury kills 90 percent of people at the scene. Bryce was hanging on by an onion skin. The doc said, "Sometime in the next 24 hours, it's going to rupture and every hour, it just gets more acute. It has to be repaired. However, we can't repair it here because he's also in a deep coma. He still has brain activity, but he has multiple brain bleeds. Beyond that, he also has two fractures, bones sticking through his skin. He'd have to be airlifted to another hospital, but he'll never survive that airlift." And then he said, "Even if he were to survive that airlift, he'd very unlikely to make it through the surgery. Even if he were to survive that surgery, he'd be so brain damaged, it wouldn't be worth it." I'm looking at this guy and Bryce is looking at this guy. Bryce says, "Maybe a 0.25 percent chance he'd make it? And the doctor looks at Bryce and said, "That sounds about right, son." Now, for a 70-year-old, it's a very different story than for a 16-year-old. So here's the cool thing. My ex-husband is a medical malpractice trial attorney. That whole side of the family are doctors, so Bryce has grown up around all these doctors and didn't have them up on some pedestal. He's very analytical. We're math people over here. He says, "That's not zero. We'll take those odds." So I looked at the doctor and I said, "We're overruling you. and time is of the essence and you need to get on this." And then my ex-husband started in on all the medical legal stuff. And so, this doc got on it and I read later in the chart that he was very upset with us because he told us Grant was going to die on the way. I said, "He's dying here or on the way, is that correct?" "Yes," he said. "We'll pick on the way," I said. Grant was airlifted to harbor UCLA. We drove there, we had no idea what we were going to see. We had no idea if he'd make the airlift. We get there. We walk in to the E.R. There's was a surgeon there, an amazing human being. He accepted the case at midnight. He assembled five surgical teams between midnight and 5:00 a.m. He got a stent that was no longer available but had been used in a study. It was not even approved for kids. He said, "I figured I'd ask for forgiveness." I walk in and he says, "Are you the mom? You don't need to worry about this. I've totally got this. I do this all the time. Let me take you to where I'm going to do the surgery, show you everything that's going to happen, then I'll take you to the waiting room and I'll come get you in a couple hours when it's all done." There were five surgical teams getting Grant prepped for surgery when I walked in. The ortho team, the neuro team, in fact there were two ortho teams because he's fractured both femurs and had to have them rodded. And then they had the trauma team, they had the pediatric trauma team and they had the cardiothoracic team. So, they had all these people and he gets me out of there, which was good. I go sit in the waiting room. A few hours later he comes and says, "Right. It's fixed. It's all fine. All good." Now, I have no idea if he'll ever wake up. So, you're thrilled and then not thrilled. And then we go see the neuro team, who are completely doom and gloom. I walked in and they're telling us they don't know if he'll ever wake up. He's got all these injuries. He's got brain activity, but he's in the deepest coma — level nine. Blah, blah, blah, blah, blah. I walk in and see my son. I can literally only hold two fingers. He's got road rash covering anything that's not in the cast and I'm holding these two fingers. There's the ventilator going. There's tubes coming out of his brain to monitor pressure. He's beeping. I said, "Grant, we're here and I love you so much." I'm holding these two fingers. "And your brother Bryce loves you so much." I feel this little squeeze. Now, he's in the deep coma. That's not happening, right? I said, "And your grandma loves you so much," and I feel nothing. And then I said, "Your girlfriend, Mackenzie, loves you so much," and he squeezed my fingers and lifted them off the bed. And I looked at him and I said, "All right. Your name means warrior. You're going to be one hundred and ten percent. I got my part. I'm going to bring in the troops. I can bring in the best people to help you, but you have to fight. That's what your name means. You have to fight. We've all got this. We're all here." Doctors would tell me "He's not going to wake up. Oh, he'll never walk again" and I'd take them out of the room so he would never hear that. I knew we could hear it and I kept telling him how he's going to be a hundred and ten percent. I had friends coming from the first night in the hospital. We had people doing acupressure and energy healing. When you have something like this happen, every religion's relevant. People were sending me scrolls and holy water. I said, "Bring it all. We're doing it all." I started progesterone cream and we started fish oil. I just decided I was going to do whatever it took. I experienced a peace of mind that you have when you know you have something to do and you have hope. I would just watch for signs that he was improving and I could find them. Sometimes it would just be that he fluttered his eyelashes or twitched his nose or sighed. But I could tell he was in there. And sure enough, he told me later that the great man came and asked him if he wanted to live or die, that it was really great on the other side, that there was no time there and everything was easy, talking to other people in the family — and all the stuff you always hear about near-death experiences. Grant said to me, "But I kept hearing you talking so I decided to stay here."

Wylde: Amazing. Just incredible. If you don't mind, tell us more about how you used omega-3 in Grant's recovery.

Virgin: It was very frustrating. I had all the literature pertaining to omega-3s and recovery from brain trauma. I took it into the hospital but they weren't enthusiastic. Their whole fear was that fish oil would cause bleeding. I said, "Forget it. I know my risk-reward here." The thing is, first, he wasn't bleeding anymore, and second, there is zero evidence that fish oil increases bleed time. But they would only allow him to receive two grams of oil through his feeding tube. But before his accident he'd been on five grams of fish oil for his bi-polar condition. That is so important because the DHA in fish oil is neuro-protective. One of the things that allowed him to survive this trauma was having that DHA in his brain. If you sit around the dinner table and ask people if they've ever hit their head, who hasn't hit their head? And they'll probably hit it again. So why wouldn't we be taking omega-3 essential fatty acids? Anyway, Grant spit out his feeding tube one day and didn't go back to it. As far as I was concerned, it was now game on. That's when I cranked up his omega-3 essential fatty acids and had a whole lab going on in the back of his room and — bam! — he went from not talking to talking. Granted, you can't knock someone on the head and give them omega-3 essential fatty acids and then compare that with knocking someone in the head and not giving them supplemental omega-3 essential fatty acids, but when you look at the risk-reward picture, if there's not any risk and there's a huge potential reward, I don't understand why you wouldn't do it.

Wylde: I think you've hit the nail on the head. It's the fact that Grant's brain was saturated with DHA that's so important. What would you advise as pertains to daily supplements of omega-3 essential fatty acids?

Virgin: This is tricky because it depends on the individual diet. If a person's diet is high in omega-6s and saturated fats and low in omega-3s, they'll need more omega-3s in order to crowd the other fats out. On the other hand, if you live in Iceland, where they eat four times more fish than in any other country – and it's also one of the happiest and healthiest countries in the world – then you probably don't need to supplement. You're getting it from your diet. But most people aren't getting this amount of fish – and clean fish – in their diet, so I'd say, absent testing, that a minimum two grams a day of a high-quality professional-grade omega-3 is good. Then ideally, you'll do your fatty acid profile – your omega-3, 6 and 9s. This is looking at you're omega-3 index. You're looking at your systemic inflammation and you're looking at your oxidative stress. Then you can really pinpoint it and consider supplementation and decide if you need more omega-3 essential fatty acids in your diet. I've got to do a shout out to Vital Choice, who sent me salmon that I would bring into the hospital for Grant. One of the first words he said was "disgusting" – it was about the hospital food. I didn't let him have hospital food. I brought him healthy stuff. Whole Foods shipped me stuff. Vital Choice shipped me stuff.

Wylde: Great products. Any other JJ Virgin favorite supplements for brain health?

Virgin: Curcumin, vitamin D with K And then the obvious suspects of brain nutrients. Things like ginkgo biloba... to be honest the list is long. I've got so many things that I've got Grant on – anything that's a potential brain nutrient – because I figure I'd rather have him over-nutritioned than under.

Wylde: And how's he doing?

Virgin: He's doing amazingly well these days. He's better than before the accident in so many ways. He has the knowledge he gained going through that accident, the knowledge that you have when you go to the other side, which you and I will never understand, even if he tries to put it into words. But he also has more empathy for people and just better understanding of himself. He understands better now what's going on with his bipolar disorder. We have to watch things because when you have that level of a brain injury, where you're basically dead in the street, and you come out of a coma — they told me it would be ugly but they didn't explain it would be ugly for years. He didn't speak for a week. He didn't make any eye contact. He just stared off into space, moved his arm back and forth. It took him months to come to even a point of being able to say anything more than let's go, when he wanted to leave the hospital. He had to learn his name and learn how to brush his teeth, how to go to the bathroom, how to eat — all over again. It was a long journey. And along that way, one of the big things they don't tell you about brain injuries is that he could become super suicidal. It was very scary. I remember at one point him saying he was just going to go out and get hit by a car again, and I'm jumping him — this six-foot, 200-pound, dude — and saying, "No! You're not doing that! Not after all we've gone through!"

18

BABY BRAIN

from an interview with Dr. Bill Sears

The number one thing I want pregnant women to do, is eat smart foods and supplement with the top nutrient omega-3 fatty acids

~ Dr. Bill Sears

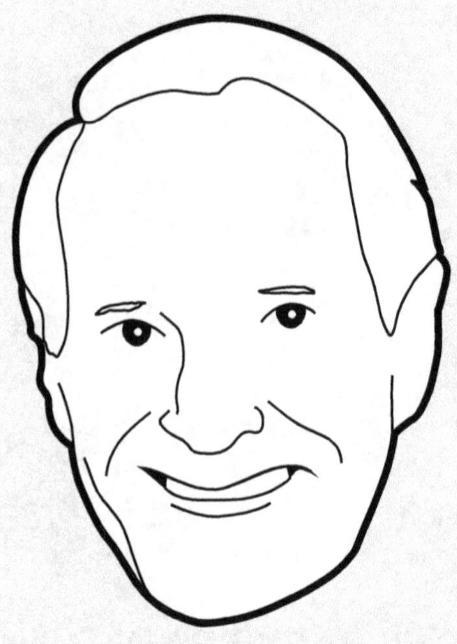

DR. BILL **SEARS**

Dr. Bill Sears is Americas favorite pediatrician and has been advising busy parents on how to raise healthier families for over 40 years. He received his medical training at Harvard Medical School's Children's Hospital in Boston and The Hospital for Sick Children in Toronto, the world's largest children's hospital, where he was associate ward chief of the newborn intensive care unit before serving as the chief of pediatrics at Toronto Western Hospital, a teaching hospital of the University of Toronto. He has served as a professor of pediatrics at the University of Toronto, University of South Carolina, University of Southern California School of Medicine, and University of California: Irvine. As a father of 8 children, he coached Little League sports for 20 years, and together with his wife Martha has written more than 40 best-selling books and countless articles on nutrition, parenting, and healthy aging. He serves as a health consultant for magazines, TV, radio and other media, and his AskDrSears.com website is one of the most popular health and parenting sites.

Wylde: What have you, Dr. Bill Sears, done for your brain today?

Sears: The first thing I did for my brain today when I woke up — I call this brightening my day — as soon as I got out of bed, I looked outside and let the natural sunlight come into my eyes. The eyes are windows to your brain. That's the number one piece of advice for brain health from Mom, the most trusted advisor in the world: Go outside and play.

Wylde: Great advice. We live in an unnatural world these days. We go to bed too late with too many lights on and do all kinds of crazy things with artificial light and then we don't get enough light in the morning. Okay, so as North America's most trusted pediatrician. you've seen tens of thousands of babies over the years in clinical practice. What can you tell a reader based on that career?

Sears: Let's imagine that you and your wife are expecting your first baby and you are what we call in my medical practice "high investors". That means that you want to invest early in life in the greatest things you can do for your child's brain development, things that will have the most lasting effect. And that begins at pregnancy. So the first thing I do, I give such parents a list. I say, "The number one thing I want you to do in pregnancy is eat smart foods and the top nutrient is omega-3 fatty acids." We find when we're talking to parents, we have to make it fun and simple. I say to them, "You're growing a little fat head inside. Your baby's brain at 60 percent fat and your baby's brain is growing faster in that last three months of pregnancy than any time in your baby's life. The fathead needs smart fats." So I have all the pregnant moms take at least a gram a day of omega-3s. It's better to eat wild salmon, but sometimes during pregnancy, mothers can't stomach it. As a show-me-the-science doctor, I measure the omega-3 red blood cell index in my pregnant patients, make sure they're up to 8 percent, and put them on a gram a day. Then I have them come in a month later and I measure the omega-3 index again and sometimes I have to increase it to two grams a day. Number two, I advise during pregnancy to avoid stress. Easier said than done, especially for a male. We all get stressed but prolonged, unresolved stress raises the level of cortisol, the stress hormone. Sometimes it's good stress, sometimes it isn't. But when a baby's vulnerable brain is exposed to stress hormone levels that are too high, too long, especially after birth — the term is "glucocorticoid neurotoxicity" — it wears out the growing brain. And number three is, "Breast feed your baby as long as you can and as often as you can." There's no smarter milk to raise a smarter brain than momma's milk and there are several nutrients in mother's milk that nobody can make. The baby needs the human milk olgosacchirides to feed that the baby's microbiome, its "second brain", its "gut brain". The mother's touch and interaction dramatically lower stress hormone levels. I've watched nursing moms in my office and when my wife was breastfeeding our children. The peace and tranquillity in a breastfeeding pair is unparalleled.

Wylde: And I'm assuming you're going to suggest that, depending on their measured index, that mothers continue to consume that gram or two of omega-3 index during breastfeeding in order to to impart that DHA to the baby.

Sears: In fact, I give them almost a prescription for wild salmon. "Hold up your fist," I say. "Three fistfuls per week." I tell them where to get wild Alaskan salmon and I give them a list of what I call "smart foods". My "smart seven": salmon, eggs, avocados, nuts, berries, greens and olive oil. I want them to eat all of those while they're breastfeeding to have the good fats in their milk. Then when they come in for their six-month check-up, we have what we call the "fathead talk". Remember the old days when we used to give our babies rice cereal because we didn't know any better? Rice has iron in it, which is good for the brain, but no fat. We learn a lot from Mother Nature because Mother Nature doesn't change her mind all the time. If breast milk is 40 to 50 percent fat and baby's brain is 60 percent fat, it makes good sense to feed babies a smart fat diet instead of a low fat diet.

And so the first food we start with at six months is avocados. It's great fun — great pictures — all the little green faces. And then we have salmon at seven months, a little fingertip full of mushy pieces of salmon. I want the first foods that little baby tastes to be avocados and salmon. That's called "shaping the creative center in the brain" or just "shaping young tastes". Those are the three magic words of infant feeding, of smart infant feeding.

Wylde: Got it. So just to go back a step, you yourself were a tremendous influence, if not be most influential person, in getting DHA and omega-3s into infant formula. If if a mother just simply can't breastfeed, is there something that you recommend, something that is second best to breastfeeding?

Sears: Yes, and this will surprise your readers. The World Health Organization a year ago came out with a statement that shocked the baby feeding world. They said that the first choice should always be breast milk, the second choice should be donor milk. And the third choice infant formula. This is all new. Following that, milk banks are spreading all over the place.

There are medical conditions in which moms simply cannot produce enough milk. So in my office, when we have a mom come in and say, "I just can't do it. I need more." I say, "Well, do you have a few friends who would like to become milk moms?" And they look at me. What do you mean by that?" I explain that I mean donor milk from people they know and trust. Twenty five years ago, our eighth child was adopted and she came into our life as a new-born. Just because she was adopted, we knew she shouldn't be deprived. In my office I had six breast pumps in a side room and when moms would come in for the check and say, "I'm leaking so much." I'd say, "Oh, really? Step in the other room." Lauren, our baby, had 35 milk moms. She Keeps in touch with some of those moms. It's not only good for the baby, but can you imagine how good a donor mom feels? Contributing part of herself to help that baby's brain be smarter? The modern formulas are actually much better than they were before they now include DHA and they're starting to put in more probiotics and human milk oligosacharides. They're trying to duplicate. The current standard formulas are certainly much better and much closer to human milk than they've ever been. So those are the three choices.

Wylde: You mentioned a few times how we're coming to learn about better formulas, and coming to understand the gut brain connection and the microbiome and t how this impacts our brain. And you also wrote the book, ***Dr. Poo***. So what were the most important takeaways from that? What is it that we need to know, especially as it relates to pregnant nursing moms and the post-natal gut brain?

Sears: The person who wrote the foreword to ***Dr. Poo***, is a well known clinician in Canada — Bryce Wylde, my favorite naturopath up there. We wrote *Dr Poo* because there's so many intestinal problems in kids and the term microbiome was coming out and nobody understood what it meant. So my role is kind of making science simple and fun. And for example, my favorite in the *Dr Poo* book is where we have a baby breastfeeding from mom and the baby's gut says, I love MOM, which stands for milk-oriented microbiota. There are special nutrients in mother's milk that help grow the baby's gut garden. The term garden I use a lot in my medical practice and I had to help patients understand what we're talking about when we talk about the "head brain" and the "gut brain". I tell them "I want you to think of your baby's head brain and gut brain. Think of the second brain as the greatest garden ever grown. What do you need to do if you want your garden to grow? First, you need to feed and fertilizer it — smart foods. Secondly, you need to irrigate it. And what irrigates the brain garden? Blood flow. And what makes blood flow faster? More movement. And thirdly, you need to keep the weeds and the pests out by keeping stress down. Just giving them those three simple tools: how you feed your garden, how you irrigate it and how you keep the pests and weeds out.

Wylde: In the process of writing this book, I've learned about neuroplasticity, neurogenesis. You're also writing a book right now about brain health. What new revelations can you share, having gone through the process of writing the book on brain health?

Sears: Well, the first thing I learned was, when do you think Alzheimer's begins? If you had to pick an age.

Wylde: from what I understand it's about 30 years prior to diagnosis.

Sears: Exactly right. I surprised my patients by saying Alzheimer's begins in adolescence. Alzheimer's begins when you're starting to prune away all the the plants in your brain garden you may not use and replace them with plants you're going to use. But if you feed the brain during those precious times where the brain is growing the fastest, which is pregnancy, the first five years, and during teen years, those are what I call my three top childhood times when the brain is most vulnerable to change. And that's when we need to be feeding and taking care of our brains. So that's when Sears' Alzheimer's Prevention begins. The brain can heal itself at any age. But the older we get, the less able we are to heal the brain. We used to be taught — you've probably been taught that too — that once you reach a certain age like 25, 30, the brain doesn't make any new cells. Well, that's wrong. Now we know that the brain can regenerate and regrow healthy brain cells at any age. Yet the older we are, the more difficult neural regeneration and neuroplasticity become. And that's why in our book we stress prevention so much. This figure will just astonish you. Drug companies have spent 84 billion dollars on pharmaceuticals to treat Alzheimer's and they've failed. But what Dr. Mom said, was "Eat more fruits, vegetables and seafood and go outside and play." That right there, in nutshell, is the best medicine for the brain at any age. It has the most science behind it.

Wylde: Great. Get off those darn devices. And does all this positive talk about cannabis concern you at all? It may be leading some kids astray and especially during those formative years. Does that concern you at all?

Sears: Oh, very much. You hit a magic dial inside me right now, because we pediatricians come out with the statement that this is one of the most concerning experiments of mankind that we've ever noticed in our years of practice. This is one big experiment and we're afraid how it's going to turn out, because nobody is addressing the fact that we do not know the long-term effects. And I think sometimes we just have to go back to the rule of common sense. If you mess with the greatest hardwiring and software that's ever, ever been produced — the human brain — if you mess with that in a way that's artificial and it's not designed for, it can't be good for the brain in the long run. And here's what I think happens. The brain makes natural antidepressants. It makes cannabinoids, natural feel-good, happy hormones. All this our brains make. But when your brain makes its own medicines and then you take other medicines, say an opioid or cannabis pill, over time the brain says, "Hey, you take them so I don't have to make them, right? I'll just go on vacation a bit because you're taking them. Well, over time, then the effect wears out – it's called "down regulation" – the effect of the artificial ones wear out, prompting the brain to make more of it, which does two things. It wears out the brain or the brain becomes increasingly resistant to these artificial ones. So you have to take a higher dose to get the same effects, which means higher side effects. It's a downward spiral, which we doctors call the hole, and the hole is: when you have a problem and you're taking these artificial medicines, is the problem you're having due to the side effect of the medicine or is it your brain? And we don't know. So this cannabis thing is a great experiment. I've had patients who do very, very well on the cannabis oil – short term – but when I give them a prescription for any brain medicine, I say. "I'm writing you a prescription for the pills. However, we're going to have a target here: three to six months down the road. I'm going to give you a list of skills to build up your own brain medicines. So as you go up with the skills, I'm going to hold you accountable. As you go up with the skills, we're going to go down slowly and gradually with the pills. Now, maybe at some point you'll need pills and skills. However, you're never, never, ever treat the brain with only pills. It's always pills and skills – or skills only.

Wylde: But if this is an experiment, should it happen during the formative years? And so perhaps your advice might be to not even go there unless it's under the supervision of a doctor or a pediatrician or certainly not before, say, 25 or some date where we know the brain is perhaps evolved enough that it can handle a little bit of these cannabis derived CBD and then the THC chemicals?

Sears: Yes, I totally agree. That should only be done under supervision of a trained professional medical professional who has experience and knowledge. And another thing: pediatricians are seeing more and more stress related illness and mental unwellness at younger ages than we've ever seen before, a higher incidence of depression and anxiety at younger ages. In the last few years, we've started teaching meditation and stress management techniques between five and seven years of age. From five to ten is your window. After that, the children start rebelling. Between five and 10 most kids will just accept what mom and dad tell them. I have the parents or caregivers every night lie down and help their child go off to sleep. As they drift off to sleep, we have them repeat. "I am smart. I am funny. I am a good soccer player. I am a good hockey player. I have a good mom and dad. I am. I am." And they drift off to sleep. It's called raising a grateful brain. You are implanting in that brain, that growing brain, a gratitude center. And that gratitude center will offset the stress center. And then when they wake up in the morning, I am, I am, I am. The way you start today programs the brain to behave that way during the day and the way you end the day programs the brain to get a good night's sleep. And then when they're eight or nine or even teenagers, have them put on the wallpaper on their cell phone and draw big pictures on their bedroom mirror. Five things I like about me. I like my hair. I like my eyes. I like my skin. I like my school. I like my boyfriend. Just so they don't go to bed worrying. They don't get up worrying. And they replay that attitude of gratitude. Life does suck sometimes and as soon as that happens, you quickly switch on your gratitude center with what you like about yourself before the worry wart and before the worry center in your brain has a chance to infect the whole brain. Nip it in the bud.

Wylde: You're so right. Taming that default mode network. Now, tell me again the name of your book that's coming out — this latest one on brain health?

Sears: It's called ***The Healthy Brain Book***. And the subtitle is ***"An All Ages Guide to a Calmer, Happier, Sharper You"***

19

4/20

from an interview with Dr. Guy Chamberland

The biggest claim for CBD I would warn people about is pain relief. There's no evidence that CBD is effective for that. I'm not trying to mock CBD, but if I look at it as a herbalist, I would tell you the plant didn't necessarily want its ingredients to be isolated.

~ Dr. Guy Chamberland

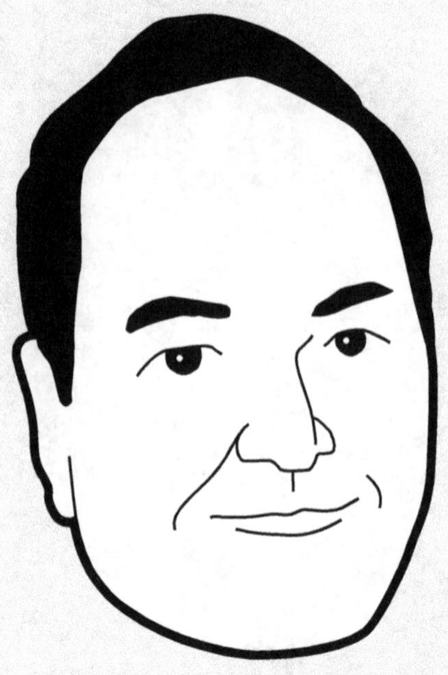

DR. GUY **CHAMBERLAND**

Dr. Guy Chamberland Ph.D. is a Master Herbalist and Chief Executive Officer and Chief Scientific Officer of Tetra Bio-Pharma, a Canadian-based global leader in the discovery and development of cannabinoid-derived pharmaceutical products. In assuming leadership of Tetra Bio-Pharma in 2018, Chamberland was instrumental in differentiating Tetra's approach to exploring the potential therapeutic uses of cannabis by adopting a pharmaceutical pathway built on rigorous standards that meet the inclusion requirements of regulators, medical bodies, and payors. He is an acknowledged expert in the biopharmaceutical space with more than two decades of experience in drug development for the North American pharmaceutical industry, particularly in regulatory affairs and the development and management of clinical research protocols and clinical studies for botanical medicines. He is also a prolific contributor to the field of botanical medicine, publishing, lecturing and conducting continuing education workshops for health professionals on the use of plants in the treatment of pain, anxiety, insomnia, and wound healing.

Wylde: Guy, tell me a bit about you and your professional background.

Chamberland: I began my career in drug safety, basically convincing the FDA and Health Canada that specific new molecules were safe, that all the regulatory requirements were there. I've always worked with a lot of startup companies in pharma and many of these were affiliated with universities. So to start things on the right foot you have to go into research early in the process. I've never actually touched a simple synthetic drug mainly because I have a PhD in toxicology and always ended up inheriting the most complex molecules, things that wouldn't fit in the regulations or had safety issues. Over the years, I developed an expertise in what we can call jurisdictional regulatory affairs and that's what brought me to cannabis. As a passion on the side I teach herbal medicine at a naturopathic college and I strongly believe in herbals, which are underused in medical practice. Cannabis was great from that point of view because I could use some of my knowledge as a herbalist to help move cannabis products forward. Tetra Bio Pharma Inc is where I am now as CEO. Tetra wanted somebody strong on the jurisdictional side, basically a toxicologist who was comfortable working with the safety issues of a new molecular entity.

Wylde: For my readers, Tetra Biopharma has no vested interest in the production side. You're strictly research analytics.

Chamberland: Correct. We're basically a tech company developing cannabinoids as prescription drugs. We're following the regular path that a drug must to get approval. It involves studying how cannabis works because how can you develop a cannabinoid drug if you don't understand it? That's where my herbal background came in. We only develop cannabinoid drugs. We don't sell medical cannabis and we don't touch the recreational market. You could say we're not even favorably disposed towards it.

Wylde: Can you tell us in the simplest terms what we are learning generally about the endocannabinoid system?

Chamberland: There is a lot known in animals but we're just beginning to understand what this means in humans. To give you the best example, there's a cannabinoid drug approved for epilepsy. It works great. Doses are relatively low. But if you talk to a pain doctor who's using medical cannabis oil, they may have to move a patient rapidly into the 500mg dose and up to a gram a day. It's not just bioavailability issues that interfere with its efficacy. It's because there's a hell of a difference in the way the cannabinoid system responds in various conditions. Epilepsy involves lower doses, pain involves much higher doses. Although you could say pain is a neurological condition, the receptors behave very differently in epilepsy than in conditions such as anxiety. These are things we're all discovering.

Wylde: The endocannabinoid system, as we understand it, is limited to the two receptors that we know: the CBD1 and CBD2. How many others are there at play in the human body at this point?

Chamberland: There've been more found in animals — from what I understand from the pharmacologists, up to CDB3 and CDB4, but these have not been found in humans to date. I will say one thing: as a company, we've done multiple clinical trials, actually competed for clinical trials with cannabis, not cannabinoids. But as a professor of herbal medicine, I look at the traditional knowledge known for thousands of years, although it wasn't expressed in the same terms as today, and realize we haven't actually discovered anything.

Wylde: Give us some examples.

Chamberland: All the side effects were described in the literature, the hallucinations were known two thousand seven hundred years before Christ.

They were published in official documents before 1800 B.C. Effectiveness for neuralgia, ear pain, headaches, and as muscle relaxants — all goes back to and prior to that time. It was known way back that cannabis encouraged sleep by targeting restlessness. In 1899, it was published in medical textbooks that in cases where an immediate effect is desired with drugs, they should be smoked. Cmax is achieved in five minutes. Normal drug delivery can never achieve that. It takes one to three hours to reach the Cmax. The 1927 Material Medical and Pharmacology, written by David Culbreth, and the American Materia Medica, all are witness to the fact that what we've really done is prove that what's been known for the last 4000 years is true.

Wylde: You're reminding me of that meme — I'm sure you've come across from media or online — the one about 4000 years of medicine. It's 2000 B.C.: "Here. Eat this root." It's 1000 A.D.: "That root is heathen! Say this prayer!" Sometime around the 1800 A.D.: "That prayer is superstition. Drink this potion!" 1935. "That potion is snake oil. Swallow this pill." Maybe three decades ago: "That pill is ineffective. Take this antibiotic." Today: "That antibiotic is poison. Eat this root!"

Chamberland: Exactly.

Wylde: So let's talk about the safety/efficacy aspect. There's a lot of talk about vaping, a lot of talk about administration routes. What can you tell us about both as it pertains to THC and CBD?

Chamberland: Well, before we invested in developing synthetic cannabinoids, I needed to understand why for thousands of years people said smoking cannabis worked. And I'll tell you why. The first synthetic THC drug was approved by the FDA in 1985, which meant they'd been studying it for more than five years before that. That drug has never been approved for pain, but was approved for nausea in cancer and some eating disorders in some patients, but never anything for pain.

Since then, Nabilone was approved, which is a synthetic derivative of THC with one tenth stronger affinity for the receptors. It failed against placebo for pain.

Dronabinol, which is a synthetic THC, failed. Then came Sativex, developed by G.W, which an extract of THC plus CBD. And from what I understand, in more than three clinical trials, it has failed in pain. So you sit there as a drug developer and you say, okay, in the modern literature, multiple surveys always rate it in terms of relief superior to even fentanyl and morphine. Yet in all trials, the oral stuff never works. So, early days, I told my company Tetra that they first needed to understand how smoking works for drug delivery, because if we committed to the research, we could decide to allow those patients who want compassionate use to have access to a pharmaceutical-type product. But ultimately my question was, why do these cannabis drugs fail against placebo? I needed to know that because if I invest millions of dollars in a pain drug, I don't want it to fail. Well, we discovered why it worked and it was really amazing. We realized that THC is ***not*** really a direct analgesic. It's more indirect. You can actually find it in the patient literature of Marinol and even Nabilone. The patient gets pain relief because as the restful sleep comes in, the patient's threshold for pain goes up. That's what we explained to Health Canada. We told them, THC's not really an analgesic, though over time it will have that effect. But we believe it works for patients because patients for thousands of years have used this therapy to relieve them of their suffering through improved sleep. Health Canada said, "If you can prove that we'll approve the drug."

Wylde: Well, how do you prove a secondary and indirect pathway? Getting the body to do better what it does on its own has been the age-old adage of natural herbal medicine. But how would you prove that?

Chamberland: We renegotiated. We went after a special quality-of-life criteria for proving the impact on the person. The agency actually wanted that as its primary endpoint when they understood what we were telling them. We said, "If you look at the clinical data file, you'll see that it's really, really clear that patients report that pain is not really gone, but it doesn't bother them anymore. And you can actually see that in the patient's file. It's associated with the high, so you could say that the actual endpoint is being high. And that's why it works and that's what people with cancer, terminal cancer, that's what they're looking for. Some of them leave the doctor's office with the bad news of a malignant cancer that's not responding to any therapy. They may not actually be suicidal, but they don't want to live anymore. Then, consuming the cannabis by inhalation, they regain the desire to live and the brain can do a lot more to heal the body.

Wylde: Are we considering things like THC and CBD and the influence of cannabis on the brain to be basically retraining the brain?

Chamberland: I don't know if you could ever actually ***prove*** that, but are the pain effects of cannabis related to its psychoactive nature? Yes. For me, if you lose that psychoactive nature, you're going to lose he drug's efficacy. So just as you're saying, the psychoactive nature of cannabis is retraining the brain. I don't know how we can prove that in humans but proving that the psychoactive nature of cannabis is the key to successfully treating a patient – that's more doable.

Wylde: Right. So far, this is what we've established through clinical research: safety, efficacy and dose – depending on what you're using it for. And of course the best format to take it in, which is vapor or smoke. Is that correct?

Chamberland: Well, yes. But two caveats. We were able to show in healthy volunteers that if you've never consumed cannabis before in your life and I hit you, for example, with 25 milligrams of THC by inhalation, about 50 percent will be absorbed by your body, going straight to your brain, and you're possibly going to faint. About 20 percent of people will faint. And that effect is not coming from the heart. There's no hypotension. The patients we studied were on Holter monitors with an ECG and there was a physician present. The effect is actually coming from a reaction in the brain – psychiatrists call it a defensive reaction– to an incoming vasodilator, as though the brain was shutting down. So, what was really interesting was that the subjects lost their ability to speak and lost a lot of their memory and there was a direct correlation between these adverse events and the blood plasma level of THC. Now what was even more interesting is that, if we slowly introduced volunteers to the drug, we eliminated all of those risks, all of the side effects or reduced the side effects to a point where it was very safe to consume cannabis by inhalation. So, the receptors seemed to have adapted very fast. An SSRI drug, by contrast, sometimes requires months before the body adapts well. The cannabis requires less than a week. And we were able to show that with the first doses there is a negative impact on cognitive function, but the patient adapts and you don't observe this negative response anymore. So there's great potential from a therapeutic point of view and, when its introduction is gradual, you can actually get a very safe drug on the market.

Wylde: Provided you help them to develop tolerance.

Chamberland: Most drugs, you don't do that. You just put the patient on it and get them to tolerate the side effects.

Wylde: And the side effects, the significant ones that you're alluding to a few minutes ago, these are what are affectionately referred to as "greening out".

Chamberland: Yes. You could call it that. The side effects are a shutting down of the brain, a defensive move because the drug is coming in too fast. Patients are unable to tell you what day it is or even talk. But give them three or four days, increasing the dose every day, and you can hit them with 25, 75 milligrams in one shot and they can tolerate the whole damn thing.

Wylde: Let me switch track and ask you about the status of regulations. in both Canada and the U.S. — not just for rolled marijuana, but these different delivery systems and formats, the THC to CBD and so on. Because so many people are confused.

Chamberland: I'll start with Canada. So in Canada, they have a recreational market, an adult-use market to be polite, and that market is actually one that doesn't fall under the drug regulations because of all of the safety implications of having something tolerated under the Food and Drug Act. So Health Canada created special cannabis regulations, which put THC to CBD on the prescription drug list. And this is the part that most people don't understand. The fact that they're on the prescription drug list means you cannot have THC to CBD as a "wellness product" on the market. And that's a bad thing for many industries and people such as herbalists like myself, who would have wanted to create new products in combination with other herbs because we understand the synergies between them. But the regulations don't allow that, nor allow cannabis to transition off the prescription drug list. The regulators' idea is that it has to remain a prescription drug product because it can only be used safely under the care of a physician, which is perfectly logical, except that it ***isn't*** under the care of a physician in a direct market and that's why it's not under the Drug Act. The industry lobbies a lot for the regulators to consider opening a wellness market but the challenge facing them now is that public hearings suggested a significant side effect — liver toxicity. What dose can you give that would be safe as a food? Now in the States, it ***is*** classified as a food supplement. The pertinent laws are about food, not drugs. What they'd have to do there is declare it a kind of grass and then add it to some vitamin supplements. In the United States, under federal law right now, anything that contains THC or some type of cannabinoid is a drug and requires drug approval just like any other drug. So under U.S. federal law right now, all the cannabis products are basically illegal. I doubt the FDA is going to change all of that. How will the FDA deal with opening up the wellness market? I suspect they'll probably be more business sensitive than Canada. I think they're going to open up the pathway through a "new dietary ingredients notification" path, and initially leave the responsibility to manufacturers to produce the safety data to defend the supplement and the claims to assure they've got the actual evidence. And they'll probably leave it to the lawyers to figure it out. I've got a feeling we'll get a lot of surprises. A lot of people ask, will it be a controlled substance or not? So the answer to that is, after the Farmers' Bill, CBD became "non-schedule", so it's no longer a controlled substance. That said, you cannot sell it as a supplement because the Senate and the Farmers' Bill reserved the responsibility for approving CBD to the FDA.

Wylde: Meanwhile, a lot of formulators have moved away from the cannabis plant and are looking at other pseudo-agonists. Do you feel that there may in the supplement world be a way to supplement, whether it's for the brain or other systems in the body, to supplement the endocannabinoid system without using cannabis, CBD or THC? For example, ingredients like PDA or select herbs that do engage the endocannabinoid system?

Chamberland: We have several products that are approved that act on CBD2. To answer your question, yes. We also work with PDA. We target other natural molecules that will act on those receptors. So the short answer is yes.

Wylde: As you know, not all sources are equivalent. Where raw materials come from, for example, even if they were regulated (which they aren't in many respects), is a problem and not all products are necessarily safe, or necessarily effective, or standardized. And when I talk about safety, I'm not talking about safety of THC as a pure ingredient; I'm talking about pesticides and heavy metals. What can you tell people who are consuming either recreationally or addressing clinical concerns? What can you tell them about doing their due diligence to assure they have a clean and effective product?

Chamberland: As a company, we discovered the problem of microtoxins in the cannabis product. We were seeking to demonstrate the lack of toxins when we actually found them. These toxins have never been an issue in herbalism because herbalists don't grow a ton of the material. The challenge of these microtoxin fungi is storage because they're present in all plants that are grown in the soil. But as herbalists we do a lot of wild crafting, we don't store for months or years, and we don't use pesticides. But for producers the challenge of microtoxins is that you're kind of stuck between a regulation that doesn't allow you to use pesticides and the growth of fungal microtoxins. A video that I saw about how GW manufactures a pure botanical product seemed to show that they had developed a special rapid drying system and remove the moisture. To me, that would be to avoid fungal growth, essentially a storage problem.

Wylde: So there are things that people should indeed be considering, certainly when they're consuming it chronically. Is your company creating any sort of list of cleanest raw materials?

Chamberland: We developed all the tools to identify toxins before you cultivate the plants. We want to know where the toxins are, and if they're there, then we can find ways to avoid increasing the amount of toxin. We've been asked by some research analysts for access to tests we've developed. We're certainly not against that because that's not our core business. We created a private company associated with Thorne Research in the United States, probably the strictest company when it comes to purity in quality supplements. The fit was perfect, their vision and expertise on quality. They test for hundreds of impurities in all their products. From what I understand from them, there's a huge difference in multiple natural ingredients and sources. Most people don't realize that when they buy a product off the shelf, even a brand that may be well known, they have no clue about the quality.

Wylde: Thorne has been committed from the mid-eighties, as I understand it, to not just purity, but creating products that are hypoallergenic. A lot of folks that are taking supplements are looking to relieve certain symptoms but sometimes impure products can cause the very symptoms that they're looking to relieve. I attend the major trade shows and supply shows and over the last three or four years, it just seems like you can find CBD on the product labels of virtually everything. They're often very deceiving but from what I understand, CBD is going to soon become a $22 billion industry. It's everywhere. It's in formulations, lotions and potions, coffee lattes, food products and pet products. Some strong part of this has to just be a bit of a craze. So here's my question to you. What are some of the unfounded health claims that you've seen that just make you cringe? What is CBD just ***not*** good for while being touted and promoted as helpful?

Chamberland: The biggest one I would warn people about is pain relief. There's no evidence that CBD is effective for that. I'm not trying to mock CBD, but if I look at it as a herbalist, I would tell you the plant didn't necessarily want its ingredients to be isolated. Traditionally plant-based therapies work best when you consume a whole plant rather than a single type of molecule from that plant. There are multiple examples in the literature to prove that point. So for me, I tell people, be careful. I also make the distinction between what we would call the self-care market and the pharmaceutical market. In the self-care market, you have a condition like anxiety and you decide to treat yourself and you respond. That's perfect. But for sick patients taking narcotics, you can't just switch over. The saddest part about the medical cannabis regulations when they came out was that these regulations still did not give patients what they wanted when they went to the Supreme Court of Canada. What the patients asked for when they went to the Supreme Court was to have access to medical cannabis, not to buy it but to have their physician prescribe it. They wanted their pharmacists to hold their hand and be sure they didn't intoxicate themselves with other things. They wanted naturopathic doctors to guide them and say, no, you can't take this St. John's Wort or you can't experiment with this other product. That's where I think the whole system failed and that's why I've told people, if you're taking it for a mild, occasional insomnia, fine. Taking it for a real condition? Consult your health care practitioner. And watch the brand: some companies are pure hype. Tetra Biopharma is moving into the wellness market as a strong believer in researched evidence. Our venture with Thorne brings us into association with another company, Longevity, that does multiomics for the self-care market. So if you're a patient and you want to take a particular supplement, you see your health care practitioner and Longevity can do testing. They also run clinical trials and can provide you with the results. The multiomics may suggest that such-and-such is the best supplement and may help you with your condition because you share a certain profile with multiple patients. The great thing is that after months of therapy, you do the test and see how likely it is that it's actually working for you. That by the way is where our health care market has to go. Physicians need to start doing these tests to help their patients engage. What I tell some people is that if I help you get a better — call it a placebo effect, if you like — get the brain to kick in more strongly, you're going to have a better chance to respond.

20

THE MEDICINE HUNTER

From an interview with Chris Kilham

The chemical explanation is not separate from the spiritual explanation is not separate from the energetic explanation. All of these factors coexist peacefully together.

~ *Chris Kilham*

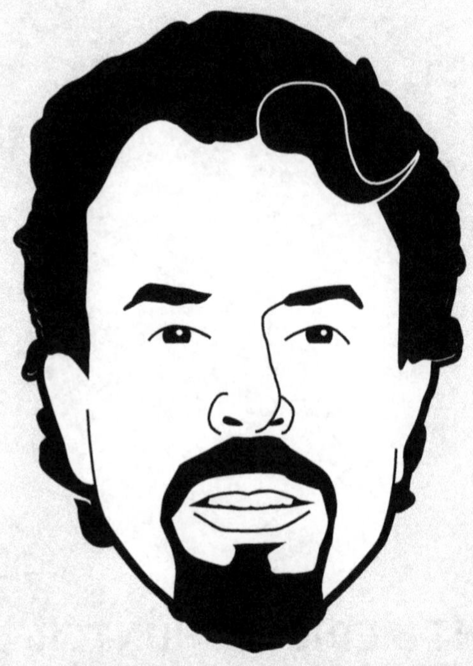

CHRIS **KILHAM**

Chris Kilham is a medicine hunter, ethnobotanist, author, and educator. The founder of Medicine Hunter Inc., he has conducted medicinal plant research in over 45 countries. He also works to bridge worlds, regularly sharing information about other cultures through presentations and media. CNN calls Chris "The Indiana Jones of natural medicine". He has appeared on over 1500 radio programs and more than 500 TV programs worldwide, with features in The New York Times, ABC News Nightline, Newsweek, The Dr. Oz Show, NBC Nightly News, and Good Morning America.

Wylde: What have you, Chris Kilham, done for your brain today?

Kilham: What I've done for my brain today is some meditation, two hours of yoga, plenty of coffee and good thoughts.

Wylde: Plenty of coffee. How much is good for you?

Kilham: I'm a rapid caffeine metabolizer. So usually I drink probably on average four large cups of strong coffee every day. I can drink a double espresso and go to bed. I'm one of those. And you know, I have to say that of the nootropics, there's nothing as cheap and fast and reliable as coffee.

Wylde: As a botanical expert, and coffee falls in that realm, what should we be looking for in our cup of Joe or its source?

Kilham: Certainly you want organic coffee. You don't want to be sucking down agro-poisons and there's no reason for that. Secondly, you want a flavor of coffee you really enjoy. I like the heavy coffees — Kenya Double-A, Papua New Guinea, Sumatra, those kinds. Some people like lighter coffees. But drink it as concentrated as you can. Coffee is the number one source of dietary antioxidants in the American diet. And when you drink a cup of coffee in the morning, it's like slugging down a whopping load of herbal extracts. The chlorogenic acids, for which there is a massive global body of science going back decades, have proved to be among the most beneficial compounds in any foods we know. When you look at the epidemiological studies on coffee — and we're talking 20, 30, 40, 50, 60 thousand people over 5, 10, 15, 20 years. — we're talking big studies here — lots of reduced rates of disease are directly trackable to how many cups of coffee you drink a day.

Wylde: It could be important to determine your genomic status as it relates to how much coffee you're drinking?

Kilham: You can find out how much coffee works for you by drinking it. I have a biological mechanism that is so delightfully wonderful — I don't know how it happened — I can drink coffee and then at a certain point I'll take a sip and it's sour. And I go, you know, that's enough. I'm done. It's like the sour taste means "You're saturated, buddy. Put it down." I rarely get to that, but when I do get to that, I get it so instantaneously, it's like eating an apple and then all of a sudden you get a mouthful of walnuts and you go, "I'm done."

Wylde: You meditate. How much time you spend meditating?

Kilham: Mostly my wife and I meditate at night, so our dedicated meditation time is probably averaging not more than a half hour at night. But I do some meditation in the morning, too, and I always do about two hours of yoga in the morning. And that really just helps me to, you know, stay alive.

Wylde: So they call you the medicine hunter, right? You travel the globe seeking out traditional remedies, botanicals that may confer human health benefit. This is a hard question, because I'm sure you've had so many in the field, but just a few of your highlights in your travels,.

Kilham: The great experiences that I've had have been for the most part with projects that I've visited repetitively. So, for example, I spent about 10 years working in Vanuatu, South Pacific from 1995 to 2005 with kava and a topical oil called tamanu oil and during that time, I became an honorary chief. I became their diplomat to the United States over the years. We fire walked in these massive, terrifying Polynesian rituals every year for six years. I made one of the best friends of my life. He's dead now but people would meet us and they would go, "Whoa, what is it about you two?" We just had this thing. I've had a similar experience in Peru with another dear friend that I met in '98 with whom I've worked all over the Andes and the Amazon. And, you know, we visited and stayed in endless native villages. We ran a dental boat that provided free dentistry all around the Amazon. I've had amazing projects in Siberia and Congo and Syria and all over the place. Where I make the strongest people connections and where I make the strongest friendships, those are the places that I think of most warmly.

Wylde: How cool is that — that the plant life, the topography, the flora, the fauna, the herb is what first brought you together with those people.

Kilham: Especially when you go to cultures where plant medicines are key and critical and really integrated into their lives, when you go and you say, "I'm very keenly interested in your plant medicines and I would love for you to teach me more" instead of "I'm the big expert and I know all this wonderful shit and I'm here to..." — you know, whatever it is that people do and say when they think that they are the center of everything. When you do that, these people's relationship with the plants is so big, they stop doing what they're doing. "We'll go around with you for a few days," they say. You say, "Don't you have to, like, earn a living and feed your family?" "It's all good," they say. And because t they're incredibly close to the plant, and especially when you go for a key plant like kava in the South Pacific, maca root the Peruvian Andes, ***Schizandra chinensis*** in northern China, then they say, "You're interested in the thing that we honor the most." So it's like saying, "I love your grandmother," right? What sort of heartless bastard doesn't care about their grandmother? Going to these cultures respectfully and with great appreciation for whom they are and letting them know that I'm interested in their plants, has afforded me access to people, places and circumstances I would never have gotten otherwise.

Wylde: You mentioned rites of passage, fire walking, you mentioned culture, you mentioned experience. Are these all equally as important to you as the mechanisms of action and the ethno-botanical characters of the various plants?

Kilham: More so. If I go to Vanuatu for kava, my purpose in being there is to work with kava to enhance kava's fortune in the world and to learn how we can build on it. But the reward for me is the people, the friendships. "Sure, I'll stay at your house. Thank you." In two instances, they ***built*** me a house. In Vanuatu, on Santo Island — I was going there often — they said, "We're going to build him a house." So they built me a small, two-storey house overlooking the Pacific Ocean. And then in a village that I took my wife to a few years ago, they thought, "We just can't have them come stay anywhere. We've got to build them a house because he's gonna be here for a week." I haven't been back for a few years, but their way of showing love and appreciation, it's almost heartbreaking, the hospitality and the graciousness and the generosity that I've experienced among people who don't really have much materially. On the other hand, they have community, they have family, they have friendships, they have great times, which is worth everything. And I take that as at least partly reflective of their being more attuned to nature. But it's not idyllic – we're not talking idyllic situations anywhere – but I really noticed that, you know, I've never had a wealthy friend build me a house.

Wylde: You mentioned schizandra. But you revere ayahuasca. You call it perhaps one of the greatest natural healing agents. Tell us about ayahuasca.

Kilham: Ayahuasca is, as people may or may not know, a very profoundly psychoactive potion that is made in the Amazon. And it's the only psychedelic that requires two plants: a vine and a leaf. And the chemistry of how those two were chosen among eighty thousand plants in the Amazon remains a mystery to everybody. But the native people say, "Well, obviously the plants told us. I mean, don't they talk to you?" They're kind of dumbfounded that we haven't figured that out. "You really think this is trial and error?" they ask. "Are you serious? You're kidding me, right?" And it's traditionally taken ceremonially. It's something that is for healing and that healing may be mental, emotional, spiritual, physical. I have personally seen hundreds of people suffering trauma, sexual abuse, chronic illnesses – stomach aches that they've had for fifteen years, backaches they've had forever, sleeplessness they've had forever – achieve significant resolution of many of these things as a result of being in one or two or three or several ayahuasca ceremonies. It's very intense. It's not for everybody. It can be scary. I wrote a book called *The Ayahuasca Test Pilots Handbook*, which is basically what you want to know about if this is something that you want to embark on. I became aware of it in 1975 but didn't really drink it until about 13 years ago or so after the death of my mother and have subsequently become an advocate of it. The psychedelics – if you think of ayahuasca, peyote, San Pedro, magic mushrooms and iboga from Africa – they occupy the highest possible positions in the cultures in which they're employed and from which they derive. This is because of their spectacular capacity to heal. Much of it doesn't make sense. You might have a night in which you're having just the weirdest visions ever. They don't really seem to make sense, and then the next day you notice that the stomach ache that you've been carrying for seven years is gone. And you say, "Well, there was nothing really that tipped me off." Or maybe there's something very direct. So, I have profound regard for it. This is not for recreational drug use. You can't drink ayahuasca and play naked Frisbee on the beach. That's not going to work. But for people who want real feeling from things and maybe they've tried a lot of other things and haven't been successful, they often find really satisfactory healing and relief with ayahuasca. So I'm a big fan.

Wylde: But MDMA and LSD and magic mushrooms. Does ayahuasca compare with these?

Kilham: Ayahuasca is hard. It's rougher. Magic mushrooms are mostly friendly and we see phenomenal science — for example, with the Johns Hopkins University Medical Center studies using psilocybin, where terminal cancer patients lost their fear of death, lost their anxiety about that, which is amazing. That's compassionate medicine. But from my experience, I would put ayahuasca at the top, though there are people who would do the same with peyote. I would say, look, I've been sitting in prayer services for years and seeing the same healings. So I don't I don't think it's really necessary to assign the top position. I mean, I have friends who work in the African iboga communities and for them, that's it, that's the big kahuna. Often, it's just a matter of what touches your heart. Maybe you meet fifteen people and one just really turns you on like crazy. Why? What are the thousands of factors that add up to that?

Wylde: It sounds like the most desirable outcome from a hallucinogenic experience may be the alleviation of a physical ailment or helping an individual come to terms with death, or managing depression or whatever. But can a hallucinogenic experience be so all-encompassing?

Kilham: Well, yes, these are immersive experiences. They get you down to your toenails. They leave nothing out. And the thoroughness of it, the intensity of it can be very challenging for some people. It can be overwhelming, but on the other hand, it can be spectacular. I've really come to accept the whole concept of mystic healing. Mystical experiences by nature are healing experiences. And when you look at, for example, the Johns Hopkins psilocybin studies, what they show is that the people who got the best results in terms of accepting where they were in their transition to death were the people who had the most profound spiritual experiences. So, I think that mystic healing is a key thing that we're really just still coming to terms with.

Wylde: So in your view, this experience is not some kind of meaningless biochemical projection, a bunch of novel chemicals firing more than usual for that moment in time.

Kilham: It happens that way, too. The chemical explanation is not separate from the spiritual explanation which is not separate from the energetic explanation. All of these factors coexist peacefully together. Is ayahuasca a physiological medicine? Absolutely. Can you say it's an energetic medicine? Absolutely. Can you say there are spiritual dimensions? Absolutely. A quick story. I got interested in ashwagandha in 1972. I bought a copy of an imponderably immense 2500-year old text on Ayurveda, the Indian medicine tradition. I confess I didn't read every word, but I read a lot of it, and when I got to ashwagandha, I was amazed. And it just happened that an Ayurvedic physician was coming to Boston around that same time and I went to see him and we talked for a while and then he gave me these little brown pills made of ashwagandha. I took them and had this really positive experience. I subsequently went to India many times, and each time I would investigate ashwagandha to some extent. I knew it was number one among the seven and a half thousand botanicals used in the Ayurvedic system. When I first started investigating it, it was in danger of being over harvested in the wild to extinction. Now it's very widely cultivated and I got to know a company, called KSM 66 Ashwagandha, who manufacture it. I saw their organic cultivation, the green technology extraction, the human clinical studies — that did it for me. With regards to stress especially, we see up to almost twenty-eight percent reduction in serum cortisol with KSM 66 over about eight weeks. That's pretty remarkable. As I like to say, with ashwagandha it's like getting off of an angry horse. Part is what you do notice — the extra energy, the stamina, the endurance — but a lot of it is what is ***gone***. "I'm just not wired. I've got all the energy in the world. I'm sleeping like a baby. Sex life is good. All that. But I'm just not wired." When I was a kid, we understood stress to be a nuisance.

Now we know that stress physically damages every organ system in the body, sometimes beyond the capacity of that system to repair itself. Stress can and will kill you if it goes unchecked. And so for me, anything, whether it's meditation or ashwagandha — anything that can reduce stress and help you to manage your life better so that you're in control, you're not just ripped to the eyeballs with tension — that's a tremendous gift to humanity.

Wylde: A key operative term being "manage", not "cope"; coping is just sort of ignoring and maybe doing the best you possibly can that day. You said one of the things you appreciate about KSM 66 Ashwagandha in particular is its sustainability, its purity and the water processing.

Kilham: Actually, there are two extracts, one is a traditional buffalo milk and water extract, which is how it's done in Ayurvedic medicine, the other a vegan beverage using just water. **Wylde**: What about standardization of this product?

Kilham: With KSM 66 Ashwagandha, the primary agents that are novel to the herb are standardized to five percent. And we know that the clinical dose, at least the dose that is proven effective in studies for cognitive function, for cardio-respiratory endurance and stamina, for stress, for sleep, for sexual purposes, is six hundred milligrams of the extract.

Wylde: Will 300 work?

Kilham: I don't know. Maybe. 400? I don't know. But we know that 600 works. The smart supplement manufacturers — and there aren't that many of them — say, "What are the clinical results? The clinical trials are using x amount of the botanical. OK. Well, then that's what we'll use and we'll use the one that's clinically tested." That's because it isn't the case that all extracts are the same. There are huge differences with extracts. There can be huge differences in the profile of the six, seven, eight hundred compounds in a finished product. So, I'm well satisfied that KSM 66 Ashwagandha is one of the great extracts.

21

BRINGING HOME THE BROCCOLI

From an interview with Dr. David Jenkins

Plant-based foods can have a drug-like effect.

~ Dr. David Jenkins

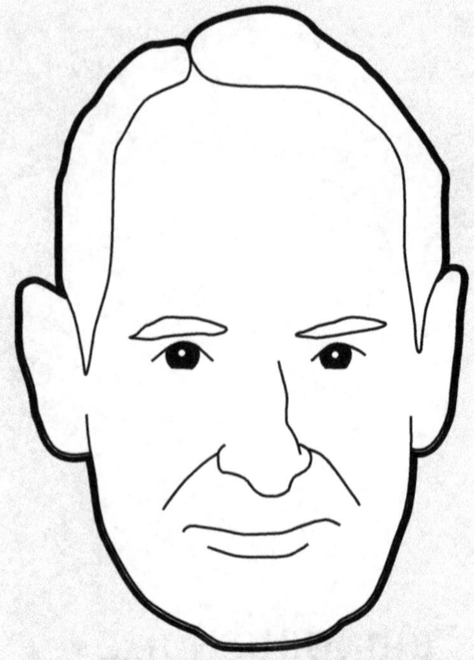

DR. DAVID **JENKINS**

Dr. David Jenkins is an Oxford University alumni and currently a Professor in both the Departments of Nutritional Sciences and Medicine, Faculty of Medicine, University of Toronto. He is a Staff Physician in the Division of Endocrinology and Metabolism, the Director of the Clinical Nutrition and Risk Factor Modification Center, and a Scientist in the Li Ka Shing Knowledge Institute of St. Michael's Hospital. He led the team that first defined and explored the concept of the glycemic index of foods. He was also the first to demonstrate the breadth of metabolic effects of viscous soluble fiber (as found in fruit, certain beans, oats barley) on blood glucose and cholesterol lowering of relevance to prevention and treatment of diabetes and heart disease.

Wylde: What have you, Dr. David Jenkins, done for your brain today?

Jenkins: Not a great deal. I probably hit the wall too hard too many times, I think, probably got too stressed over many trivial issues, which I'm sure doesn't help the brain at all. They say that keeping the brain active is good, but I think you can probably overactivate it.

Wylde: So will you be doing some sort of meditation later?

Jenkins: No. If I was allowed to, I'd probably go for a swim. I used to run. I think that was probably good for brain health, but my legs gave out and, as with so many older people, my knees started playing up. I had to take to the water because it's more congenial for the joints. I'm a neophyte swimmer. I was never much of a swimmer when I was younger though I enjoyed the water. Now it's my source of exercise.

Wylde: Your research has been largely focused throughout your career on sugar and the glycemic index. Besides the association most people make to diabetes, why is sugar so harmful?

Jenkins: We think that sugar – high levels of glucose – really high levels of any nutrient -- may not be good for brain health. Obviously, glucose can get into the brain quickly so it's probably good for you when you need to take an exam. You don't want to take an exam with low blood sugar. But it has to be kept within range. When you go to high blood sugar, especially with diabetes, you get neurological dysfunction. So high sugars tend to be not a good idea – possibly by glycating proteins, but possibly by other mechanisms, probably by pro-oxidant activity. Chronic high blood sugar levels tend not to be good for the brain or the nervous system in general.

Wylde: So we've come to be very conscious of type-1 diabetes and type-2 diabetes. But now researchers like yourself are talking about a type-3 diabetes. Can you comment on that?

Jenkins: Well, I'm not sure that I would use the term type-3 diabetes. We've got type 2 and type 1 and we've got other diabetes: gestational diabetes and drug-induced diabetes, as can occur with steroids. After that, I would go to the metabolic syndrome, which I think is probably the more important concept, because, although obviously the metabolic syndrome is associated with diabetes itself, we can get a lot of the disorders that you get with diabetes without the pancreas actually failing sufficiently to cause diabetes.

Wylde: What can you tell us about the latest research on why plant-based diets are so healthy?

Jenkins: There are a number of things. They lower the serum cholesterol, which is a big problem in terms of cardiovascular disease and possibly other diseases, too. Some of the cancers may relate to altered cholesterol metabolism. So I think plants are a good thing because of the fiber content, because of the nature of their fatty acids and even the nature of their protein. These factors all contribute, I think, to a lower risk of cardiovascular disease, and lower LDL cholesterol levels. So those are good points in their favour. Also, because plant foods tend to be water rich, the bulk provided by these diets tends to make them more satiating.

Wylde: You're actually known for saying that plant-based foods can have a drug-like effect on the body. Explain that for our readers.

Jenkins: Plant-based foods can have a drug-like effect. If you combine them in the right quantities, you can get foods that lower cholesterol to the same extent as an early statin drug. The portfolio diet that we put together many years ago and are still developing seems to be a good diet in terms of lowering the cholesterol level in a drug-like fashion. Even the "dash" diet, which is a very moderate diet, can lower blood pressure, and can possibly lower it to the same extent as doubling the dose of a standard blood-pressure-lowering medication. I do think that there are drug-like effects available through diet and if you take diets for a lifetime, then you may get lifetime benefits.

Wylde: Some people actually consider cholesterols to be controversial, as if it may be it's a myth. In your opinion, cholesterol actually does contribute to heart disease, as you mentioned, maybe even cancer. In your opinion, cholesterol and its contribution to disease is not a controversial topic.

Jenkins: Many things are controversial. I mean, the Flat Earth Society considers the shape of the Earth to be controversial. There are lots of people who think that climate change is controversial. They want to look at the Northwest Passage — it's opening up. A lot of things are controversial to people who haven't thought about them greatly.

Wylde: As it pertains to cholesterol, it's irrefutable in your mind that high LDL, high oxidized cholesterol, small particle size, all of these things significantly contribute to the human disease condition.

Jenkins: I think they contribute to the human disease condition, just as you say. If someone says that they're the only things that contribute — obviously, that's controversial. One would say that there are many things that are possibly useful, but lowering cholesterol — and keeping it down as much as you can — is a good idea.

Wylde: Would you say perhaps that what's healthy for your heart and cardiovascular system at large is also healthy for the brain?

Jenkins: Well, I think the brain is supplied by the cardiovascular system and it's pretty difficult to dissociate the two.

Wylde: You coined the term "glycemic index" and it's the focus of a tremendous body of work you've put forth. Can you clarify for our readers the difference between glycemic index and glycemic load as they pertain to foods?

Jenkins: The glycemic index relates to the classification of the food, and it just says that the carbohydrate in that food is very readily available or not readily available in terms of its ability to raise the blood glucose. The glycemic load says, "Well, that's good, but how much carbohydrate is that?" So, for example, carbohydrates in some foods may be quite readily available, but they don't have much carbohydrate. The carbohydrates, for example, in a cabbage — if you cook it well — is quite readily available. But don't feel bad about eating cabbage: there's very little carbohydrate in the cabbage, so it won't raise your blood glucose that much even if it raises it relatively quickly. So that's the beauty of the glycemic load concept. It tells you how much of a glycemic rise you'll get from a particular food. The glycemic index will tell you what sort of foods you might want to put together in your diet on the basis of their low index.

Wylde: Are there any tests that family physicians should be running with their patients on their annual physical to go beyond fats and sugar and hemoglobin? Are there other tests, whether they're physical or blood tests or any other sort of assessment, that you believe physicians should be looking at their patients for?

Jenkins: They're going to do their blood pressure, their cholesterol, their HDL — all the usual things. One thing they may not do is look at the patient's waist. Waist measurement is a good predictor. It can be adjusted according to the hip size or the height, but even the waist-chest measurement itself is difficult but useful.

Wylde: Is there an information link or a reference that readers could use to ask their family doctors to test them that way?

Jenkins: Well, I think it's a little bit contentious, as I say, but a lot of big studies reference waist size. Some measure it at the narrowest portion of the torso. Others measure it at the umbilicus. These measures are taken when the patient's lying down because then the body spreads out. And you can measure it at the umbilicus at that point because otherwise you find the umbilicus very often sags quite low in those who are large.

Wylde: And what we're referring to here, of course, is the belly fat acting like an organ and correlated with pre-diabetes and metabolic syndrome. I love that waist-size test because it's so accessible and easy to perform. And I hope doctors do get into the practice of that and correlate it back to blood work and perhaps incentivize their patients in some ways to drop that central obesity. So this leads into my next question about health benefits. You're a huge champion of soluble fiber and, along with probiotics, it's on everyone's mind when it comes to cholesterol. What about the difference between insoluble and soluble fiber and how can we achieve optimal soluble fiber levels through a plant-based diet?

Jenkins: I must say, I'm always worried by the term "soluble fiber". I think what we're really talking about is viscous fiber or sticky fiber. Sticky fibers are certainly important and you find them in things like oatmeal. They're one of the things that makes porridge sticky. You find it in things like barley, which people could substitute for rice if they wanted. Barley is a food with beta glucan and is very good in stews and soups provided you have the whole barley. If you've ever tried barley it has a sort of crunchiness to it. That's partly the protection of the carbohydrate by the viscous fibre. Vegetables like okra are also rich in sticky fibre. If you've ever boiled eggplant, you'll find it's got a syrupy water at the bottom. That's sticky fibre. Persimmon has it too. All these foods are good for that reason and may contribute to lowering cholesterol. And psyllium — a teaspoon or two a day for people who can't get a lot of fibre through their diet — is not a bad thing.

Wylde: Is it oversimplifying to say sticky fiber equals beta glucan equals cardiovascular health?

Jenkins: Sticky fibers equal beta glucan equals pectin equals galactomanan equals a lot of different types of viscous fibre. They're only a relatively few foods that contain viscous fibre. Wheat bran isn't one of them.

Wylde: What's your take on something that's become quite a craze — there are a whole bunch of crazes and we've already talked a little bit about controversy — the lectin-free diet, including gluten. What's your view on that?

Jenkins: Well, I think lectins may cause problems, but on the other hand, they're found in very good foods. So if you elect for a lectin-free diet, you could end up depriving yourself of a lot of healthy foods. If one cooks one's foods well, one may reduce some of the impact. Fruits and vegetables are not of much concern for lectins. People are really thinking of the cereals and legumes. But cereals should be cooked. Legumes should be cooked. Societies around the world that consume a lot of home-grown cereals and legumes often have very good longevity. So I think the lectin story is an interesting one but I wouldn't get fixated on it.

Wylde: If you were stuck on an island and you weren't able to access your plant based diet, but you were given a choice of one of three other diets: a paleo diet, a strict vegan diet or a keto-based diet, which one would you choose?

Jenkins: I'd choose the vegan diet..

Wylde: Tell us a little bit more about your portfolio diet and why that's so helpful for people.

Jenkins: It contains viscous fibers. It contains plant proteins. It contains foods that are generally known to lower cholesterol such as nuts, tofu and soya proteins.

Wylde: Is it more expensive to eat this way?

Jenkins: It's not cheap. This is true. I think it can be made reasonably inexpensive, but it takes a lot of thought. It's much easier to just run out and get a burger from McDonald's. I'm afraid that's where we've gone with food.

Wylde: Your breakfast today, what did that look like?

Jenkins: My breakfast today was some tofu and some wholemeal bread, an apple and a pear and some soy milk.

Wylde: Do you believe you personally and others generally should be supplementing their diet?

Jenkins: We don't see a great benefit from supplements if you're consuming a reasonable diet. I think that's the key issue. B12, for very strict vegans, may be an issue, and they can get that from basically vegan sources as a supplement. So that's fine. You can get a vegan B12. B12 generally is made by bacteria. So you can say it's a vegan food, but you don't need much of it. You really don't need much B12 unless you're old and on the way to pernicious anemia. But that's a different situation. In general, on a good healthy diet with fruit, vegetables and cereals, legumes, nuts and seeds, you're not going to need anything. You should be fine. Apart from your B12 status, which you can determine by visiting your family physician on a yearly basis to make sure that you're staying in range.

Wylde: Any thoughts on algal DHA, for example, for brain and heart health?

Jenkins: It's interesting. Sounds as if it could be good.

Wylde: Is there anything else that you'd share with our readership?

Jenkins: Well, I think the big thing is, you mustn't be selfish. Don't just eat for yourself. Eat for the planet.

22

BIGGER FISH TO FREE

From an interview with James Aspey

The step that most people have to take to become vegan is to simply align their actions with the belief system they already have.

~ James Aspey

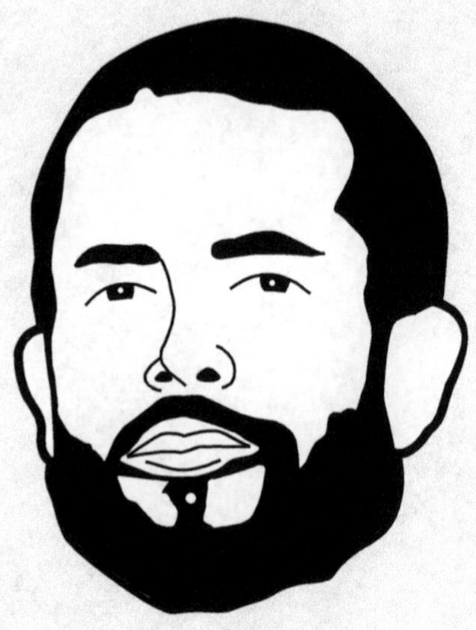

JAMES **ASPEY**

James Aspey has a lifelong mission to raise greater awareness for the planet's forgotten victims. He is an Australian animal rights activist who took a 365-day vow of silence. After an entire year without uttering a single word, he ended it on Australian national television in an iconic interview that reached millions and inspired countless people to make more conscious and compassionate lifestyle choices. Ranked #3 among the "Top 25 Most Influential Vegans" by Plant Based News, James has gone on to cycle 5000kms across Australia to prove that vegans can be fit & healthy. He got tattooed for 25 hours straight to raise $20,000 for charity. He's been featured in a multitude of prominent mainstream media outlets; given free speeches at countless schools, universities, and conferences; and attended local activism events, slaughterhouse vigils, and street outreach events all across the world.

Wylde: James Aspey, what what have you done for your ***brain*** today?

Aspey: I did a ten-minute meditation at the beginning of my morning, and in that meditation I focused on observing the physical sensations of my body and accepting each sensation, whether uncomfortable or pleasant. And this is a technique that can improve focus in your brain or in your mind, reduce anxiety and increase energy levels. After that, I took my supplements, which were B_{12} and an algae-based DHA supplement.

Wylde: But you have some "grand master" experience with meditation and silent retreats. Just tell us a little bit about it that.

Aspey: I've done nine ten-day Vipassana meditation courses. You stop speaking for the entire duration of the ten days and stop interacting with other people. There's no phone. There's no TV. You don't write anything down or read. What do you do for ten to twelve hours a day? Sit on a cushion and meditate — an insight meditation. So for the first four days you are observing your breath and only your breath. And each time your mind wanders, you just bring it back to the breath, bring it back to the breath, over and over again for four days straight. Then on the fourth day, you start a different practice called Vipassana. Vipassana is equal parts equanimity, which is accepting the moment as it is — not craving good sensations, not resisting bad sensations — just being totally objective with whatever it is that comes up and just looking at it. The other part pf the technique. is just looking at the physical sensations of your body. So you start at the top of your head and scan what's happening here, what's happening there. And whatever you find, you just look at it objectively. The goal of this meditation technique is to start observing rather than reacting to the physical sensations of your body. This technique can bring a lot of inner peace and a lot of clarity in the mind and calmness. It makes you feel like you're more connected to the things that truly matter in your life, and you don't get so thrown around by those thoughts that come through and make you feel anxious, negative, stressed out, depressed. I've done it nine times, as I said, and it has been different every single time. It has been one of the most life-changing experiences of my life. I look at my life as before my first Vipassana and after my first Vipassana. After that first course, I came out of there and I felt like I had just taken off a backpack full of bricks I'd been carrying for years. I forever then had a technique to work with that was always with me and I do use every single day. That has just totally changed the energy that I have.The type of person that I now am is much closer to the person that I always strive to be, that is, a person who is compassionate, respectful, peaceful, kind. It's as though we all have this light inside of us, but over the years, we pick up different beliefs here and there and we create stories in our head that aren't necessarily true and act like a layer of filth over our lives. We still shine through but when you do Vipassana and you keep practicing this way, it feels like the layers of filth start getting removed and your light shines more and more brightly.

Wylde: The studies done on focused meditation, mindfulness-based stress reduction, Vipassana, and so forth suggest they do confer incredible health benefits. The science continues to mount. Do you think anyone can do this?

Aspey: I think that anyone can who doesn't suffer from some type of mental health issue or something like that can do it. For the vast majority of people, this is an excellent technique. It's incredibly simple, not complicated. There's no dogma behind it. You don't have to have a particular religion. You only need to focus on your breath and focus on your physical sensations and that's something that everybody has and can do. It's such a simple, repetitive activity, but the results it brings — I just couldn't believe it, because all I was doing was observing my itches and my tingles and my pain and trying to just accept them. But the way it transforms your life is absolutely shocking. During my first Vipassana meditation — it's an insight meditation — I had a idea come to me to take a year-long vow of silence to raise awareness for animals and also as an interesting personal experiment. I also had the idea to have a long break from any type of mind altering substances — alcohol, caffeine, cannabis, just everything — and I kept up that deal with myself for seven years. Because I stayed in that clear, unaltered mindset, I started planning for that vow of silence and continuing with my Vipassana two hours every day. Before I knew it, a year later, I'd started and completed that vow of silence and I don't think I ever would have gone through with that if it wasn't for continuing this Vipassana practice. It helped me stay on track, work through my own objections to it and ultimately complete it successfully.

Wylde: You didn't speak for a whole year, ultimately because animals don't have a voice.

Aspey: Yeah. When I had the idea to do this, I had recently gone vegetarian a few months prior. I'd been a huge meat eater. I was a personal trainer for seven years. I was getting vegetarians to eat meat again and literally cooking it for them. Then I became aware that we can get every essential nutrient from a plant-based diet. We can live, we can thrive, potentially live longer lives, and reduce our chances of developing many diseases on this diet – something I had never considered possible before. I always thought that we needed meat for protein, dairy for calcium, eggs for omegas, that there was simply no alternative. Learning about the health side of a plant-based diet led me to to learn about what happens to animals inside slaughterhouses and what happens to animals for us to consume animal products such as meat, dairy, eggs, leather, wool, silk, products that are tested on animals – all these kinds of things. What I saw was like watching the worst horror movie I'd ever seen except that it was real and it was happening constantly to tens of billions of land animals every single year and trillions of sea animals every single year. The question that came to my mind was: if we don't need to consume animal products to be healthy, then how do we justify this relentless and brutal treatment of them? Everything from forcibly impregnating cows to get them to lactate and stealing their babies from them once they're born, slaughtering their baby boys because they don't produce milk, slaughtering the baby chicks in the egg industry because they don't produce eggs – the many different mutilations that happen to the animals in every single one of the industries. For example, pigs get castrated without pain relief just a few days to a few weeks old. They have their teeth cut out, they have their tails cut off, they live almost always in horrendous conditions. And this is just standard legal normal practice for almost the entire world – well, really, the entire world. So what I saw with my own eyes – the animals being used in this way – coupled with the understanding that we can live and thrive on a plant based diet, made me realize that I have no excuse to ever go back to eating animal products. I can't justify it. I'm not a violent person. I would not be okay with this happening to me, so how can I cause this type of suffering to somebody else? If the world was doing this to dogs we'd all be outraged. It makes no sense to be against violence to some animals and not against the violence to equally aware pigs, for example, who are even more intelligent than dogs. Doesn't make sense to not be against that type of violence. It doesn't make sense to be completely against something like throat-slitting, and yet pay for that every single time we eat a meal with eggs, because all of those animals end up getting stabbed in the throat. They get put in gas chambers, they get electrocuted to death, horrific violence that need not exist. So when I learned that, I decided that I would no longer just be vegetarian, that I would be vegan. Being vegan is about the golden rule in action: treating others the way you'd want to be treated. And that extends to all beings and focuses on causing the least amount of harm as practically possible. Basically it is being consistent with your values of non-violence.

Wylde: You've been there, you've done that. You've been in the slaughterhouses, unlike a lot of other vegans who may not have had the stomach for it, but simply rely on white papers or documentaries. You've been there, boots on the ground. But before we go further down that rabbit hole, so to speak, what do you tell folks who think that a vegan diet simply can't supply all of the necessary protein and micronutrients?

Aspey: I would refer them to the position of the Academy of Nutrition and Dietetics, which Is an association that has over one hundred thousand scientists, nutritionists, dieticians, and they have done a meta-analysis on I believe it's over 100 studies on the vegan diet and what they have come to the conclusion of is that "it is a position of the Academy of Nutrition and Dietetics that appropriate planned vegetarian, including vegan diets, a healthful, nutritionally adequate and may provide health benefits for the prevention and treatment of certain diseases. These diets are appropriate for all stages of the lifecycle, including pregnancy, lactation, infancy, childhood, adolescence, older adulthood and athletics. Plant based diets are more environmentally sustainable than diets rich in animal products because they use fewer natural resources and are associated with much less environmental damage. Vegetarians and vegans are at reduced risk of certain health conditions, including heart disease, type-2 diabetes, hypertension, certain types of cancer and obesity." I quote this because this is the largest nutrition and dietetics association in the world and their conclusion is echoed all around the world by similar associations in Britain and the U,S, and Canada and Australia and New Zealand. Harvard has put out a similar statement. And basically the consensus is that not only can we live and thrive, but we're likely to live longer and reduce some of our most common diseases, such as heart disease. In fact, the only diet that has ever proven to reverse heart disease in the majority of patients is a whole-food plant-based diet. We have vegan athletes who are at the very top of their very demanding sport. Some of the most elite athletes on the planet are vegan, including the world-record-holding strong man, Patrik Baboumian, who is a world record holder of the yoke walk, which is where you put a insane amount of weight on your shoulders and walk forwards — I believe it's 10 meters. He also is a world record holder for holding the most weight — I think it's twenty kilos — in front of you at shoulder height with your arms almost straight for the longest amount of time. We have world record holder Scott Jurek, who broke the through-hike record for the Appalachian Trail, which is an extremely long run. We have a world-record arm wrestler. A new record was broken by a vegan woman who did the longest plank in the Guinness World Records. We have NFL players, we have UFC fighters. The list goes on. These examples basically prove that you can not only be healthy on a vegan diet but achieve excellent physical strength, power and agility. A good friend of mine, Brandon Brazier — triathlete, long distance, marathon runner —is vegan.

Wylde: Let me ask this question from a nutritional standpoint: Do you, James Aspey, supplement with anything out of a concern that a vegan diet may not cover all nutritional bases? Is there anything that you think a vegan diet might lack?

Aspey: Excellent question. Well, first of all, the difference between plant based and vegan isn't the diet. Somebody on a plant-based diet shares the exact same diet as a vegan. But the difference between plant-based and vegan is that a vegan is also making an ethical connection, that is, being vegan as a stance against the oppression and exploitation of other species. And that's why veganism can travel further than just diet, to clothing choices, etc. Me personally, yes, I definitely supplement with a couple of things. I am aware that one thing that vegans will struggle to get just through food alone is vitamin B_{12}. Before modern farming practices, we would have got enough B_{12} because it was made by a bacteria found in soil and water. But modern practices basically destroy the vast majority of B_{12}. A lot of meat eaters are getting B_{12} because the animals that they eat are also being supplemented with B_{12}, either directly injected into their bodies or having their feed supplemented. The B_{12} is filtered through their bodies and then people kill the animal and eat the body and obtain B_{12} that way. Also, it's interesting to note that a very large percentage of people who consume animal products are also B_{12} deficient. With a vegan diet, if you are eating foods such as tofu or nutritional yeast, which is a cheesy, delicious, flaky food, or you are eating other foods that are fortified with B_{12} such as vegan meat or vegan cheese or soy milk, then you can get B_{12} that way. But because B_{12} is such an important vitamin for brain health, it's advised that all vegans, and in fact all people, take B_{12} Supplement and that could be as simple as a spray under your tongue once a day. Also, there are some supplements that are strong enough that you only need to take them once to twice each week. And that is really the number one main supplement that all the doctors that I trust and follow would agree on. Other supplements that are also important and can be lacking in a vegan diet is vitamin D. That can be easily be rectified by getting enough sunlight, but if you are not getting enough sunlight because you live somewhere that doesn't have a lot of sun, then it would be advised that you take a vitamin D_3 supplement and again, vitamin D is available from vegan sources. It's also interesting to note that vitamin D deficiency is prevalent amongst not just vegans, but also people eating animal products. Lastly, it's important to supplement omega-3s for brain health unless you are eating enough chia seeds, walnuts, flax seeds, hemp seeds every day – that would just be a tablespoon of one of those choices. I personally don't eat that much every single day. I want to make sure that I'm getting a good omega-3 ratio so I take a supplement of algae-based DHA. Those are the only three that I think are important. You can definitely get enough calcium, iron and protein on a vegan diet.

Wylde: Do you happen to know what you're omega-3 index is?

Aspey: I do not.

Wylde: Sometimes achieving optimal levels requires taking suplemental algal omega-3s – which are vegan by the way. I mean, dolphins have a 17 percent index. They tend to eat a lot of fish, but ***we*** need at least 8 percent or higher for optimal health, brain function, cardiovascular function. Check out www.thelivingbrainproject.com. Switching gears real quick, what is your position on lab-based meat?

Aspey: I think that if the world switched to this new technology of lab meat, it would be hugely beneficial for our environment as animal agriculture is a leading cause of deforestation. Eighty-one percent of deforestation happens to clear land for animals to graze. Species extinction is a leading cause of habitat loss ocean dead zones, greenhouse gas emissions, water pollution and the list goes on. So, for that reason alone, I think it would be a massive step forward. But then of course, it would mean reducing the suffering and violent death of literally trillions of feeling, sensing, emotional, intelligent beings that we share this earth with. And on our health side of things, we're talking about the exact same same taste, the exact same texture, the exact same food but simply created in a lab, which means that you are avoiding many possibilities of disease outbreaks that happen in these factory farms, which is where over 95 percent of animal products come from. So that's why they call it "clean meat", because it is a clean version of the meat that currently people eat. We have E. coli outbreaks and salmonella, listeria, and all kinds of problems that can come about when these animals are raised in such cramped and filthy conditions.

Wylde: That's the stuff that we perhaps know about. I mean, what freaks me out is the stuff that we're not so aware of that may cause chronic illnesses – things like prions, the invisible stuff that we don't even feel for many months and years after being infected.

Now, I already know what your answer is going to be but I must ask it for my readers. Isn't organic grass-fed beef humane? Isn't that an alternative option to factory-based slaughterhouses?

Aspey: It is most definitely an ***alternative***, and in many ways it might be seen as a more ethical alternative, but my personal belief is that there is no ethical way to kill somebody who does not want to die. If we use humans as the example, instead of caging humans and killing them for their meat, would it be more ethical if we let them have a good life for a few years, all the creature comforts, then after that, send them to the slaughterhouse, bolt them in the head and stab them in the throat, which is what is described as humane slaughter? Would we actually describe that as humane when it came to humans, or would we describe that as a premeditated murder? I think it's obvious what we would decide. Although instead of torturing an animal in a factory farm, allowing them to roam freely and then slaughtering them is the lesser of two evils, it is still evil. The way our world is and given how abundant the choices we have are, there's no need to continue slaughtering animals. There's no need to obtain nutrients from the body parts of murdered beings anymore. There potentially was a time when that was 100 percent necessary for our survival, but that time is long gone. So organic meat is great for humans because it means many fewer chemicals, it doesn't really mean much to animals. And although free range and grass fed does mean something to animals, it does not justify the fact that they all end up in the same slaughterhouse losing their lives against their will. These animals do have an interest in living. They don't want to be killed, just as you or I don't want to. They are intelligent beings with the same emotions as us: fear and stress. Cows have friends. Pigs have a sophisticated language, body language coupled with the noises they make, and we are aware of 80 different things they are saying to each other. They're very intelligent beings and to put them through this violent practice just so that we can satisfy our desire to taste their flesh. It's not for their nutrients thast we do this because that can be done in another way. I think is a current dark stain on our civilization. I think it's it is not in alignment with the type of world we are striving to create, which is a world of respect and compassion and non-violence. I think the easiest way to figure out if something is genuinely humane or not is to imagine yourself in that situation and ask how would you like it if it was you at that slaughterhouse? Thinking you may face a bolt guns in the head and be humanely stabbed in the throat.

Wylde: In the context of humane, let's talk about organic free range. What's wrong with dairy, eggs and fish?

Aspey: Well, let's start with fish. Fish are sentient beings with pain receptors, even though a lot of people are under the impression that fish don't feel pain. That's not true. A lot of people find it hard to connect with fish because they don't really show a face with much expression and they live in a completely different environment than us. So it's just a little bit harder to relate and connect to them. But I think what helps us to relate to what we do share with fish is that we all have a heart, we all have a brain, we all feel pain. It appears that they want to avoid danger just like we do. They build, they use tools, they have families and to me, it's clear that they deserve to be treated with respect. If I don't need to cause them harm in order to survive and thrive, then I can't justify it. I believe it's wrong to hurt a pig or a dog and for the same reason I wouldn't hurt a fish. When it comes to eggs, the hens that lay eggs have been selectively bred to lay usually about one egg a day. Years ago, in nature, these chickens were laying twenty eggs a year roughly. So their bodies have been very greatly manipulated and this is causing them a lot more stress. They're not born to live a long life. They're born to live a very short life. They pump out as many eggs as possible. And then once they start slowing their production, they are sent to a slaughterhouse. If they were left to continue living they'd get all kinds of different health problems because of the way their bodies have been manipulated. But these animals are not here for us to use. In the egg industry, they shred the male chicks or gas the male chicks. We use them for their eggs, even free range organic eggs. They all end up in a slaughterhouse after living a fraction of their lives, getting killed against their will.

Dairy is one of the most horrendous industries on the planet, as far as I'm aware. Cows are caged and tied in an apparatus commonly referred to as a rape rack. A worker shoves his arm inside the anus and injects their vagina with bull semen to force them to become pregnant — without consent, of course. We have no right to invade other beings' bodies this way or force a pregnancy upon them. She gives birth. Her babies are taken from her, which is a traumatic experience. I've seen this happen with my own eyes. The mother cow cries and cries, and this can happen for days. They face the same direction they last saw their babies. Baby boys are slaughtered because they're seen as a waste product because they don't produce milk, just like in the egg industry. And the baby girls experience the same fate as their mother. They're forcibly impregnated and their babies are taken. They're used as a milk slaves every single day for their short lives of four to seven years and when their milk production starts to slow, they also are sent to the slaughterhouse, bolt gun in the head generally and stabbed in the throat. They can live 20 to 25 years in nature. And this is all for a product that is very unhealthy, contains a huge amount of cholesterol and saturated fat. The antibiotics and hormones are causing different types of disease in our body, such as heart disease and cancers, and it is unnecessary. We have so many alternatives to cow's milk.

Wylde: Can you whip out your favorite alternatives for dairy products?

Aspey: You can make it yourself in your own house with a handful of almonds or a cup of oats or cashews, or Brazil nuts. Basically, you just put a cup of your favorite nut or a cup of oats with four cups of water, blend it, strain it, and you have delicious oat milk, rice milk, coconut milk, hazelnut milk, hemp milk, cashew nut milk. They look the same — an opaque white milk — and they taste delicious. You can add a little bit of date for a bit of sweetness or some vanilla. And they're so much healthier and they are so much more environmentally friendly. And they don't cause any of the violence that animal products do cause, so it's a much better alternative that you can make in your own home that's affordable and healthy and just a better option all around.

Wylde: You endorse a 22-day vegan challenge.

Aspey: It's called Challenge 22. The idea behind the 22 days is that apparently, it takes 21 days to form a habit, so we'll do a full extra day just to be safe. The organization Challenge 22 run an e-mail program where you join a Facebook group. They send you e-mails and each day for 22 days, you have access to a registered dietitian. You have access to a group where you can ask all your questions and concerns. They send you recipes. They teach you everything you need to know about how to live vegan in a healthy and sustainable and enjoyable way. And it's totally free. And what people find is that it's so much easier than they'd expect. They're shocked at the delicious, satisfying foods that are available, all the amazing meals that can be made. A lot of people enjoy trying the vegan alternatives to meat and cheese and milk which taste the same, look the same, smell the same but are purely made from plants, which I personally think is a better option than the lab-grown made because we already have vegan meat alternatives that are basically identical and they're becoming more and more affordable and more and more closely resembling the real thing. People realize how much easier it is and how good they feel. And it's not just about feeling good in regards to health, but there's also a very good feeling to start living in a more ethical way. By far the cruellest thing that we are all contributing to society is our consumption of the bodies of animals. And there are other things we can do ethically, such as using less plastic and being careful that our clothing has come from an ethical source. But by far the most suffering from our personal choices comes from the consumption of animals. So when you start living more in alignment with who we all are, which is not violent people but good people, you really feel different on the inside. It shows in your life and it just feels right. Anyone can do it and my personal belief is that everybody ***should*** do it. I don't think cashiering animal products should be an option. I don't think it should be legal, just like slavery was once legal and then outlawed. I'm looking forward to the day when the same thing happens for other animals. Veganism should be the moral baseline and is the moral baseline for the majority of us because we're against causing unnecessary suffering. So the thing for us to do is not to create a new belief system, because that's the belief system we all already have. The step that most people have to take to become vegan is to simply align their actions with the belief system they already have. And that's a very simple, simple thing to do that seems hard until you do it and then you realize, oh, I should've done this a long time ago.

James Aspey's website is at ***jamesaspey.com*** and Instagram is @jamesaspey

23

MEAT OF THE MATTER

From an interview with Robb Wolf

The current crop of young people, the next generation, is poised to live a shorter, less healthy life than their parents. And this is the first time that this will have happened in modern history, in the 200 years of modern medicine following the scientific revolution.

~ ***Robb Wolf***

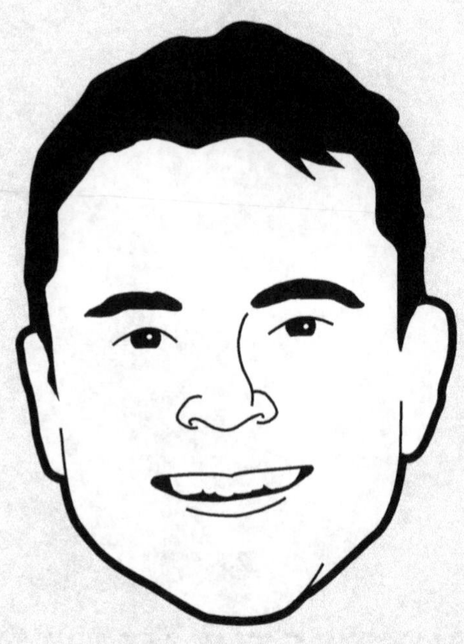

DR. ROBB **WOLF**

Robb Wolf is a former research biochemist and New York Times Best Selling author of The Paleo Solution and Wired To Eat. He has transformed the lives of hundreds of thousands of people around the world via his top-ranked iTunes podcasst, books, and seminars. Robb is a review editor for the Journal of Nutrition and Metabolism (Biomed Central) and a consultant for the Naval Special Warfare Resiliency program. He serves on the board of directors/advisors for Specialty Health Inc, the Chickasaw Nation's "Unconquered Life" initiative and a number of innovative startups with a focus on health and sustainability.

Wylde: What have you, Robb Wolf, done for your brain today?

Wolf: Well, I had a very early dinner. I do the best I can to eat early and frontload my calories early in the day. If I had my way, I'd just skip dinner altogether, but I have two small children, two girls, and so it's kind of unreasonable to sit down and do nothing with them at dinner. But I have a really small dinner and we try to eat between 4 and 5 p.m. and then I try to get in bed as early as I can. I get about a 16-hour or 18-hour fasting window most days. I started things off today with a cup of coffee, which enhances autophagy. I do a little bit of cardio on an assault bike. And that, in theory, could enhance ketone production, mitochondrial biogenesis both in my muscles and in my brain. And then I had a pretty good breakfast on the tail end of that with some good protein and some good fat.

Wylde: Great. So let's start by talking about ancestral health and why should we be paying more attention to this seemingly controversial concept.

Wolf: Ironically, it's only controversial as it relates to humans. If we were talking about parakeets or penguins or virtually any other organism on the planet. there really wouldn't be much discussion or drama around this topic and we would mainly relegate it to areas like ecology. As to humans, what were we designed to eat or how have we evolved within the ancestral health framework? There's contention over what exactly that means, but it definitely didn't mean that we had a snack aisle in middle of the supermarket with foods that were engineered to be hyper-palatable and containing substances our biology had never been exposed to. And then if we march that story forward, we have agriculture and then we have the early industrial revolution, which was a dramatic change in our food systems. But the ancestral health model really, at its core, is a kind of natural experiment. It's looking at populations before they were exposed to a modern mutation in their living style. And it's not just food. We get so wrapped around the axle of food, but it's the sleep and the community and the microbiome that we're exposed to and a ton of different things. I'll make the observation that despite not having modern medical interventions, folks that lived in this kind of ancestral life way — whether it was hunter-gatherer or horticultural or agriculturalists — by and large didn't suffer the diseases that we suffer. It wasn't just because they died young. Their children didn't develop childhood diabetes. They didn't develop childhood cancers. And this isn't just an opinion. This is well documented within the anthropological and archeological literature. So I'm just trying to ask the question, is there anything we could learn from the people who came before us with regards to diet and exercise and community and lifestyle that could help us inform what we do today so that we could add, to the best of everything that we have in the modern world, some insight from our ancestral past? And if we're being really honest, modern medicine has been very, very effective with antibiotics and the incredibly controversial and incendiary topic of vaccination. But modern surgery, emergency medicine, those things are nothing short of miraculous. But if we're really, really honest about modern medicine, after antibiotics, everything became a little bit of a shrug. Antibiotics never needed efficacy trials. It has always been obvious that they save lives, whereas we are now loading folks up on statins and I don't think that from an evolutionary perspective, people are suffering from statin deficiencies. We need tens of thousands of people to see if there's actually an effect of statins. So, we understand modern disease processes better than we ever have in history, but yet our treatments cost more and are arguably pretty ineffective compared to things like emergency medicine and antibiotics.

Wylde: So I know part of the idea is "Eat as our ancestors ate, do what our ancestors did." And we know that stressing our genome, our proteome, our microbiome does affect change. But is part of what you're saying that what we've been doing over the last perhaps hundred years or so, is too much stress, too fast?

Wolf: That's really the crux of the whole argument. It takes a certain amount of time for organisms to adapt to change and we may have reached a point at which our environment, which includes our food and our circadian rhythm, has outstripped our ability to adapt. The current crop of young people, the next generation, is poised to live a shorter, less healthy life than their parents. And this is the first time that this will have happened in modern history, in the 200 years of modern medicine following the scientific revolution. If that doesn't give folks pause I don't know what else possibly could. We have had the unbroken general march towards people living longer, living better, living healthier for the most part until now. And now, despite all of our technology and innovation and knowledge, what we are doing is so at odds with our basic biology that the next generation is likely going to live a shorter, less healthy life than their parents did.

Wylde: So scary. You've written massive amounts about the paleo, keto, and even the carnivore approach. But how different are these nutritive methods? And of course, being brain-centric as I am these days, what is the best way to eat when it comes to brain health?

Wolf: Even though I do paleo-keto interventions as kind of my home base, for me, this diet is just the template that I use to begin the process toward helping people unpack where they are in addressing whatever health problems they have or trying to improve performance. So, I don't know that there's a single intervention that's going to be best for everybody. The big pieces that I see that are universal and have a lot of nuanced individual detail are the following. Everybody has kind of an optimized glycemic load. Some people do wonderfully on a high-carb, low-fat diet. Other people do terribly. And this is some of the research that came out of the Weitzman Institute in Israel looking at personalized nutrition and the reality that, person A to person B, they might eat the same amount, the same type of carbohydrate, but yet have dramatically different blood glucose responses. The person who has a really dramatic blood glucose increase, they will do more poorly over time with their health and they will tend to overeat for a whole host of reasons. But, having said that, the appropriate glycemic load is a really important feature. And we have to be aware of immunogenic foods – things like gluten, nuts and soy, and possibly dairy and even eggs for some people – unfortunately a long and growing list of foods for which some folks have a tendency to react with an inflammatory process that can be incredibly injurious to brain health. And this is one of the things that I will actually stick a bit of a flag in the sand as validation for the ancestral health models. Back in 2001, 2002, when I was talking about that stuff and we would mention the importance of gut integrity and gut health, if someone mentioned something like "intestinal permeability", they were practically run out of town. If you looked at something like ***pub.med,***

most of the published literature at the time — and there wasn't a lot — was saying that this stuff was all hokum. If we fast forward fifteen years, intestinal permeability is the first or second "provided prompt" when you're on pub. med and looking at intestinal issues. I've got to say that the paleo-ancestral health movement was the champion of that topic and really put it on the radar. It's easy to track some of the main researchers like the Sonnenburg Lab at Stanford and the Human Gut Project studying the Hadza to the ancestral health model, which highlighted glycemic load, immunogenic food, and a nutrient-dense diet to trying to get as many vitamins, minerals, and I would say appropriate nutrients relative to our caloric load. I know that some of the dieticians and folks will cringe at this, but we'd ideally like to eat as little as possible while getting as much nutrition as possible and do all of that in a way that supports activity and bone mass and muscle mass. If we're able to do that, if we're able to eat a nutrient-dense diet that has an appropriate glycemic load for us and keep a bit of an eye towards immunogenic foods, then I think most of the neurodegenerative disease process is largely prevented.

Wylde: The known long-term fast/famine periods that our ancestors went through seem to suggest that our brains have perhaps favourably adapted to liking ketones, perhaps even better than glucose. Is that correct?

Wolf: It seems very accurate. Something that's interesting to me, is that we assume that carbohydrate is the only fuel source for the brain, which isn't accurate. Not only can ketones function as substrate for the brain, it's now looking like certain types of fatty acids can serve as fuel substrate for the brain. So, the brain is much more flexible in its fuel utilization than we've ever given it credit for. It would be just a little bit of a perceptual shift to say, well, why couldn't the brain run effectively on lipids or lipid by-products like ketones? I mean, it's somewhat heretical presently to suggest that, but it's also completely physiologically reasonable that these may be in fact a default mode for humanity. Some populations, the far northern population Inuit and some folks in Siberia have developed a CPT1 genotype modification that is not dissimilar to lactase persistence and sickle cell anemia, but it's an adaptation in these populations that on the one hand somewhat inhibits their ability to enter ketosis, but yet, on the back part of it, it deals with the up-regulation of melamine but not suppressing ketogenesis. Effectively, what happens in even these far northern populations that arguably eat the closest thing to what we would call a ketogenic diet — they have some type modifications that actually modify their production of ketones to be steady and continuous. And so it seems to be kind of a default mode for all of humanity and it's interesting, the other organisms that use ketone bodies, some of the critters with the largest brains, like manta rays, which within the fish world is arguably one of the smartest of these organisms, and it does some really remarkable, extremely deep dives into the ocean, which prevents all kinds of neurotoxic potentiality due to oxygen narcosis and nitrogen narcosis and manta rays really rely heavily on ketone bodies and it appears to modify their ability to dive deeply. Some of the best research that's been done on ketones and brain energy metabolism have been funded by the military, looking at ways to protect military personnel doing either deep dives or using rebreathers. But they're exposed to the same types of oxygen or nitrogen toxicity that other deep diving organisms face.

Wylde: So, tell us about the carnivore diet and what you have found as benefit from the modern paleo or autoimmune paleo approach.

Wolf: A good friend of mine, Dr. John Baker, wrote ***The Carnivore Die***t. You know, I was super skeptical of the whole topic for a good period of time until I started seeing folks who had either really significant gastrointestinal problems and/or diagnosed autoimmunity like lupus, rheumatoid arthritis or multiple sclerosis. These folks had done everything. They had tried the swank diet, different modification of vegan diets, different iterations of paleo, auto-immune paleo, specific carbohydrate diets — I mean, these people had turned over every stone and the last stone that they turned over was completely removing plant material — and then they got better. And I've got to be honest, it was incredibly perplexing to me. But I am the person that coined the term auto-immune paleo in my first book, ***The Paleo Solution, a***nd this topic has gone on to attract quite a lot of research. Dr. Terry Wahls, who's a professor of medicine in Iowa, just received a two million dollar grant to study the auto-immune paleo diet in multiple sclerosis patients. Again, it's really gone from the fringe of the fringe to — certainly not being mainstream, but having enough sway that it's getting well-funded for research. This carnivore approach is just fascinating because it looks at the possibility that plants in some people elicit some sort of an inflammatory response that is just injurious to them. On the flipside of this, I wouldn't be shocked if there were not people at the other end of the spectrum and just react terribly to various types of animal products. It seems almost inconceivable that we don't have a mirror image of that on the other side. This is where I simply try to be pragmatic and rely on the science as best as we can. But also, if somebody is sick and we have different tools to use — and I still am of the mind that a 30-day intervention is pretty darn safe in the grand scheme of things when we compare it to chemo and radiation and surgery and a whole host of other interventions that are used to address chronic degenerative disease — I've grudgingly become a bit of a fan of something like a carnivore-type diet. But again, it's absolutely not the first whistle-stop I would make in dietary change. There's a whole host of other places that I think folks should look first, starting with "Let's achieve your appropriate glycemic load. Let's be aware of the immunogenic foods." Yet when we speak of immunogenic foods, there are people seem to react to darn near everything that is plant-derived. And ironically, though they may do reasonably well with fruits and some things such as mushrooms, green leafy vegetables just absolutely crush them. We don't know if it's oxalates or what exactly the story is there, but just from a clinical outcome perspective, they get better by the removal of these foods.

Wylde: It speaks very potently to the idea of an individualized approach to health. I'm hoping you can comment on the genetic variations that so many of us have that relate to the inability of our immune systems to understand and process certain plant-based materials.

Wolf: You asked earlier about my perspective on an ideal diet. I think there are things that we could emulate. But I would make the case that under ideal circumstances, humans should be virtually like a garbage compactor. You should be able to throw just about anything in us and we can turn it into energy and thrive. The fact that we can't do that now is a really complex story. I mentioned antibiotics earlier. They're clearly a lifesaver, but they're also known to modify the gut microbiome in pretty profound ways. We don't really know what that means, but we know that each round of antibiotics changes things. We know that Westernised living dramatically changes our gut phenotype and genotype as to the types that are there and the way that they express themselves. And this is where it gets so remarkably complex, because when we look at the gut microbiome, we're not just considering a complex system with regards to the species there but we need to actually consider the proteomics are of these species, because a bacteria we assume is beneficial could take on a gene for producing a toxin that makes it pathogenic. So, we can't even rely on the genetic screening of these organisms. We need to get to the proteomic screening. When they first started sequencing the human genome, there was all this fanfare that it was going to change everything and it changed nothing other than a few isolated genetic polymorphisms. It's done nothing other than confuse people because we have a bunch of inactionable data. And now we have the gut microbiome, which is even more complex than our genome, and we still have just more inactionable data. But the point here that I'm trying to make is that, under ideal circumstances, humans should be able to handle a wide variety of plant material and they should probably also be able to handle a wide variety of animal material. But depending on changes in our environment that either modify our genetics or epigenetics or the genes in the variety of microorganisms in our gut or on our person, we are less robust or less resilient and we kind of operate within tighter parameters to avoid disease process.

Wylde: What's your take on lab-based meat or what some people are referring to as "shmeat" — whatever that is. Where do you think that's headed?

Wolf: The lab meat topic is really fascinating because it's couched as a sustainability boon. What is fascinating to me with that is that we have one system — nature — in which we have sunlight that falls on the earth and there are plants over two thirds of the Earth's surface — grasslands — in those grasslands is a huge variety of herbivores and carnivores and omnivores and this whole ecological cycle that defines the planet and it's essentially great, that whole system, because the sunlight — fingers crossed — is going to continue to fall as well and these organisms will keep moving forward. What people propose with this lab-grown meat is first you have to take some cells out of a not-yet-born baby cow, stick them into a vat and then into the vat you need to put a nutrient broth and the nutrient broth is derived from the outputs of industrial agriculture. So, this thing has been grown in a lab that can't be too hot, can't be too cold and needs lights and infrastructure, which maybe you put that into an old industrial building, so that's somewhat of a wash. But it's just so fascinating to me that this thing has been sold as a sustainability feature. But when you do the life-cycle analysis, which looks at all the energy and environmental inputs and outputs and compares lab-grown meat with pastured cows and pastured meat, they're not even on the same planet. Lab-grown meat is incredibly energy intensive. When the life-cycle analysis was done, the scientists said the only way that you could make that system sustainable was having a robust system of grazing animals to make sure that the crop land didn't degrade, so you could continue growing crops to feed the lab-grown meat cells. The anti-meat messaging is very simple, very sexy, elevator pitch, sound-bite-worthy material. Meat causes cancer, meat destroys the environment, lab-grown meat is better for the environment. These things are just super catchy, really compelling, and to unpack them is a kind of a mini PhD dissertation that involves ecology and physics and chemistry, and very few people have the time or the attention span to take all that stuff in. The anti-meat camp has some great points to make about industrial agriculture and whatnot, but a lot of nuance gets lost in that process

Wylde: I know you are partly on a mission to take vegans to school. I love it because it is based on science, whether it's about sustainability, lab-grown meat or micronutrient levels, but what are some of the biggest vegan misconceptions? Let's leave ethics aside, because that may or may not be an argument when it comes to industrialization and the way that animals are treated these days. But what are some of the most specific nutrient and sustainability vegan misconceptions that are perpetuated?

Wolf: I'll actually throw out a really quick ethical piece because this becomes a game of Whack-A-Mole where you'll bring up the nutritional characteristics of meat, inclusive or not to diet, and then the topic will shift to the environment. You address that and then it shifts to ethics question and keeps going in a circle. And so on the ethical side, a professor of ecology at Oregon State

University wrote a paper on the least harm principle. The least harm principle is this idea that it would be laudable to live in a way such that the least suffering possible is inflicted upon the organisms around us. And in that analysis, he looks at all of the organisms that are killed or hurt in the process of industrial agriculture. If we hold the life of a mouse equivalent to a cow because they're both mammals, then it starts getting very interesting because with industrial agriculture, which is in escapable if we are to support a largely vegan-based food system, we are usually killing far more animals in the process of doing that than if we had mainly large grazing animals on grass. And then instead of row crops, grains and legumes and whatnot, we focus on fruits, vegetables and nuts and seeds, which ironically ends up looking a whole lot like a paleo diet. When we shift gears to the ecological stability story, interestingly, what ends up looking very favorable from the long-term sustainable-food-systems perspective is something that looks a whole lot like herbivores on grass, and fruits and vegetables, even if grains and legumes are grown. And then on the health side, I think more directly to your point, we tend to see some pretty common vitamin deficiencies in vegetarians and vegans. I'm working on a book called ***Sacred Cow***, which will be out July of 2020 and we address key nutritional, environmental and ethical considerations of eating meat. So, we've dug into this pretty thoroughly. It's been four years of work and it's about a 400 page book. It would be easy to dismiss that because I'm kind of the paleo guy, just kind of supporting my bias. But there's some interesting stuff that has emerged out of this. We analyze the nutritional characteristics of pastured meat versus conventional meat and find there's not much difference. However, there's a huge difference for pastured dairy, pastured eggs, and wild-caught fish.

Wylde: Was there any look at the additional ingredients such as hormones, those that would ultimately be considered non-organic — toxins or otherwise things that end up in the animal — that you would find in conventionally raised?

Wolf: So the hormone thing is a little bit of a misnomer. Hormone therapy or hormone modification within animal products happened for a brief time in the 1970s. And then they figured out that that was a really terrible idea and really haven't done that in a very long time. But a little bit of the mythology around this is that this is a commonly occurring thing. Now, that said, what's interesting is that, within traditional cultures, they preferentially did not, for example, milk cows at certain times of their dairying cycle. And it just so happens that the period of time when they avoided milking cows was when the estrogen content was exceptionally high in the dairy. Nobody knows how they figured this stuff out. It was probably observational that they had milk at certain times and maybe there was a little bit of a qualitative difference and then they noticed maybe some negative health effects. But that's a piece of the story that isn't well accounted for. But if we just talk about nutrition, which would be vitamins, minerals, essential amino acids, essential fatty acids, there's not much of a delta there.

As to the bio-accumulation story, that could be a real deal – like atrazine, for example. But the atrazine is a product of grain production is not inherent in the animal food system other than the fact that we are feeding these animal grains. And as a byline with that, 85 to 90 percent of what the animal eats is grass, whether it's conventional or grass fed. Grass fed is actually 100 percent. Even for conventional animals, the vast majority of what they eat is grass. They do not live on grain their whole life because it would kill them. They only have a short period of time that they can eat grains in any significant amounts. And even the grains products that they eat, almost all of that literally 90, 95 percent is by-product of alcohol production. Nobody is picketing brewery's wineries and distilleries because food is being misallocated away from human consumption and into booze consumption. But it is wrong to assert that this food that ostensibly could feed humans, is being allocated to cattle. In fact, the bulk of that has already been used. It's the end product material of ethanol production.

Wylde: So what's your checklist for healthy meat for you and your family?

Wolf: When we look at just the nutrition, children that eat more animal products do better in school. People who are wealthier tend to eat more animal products. One of the big gripes I have with the vegan-centric drive is that they are telling people who are living at the margins to take their already probably paltry animal product consumption and to drop it further and it is virtually guaranteed to hamstring the neurological development of the children. So, I would make the case that folks should eat animal products that make sense for them and where they are in their budget and their philosophy. But I would be very nervous about steering clear of that for the sake of even claims around environmental sustainability. I think we have credible arguments that animals are not remotely the environmental impacts that's been suggested by many people. And then from there, if you are more affluent, if you have more disposable income, then really make an effort to support local decentralized pasture-finished farming. Even in places like Costco and Walmart, there are very, very good sources of pastured meat now that have very solidly maintained supply chains. And with the development of technologies like blockchain, we will have complete transparency in supply chain processes and if people are doing nefarious activities it's going to be immediately apparent and virtually impossible to hide. So, a lot of the ethical considerations around these topics can be addressed with the proper application of technology.

Wylde: Couldn't agree with you more. Could we perhaps agree to draw the line at gas station pepperoni?

Wolf: I tell you what. When I was moving from Reno to Texas, I did one meal out of a gas station and it was some sort of summer sausage, and I was sick from that for like six days. So now we can draw the line there.

Wylde: One last question, does Robb Wolf supplement his diet? Is there any sort of a pill or capsule that you swear by, whether it's based on personalized approach or just because you think it's a good thing to take?

Wolf: The main thing that I do in the winter, I will do a vitamin D and K drop in a ratio that looks like what we would get out of food. Day to day, I also use an electrolyte supplement called LMNT because I eat a little bit on the low carb side and my sodium needs are probably higher than normal. I do some Brazilian jujitsu and lift some weights and I just noticed that I feel so much better with appropriate electrolyte, ironically mainly focusing on sodium.

24

TOTAL RECALL

From an interview with Nelson Dellis

Memory is something that you have to work on. It's a skill and something that anyone can improve.

~ Nelson Dellis

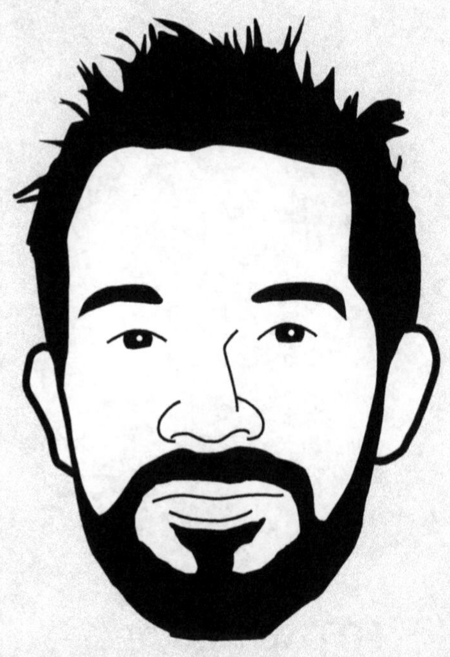

NELSON **DELLIS**

Wylde: Nelson Dellis, memory champion, what have you done for your ***brain*** today?

Dellis: A few things. I've worked out at the gym. That's kind of a big part of what I try to do every day. Some high intensity workouts for about an hour, an hour and a half. I've done a bit of my memory training, which I do when I come back from the gym, usually memorizing something timed, trying to push for my personal best in a certain category of memory competition. And then I guess there's what I had for breakfast, too. That's more of a long play, but I try to eat the right foods.

Wylde: I think what readers really want to understand from you is, what the heck is a memory athlete?

Dellis: It's a funny name given to someone who competes in a memory competition.

Some may argue that it's not athletics, but I definitely feel like I'm doing some type of mental athletics. IBasically, these competitions are testing your memory under a time domain and in various areas. What kind of information can you memorize? How quickly and accurately can you recall it?

Wylde: What would your official title be, then, within the realm of the memory athletes?

Dellis: I got a couple things I can go by. I'm officially a Grand Master of Memory, which is the kind of coveted titles you can achieve by getting certain scores at the world championships. And then I'm a four-time U.S. memory champion, meaning I've won the U.S. National Championships four times over the years. I currently hold a couple of records in the memory world. I've had records in the past, but lost them, then got them back, then lost again. But currently I have two records that are still standing.

Wylde: So you're at the gym daily and eating well. Tell us why you feel like you need to do all those things.

Dellis: For me, memory is something that you have to work on. It's a skill and something that you can improve. It's not something you're born with. So just like any other skill you'd like to perfect, you have to get any edge you can in any way possible. And so I train every day — actual memory exercises — but also the physical part of training keeps my mind sharp and the diet keeps my body healthy and my brain healthy. These all synergize together to hopefully make my brain as sharp as possible.

Wylde: Do you feel like your brain is different structurally than the average person?

Dellis: Not naturally. But maybe now because of all the training. I don't have any conclusive evidence but I'm just talking from my experience of these competitions and the world of memory that I'm so immersed in. I've never met anybody who can do the things that I can do or things that other memory athletes can do, and who claims to be just naturally able to do that. There are a very few exceptions — people who are autistic or savants, that kind of thing — but they usually can do only one thing really well, whereas we can memorize pretty much anything to a high degree of accuracy.

Wylde: Have you heard of the connectome?

Dellis: Remind me.

Wylde: We know certain brain structures are allocated to certain functions but for some time now, scientists have debunked the idea that the left brain does something specific that the right brain can't do, and vice versa. But they're coming to understand that though there are structures — the hippocampus for memory, the prefrontal cortex for higher abilities — that do certain things, perhaps as important are the connections that go to and from these areas. These connections may be what folks such as you are improving, just as working out increases your muscle strength or lean carbontration. Practicing or exercising your brain literally increases the amount of connections between one spot in your brain and another. In other words, as important as, say, the size of the hippocampus may be, the numbers of connections between the hippocampus and other actionable centers such as the temporal lobe or prefrontal cortex is just as important. The connectome consists of these connecting pathways established between the various structures.

But let's go back to why you started to consider exercising your brain, becominga memory grandmaster, or, as we could say, improving your connectome. What was the first day you realized you wanted to do that?

Dellis: It all started because of my grandmother, who was suffering from Alzheimer's. To see her go through that over the years increased my interest in the brain and then, of course, memories. She passed away in 2009 and then I started really trying to figure out ways to train my memory to another level. That's when I discovered the championship and my goal became to compete at a high level and maybe even win.

Wylde: So let's talk about the secret sauce that makes this happen. How do you turn this ambiguous information into something that is for you at least quite easily recalled? What is it that you do?

Dellis: It's pretty much the same process every time. I look at something and have to make a lot of effort. It's not something that naturally just happens even at this point. But I'm always trying to first encode the information as some picture I can imagine in my mind. That's usually half the battle. If it's something complicated like a number or a scientific formula, how am I going to turn those symbols and numbers and letters into images that are meaningful and expressive and all that? That's the first step. The second step is to then store them in some kind of structured way in my mind. There are a few different strategies but the one we typically use in competition is called the Memory Palace, which I'm sure you've heard of. We're basically taking something that's already organized in our mind, specifically a place, a place that we know well, and placing the images that we've encoded within the expanse of this memory palace. When we want to recall them, all we have to do is mentally navigate back through that palace in our mind and pick up the pieces that we left.

Wylde: And anyone can do this?

Dellis: Yeah. I've worked with kids, senior citizens, business people, men, women, people who have learning disabilities, all over the board. This is something that we all inherently do. We just haven't been aware of it.

Wylde: You wrote a book called ***Remember It***. Can we learn more about the Memory Palace and how to do that in ***Remember It***?

Dellis: Yeah, exactly. That book is all about these strategies, in way more depth, but the memory palace's definitely in there.

Wylde: Do you have sort of a perfect routine that, if you could do it every day, you would? A routine that anyone could do every day to support their brain and memory?

Dellis: If I had nothing else to do, I would probably spend a lot more time in the gym, probably doing my memory training in the gym while doing some of the physical exercises. I'd try to have my meals prepped a little better. I'm not always perfect with my diet, though leading up to competitions I get very strict. For me right now what's hitting the mark is a super-low-carb diet, and then just eliminating sugars and a lot of processed foods.

Wylde: You a fan of the keto protocol?

Dellis: Yes, that's what I'm doing for months at a time before leading up to a competition.

Wylde: If you had a favorite diet for your brain, it sounds like it would probably be keto with intermittent fasting.

Dellis: Exactly. When I started and I tried keto first time, I had no plans to fast, but it just lends itself to fasting. I don't find myself needing to eat as much and I almost always feel better when I fast for 16 hours.

Wylde: Anything you believe that we should all avoid that depletes our ability to recall effectively? Obviously avoiding smoking and the major toxins, alcohol, etc. But is there anything in particular you've come to learn through your own experience, that when you avoid that exposure or avoid doing that thing, your memory and recall improve that much more?

Dellis: For me, I have a lot of sugar in my diet when I'm not training. When I cut sugar out and I'm really mindful of what I eat — sugar isn't always obvious in some forms — I just feel amazingly sharp and less foggy in my head.

Wylde: Just to be clear, when you say sugar, you're talking about refined, processed foods. The sugar naturally found in berries and low glycemic fruits, I'm sure you would endorse, though perhaps in moderation, when you're training.

Dellis: Of course.

Wylde: Was there ever a time that when your memory failed at the worst possible moment?

Dellis: I'm not a steel trap all the time. There've been competitions where I was in the finals and I pretty much thought I had it in the bag, and then I blurted out the wrong thing. A lapse of memory. I'm specifically thinking of one instance in 2013 where it was me and another guy. We were at the finals memorizing cards and reciting them onstage and I knew I had memorized more than he had. I had both decks completely in my mind. I had rehearsed it, I knew it. And then I remember I looked out at the audience and I think over confidently thought I knew what I was about to say. And then I said the wrong card and it was over.

Wylde: Right. Do you apply mindfulness in your routines to manage stress?

Dellis: I don't meditate but I do find that when I'm training my memory, there are a lot of similarities in what I'm doing to those things people do who do meditate. I'm focusing on breath, focusing on the numbers that I'm looking at, trying to block out that inner voice that's distracting me. The more at peace I can be while I'm memorizing, the faster I'm going to get a better result.

Wylde: Earlier you said that perhaps if you had your choice, you'd work out longer and maybe do your brain training during exercise. We know that when we're exercising certain areas of our brain light up. Could it be, especially when you're preparing for competition, that you require a combination of both memory training during exercise and training when you're at rest and calm?

Dellis: You're never really calm during a competition. There's a ton of pressure. Everything's on the line. Your heart rate is through the roof and you can psych yourself out really easily. So the whole idea behind memory training while I'm working out is that I'm trying to survive these workouts. They're not exactly like a competition but my heart rate's elevated. I feel that if I can memorize while stressing my body, then when I'm sitting in a chair dealing with the stress of a competition, I'm going to find it easier.

Wylde: You've written that you came to realize that nutrition is important. But in this day and age, it's sometimes difficult to get optimal levels of certain ingredients through food. The omega-3 fatty acids are an example.

Dellis: Yes. Ever since my early days of competition in championships, there was always some kind of DHA/omega-3 sponsor and a number of products. One of these was Brain Armor, for athletes. Being someone who was big into athletics, I gravitated towards that brand and have been taking it for almost seven years now.

Wylde: I understand you've never had your omega-3 index measured. Here's an idea. When you're not in training, try doing a "wash", that is, clear the supplemental DHA out of your system for about three or four weeks, then take a baseline measure, then saturate your system with DHA for three months as you typically would be doing anyway, and then remeasure it. It's a simple blood test that measures the saturation percentage of DHA, EPA and the red blood cells. What we want to see is at least 8 percent or higher. Dolphins have 17 percent because they eat a lot of fish. The stats supporting these higher DHA/EPA levels are incredibly impressive around everything from inflammation to cardiovascular disease to dementias. Most folks in North America who are not supplementing come in around five. But by changing from five to eight, what we've seen is a decrease in all-cause mortality, with cardiovascular risk decreased by up to 90 percent. It seems that it benefits all systems, in particular the brain.

Dellis: I want to test my index, for sure.

Wylde: Meanwhile, I understand you've worked with the group that developed a language-learning app. We know that learning a new language — whether you retain it or not — is an incredible way to boost brain function and memory.

Dellis: I grew up speaking French because both my parents spoke French, but only my mother spoke Flemish Dutch. I decided I wanted to learn that language if I could learn it in a year and I partnered with this app as part of that. This app is very gamified to help you learn vocab. It doesn't teach you grammar or help you converse or anything like that. And so for the first 90 days, I tried to learn all the words in that set, which was about 2500 of the most common words in that language. It was great. I mean, it was a different kind of memory challenge than I'm used to but I'm always down for anything that challenges my mind because I know how good it is for my mind — because it's hard.. Since those 90 days some six months ago, I've been taking lessons in Flemish and trying to get some level of fluency by the end of the year. That's coming up very soon.

Wylde: Okay. Very last question. Do you believe that by doing everything you've done specifically for your brain and training and trying to win the next memory championship that you've put years on your life?

Dellis: In a good way, yes. I'll have more future years, yes. The main reason I started this was seeing my grandmother suffer. I told myself, I don't want to end up like that. What could I do now to build habits, to strengthen my brain now so that as I age I have a better chance of outliving my previous version of myself?

25

THE MEMORY PALACE

From an interview with Yanjaa Wintersoul

In certain ways, we are atrophying our capacity to recall — not necessarily memorize, because we're actually getting a lot of information input. But when it comes to retrieval, that's very different.

~ *Yanjaa Wintersoul*

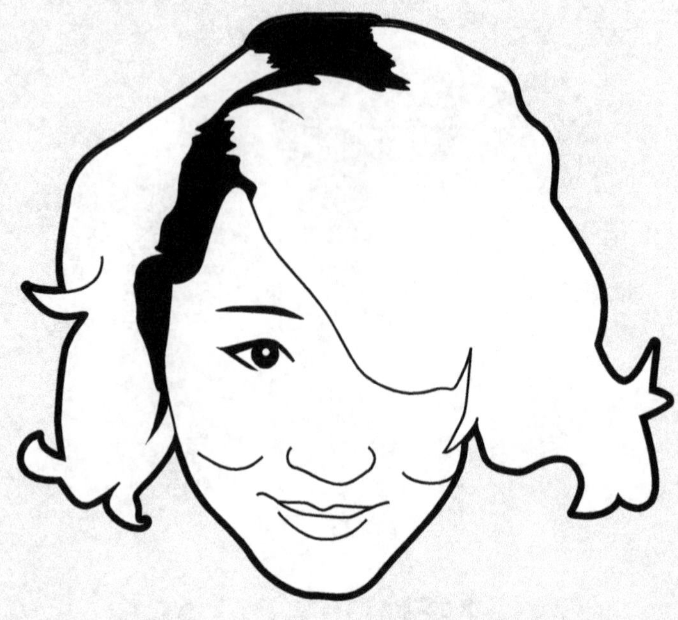

YANJAA **WINTERSOUL**

Yanjaa Wintersoul is a 23-year-old award-winning memory athlete from Mongolia. Within her first year of memory training she got the gold medal at the World Memory Championships for remembering names and faces, also winning the World Memory Championship team medal with Sweden. The following year she got the world record for the most names and faces ever remembered (187 international names in 15 minutes) and was the eighth person in history to achieve an International Grandmaster of Memory (which includes memorizing more than 1000 random digits in under an hour) at her second World Memory Championships.

Wylde: Yanjaa Wintersoul, memory champion, what have you done for your ***brain*** today?

Wintersoul: I took my dog out for a walk and I took the first ten hours of the day in complete silence

Wylde: Those two things resonate with me very well. So tell our readers what a memory athlete is.

Wintersoul: A memory athlete competes in the domain of mental prowess to determine who can memorize the most in a set amount of time.

Wylde: So was there a particular age or time when you realized that you had this special gift to memorize a lot of different things at once?

Wintersoul: I don't think I was born with an awesome memory, but I realized during business school that I needed to find some way to graduate faster because it wasn't really my wish to go to business school. I was studying two years overlapping in one year, and during that time I found this book on memory techniques. The first semester, I was terrible at school, which is why I was trying to find a shortcut so I could leave.

Wylde: So this was later in life. You didn't grow up swatting people away who were trying to study you as a specimen of memory prowess.

Wintersoul: No, actually, I was bullied by teachers a lot because I'd forget what we had just learned. I would forget that we even had a certain type of homework. I failed the third level of English in high school because – even though my English at the time was very good for a high school student – I had forgotten to send in any homework. I had done it. I just forgot to submit it. So memory didn't come naturally to me at all.

Wylde: I am aware that most studies show that memory champions and athletes don't necessarily have hippocampal structural changes. But, what makes your brain different or what makes what you *do* with your brain so different?

Wintersoul: I usually liken memory techniques to reading. In the 15th or 14th century, reading was a kind of a privilege. Only the priests and people in the well-educated upper classes were taught how to read and write. Everyone else just had to listen to what the elite read to them. It was seen as a low key form of magic. But anyone could learn it in the same way that memory techniques are something possible for everyone today. We simply haven't been taught the proper ways to learn how to memorize. Right now, at this present moment, it seems like what I do is magic. But, I simply learned it from reading a book *Moonwalking With Einstein* by Joshua Foer, just an average guy though an excellent journalist. I thought, "I'm a student who barely graduated high school and middle school yet still learned Mongolian, English and Swedish. Maybe I could do it, too. I tried the memory techniques after reading the book and it went pretty well.

Wylde: So it's the same for a memory athlete as any other athlete? The more you practice, the more you train, the better you become?

Wintersoul: Of course, I think a lot of the research is very domain specific. But there have been some basic studies that have shown that it's better for battling anxiety and depression than mindfulness training. Now, these aren't very well funded studies, although I would say they're very well executed studies in Finland and Sweden and University of Texas. Austin. They show that basic memory training is better for lessening depression and anxiety. The weird things we do in memory competitions — for example, remembering "binary digits", as the discipline is called — wouldn't be applicable for anything else in life. But what I found is that it's actually more like going to the gym. Every athlete goes to the gym regardless of their sport. And in the same way, even though binary digits is such a specific thing, it is helpful for my overall mental health and my overall memory skills. You don't see a pitcher go out onto the field and start doing push-ups. In the same way, in my day to day life, I don't try to impress, say, recruiters with my skills in remembering binary digits. But it does have overall applications.

Wylde: So about memorizing these binary digits — strings of ones and zeros. Are you literally memorizing scripts like a computer would?

Wintersoul: Not in the same way as a computer would, but that is what we are doing. And I think the current record for a 30-minute "binary digits", a longer discipline that we have here, is over 6500. So there is someone in the world who can memorize more than 6500 binary digits in 30 minutes.

Wylde: We understand now that the brain is neuroplastic, that we have neurogenesis going on in certain areas of the brain such as the hippocampus. Nerve cells are disconnecting, reconnecting all over the brain as well as new nerve cells are growing. What neuroscientists realize now is that neurons that fire together wire together. You don't use it, you lose it, but the more you use it, the more solidified or easier the access you have to those areas. Maybe what is happening is that you're strengthening this particular connection between areas in your brain that work to improve recall.

Wintersoul: You're also developing that procedural habit of trying to retrieve what you have lost. In competitions, one third of the memorizing is memorizing, but two thirds is actually given to recall. So in the example of 1s and 0s, we're given 30 minutes to memorize, but we're given an hour to write it all down. Those of us who are good are spending an hour trying to remember what we saw, what we have read, what we have memorized. And that's something most people don't do anymore because we're so used to just looking stuff up — "What's that actor's name, the guy with the thing, with the hair?" — instead of trying to think, "Oh, it starts with a C — something like Cooper? Cooper? No, no, no." Instead of digging deeper into the tip-of-the-tongue syndrome, we just go, "Oh, let me google it."

Wylde: Since the inception of the internet, do you think we've become memory lazy?

Wintersoul: Yeah, I think in certain ways we are atrophying our capacity to recall — not necessarily memorize, because we're actually getting a lot of information input. But when it comes to retrieval, that's very different. So people will say, "I can recognize the face". Recognition is easy, but can you reproduce? Some people will say, "I'm so good with faces but not names". But names require retrieval and recognition doesn't.

Wylde: In your Netflix feature ***Memory Games***, you and some of your colleagues spoke about the concept of the Memory Palace. That was really neat. Can you tell our readers what this means?

Wintersoul: The Memory Palace is a technique by which we encode the new information with old information, which is the whole idea of memory techniques and learning. Something that we're never taught in school is that the more you know, the easier it is to know, but if you have no solid foundation to relate the new knowledge to, it's very hard to make sense of it. We use this thing called the Memory Palace to connect new things to a place that we're already familiar with. So we're trying to learn new things that we don't know with things that we already know. The Memory Palace is a pre-determined route or path through a physical location or a place that we've already been in. So the best example is usually starting with someplace in your mind that you know very well, such as your bedroom or your childhood home. You know it inside out and you wouldn't get lost in this "palace". We kind of put the binary digits, the decks of cards, the random numbers and words so that we know the order of them. And we do that because we are very visual and spatial learners and so it allows us to connect what we don't know with what we already know.

Wylde: My wife would love hearing this because when she was in dental school she'd make these elaborate pictures to memorize drug pathways and drug indications and contraindications. She'd associate these things with silly pictures of people that she knew. It sounds exactly like the Memory Palace.

Wintersoul: It is.

Wylde: Do you have a daily routine that you think helps you maintain your memory?

Wintersoul: The most basic trick I try to do is when I feel like I have something on the tip of my tongue, I just try to remember it instead of looking on my phone. This actually does help people in the beginning. When people ask me about memory, I usually try to give simple advice because I'm not expecting anyone to spend three hours a day like I do when I'm in competition mode. Other tips are that I try to move my body and I try to sleep. Sleep is probably the most important thing that I do because sleep helps filter out the unnecessary memories from the necessary memories. It's kind of like your spam filter. It consolidates memories and if you don't get enough sleep, you might be experiencing new things, but you're not really encoding them well. Sleep is the way we make short-term memories into long-term ones. Also I try to eat well and hang out with friends because we are really tribal, social animals and I think we kind of forget that now that we're in this individualistic society. It's not good for our brain health to be so separated from each other.

Wylde: That's how we evolved to learn things. We passed the stories down generation to generation. We may read Robert Munch books or Dr. Seuss to our children today but there are really few internal family stories that can be passed over the centuries.

Wintersoul: Here's another tip. University of Texas, Austin – and some other universities and institutes have tried to replicate this – did a study about putting your phone away. They've shown that just having your phone on you is a distraction – and having your phone on your desk while you're working is worse – because you're constantly and subconsciously thinking about other things that you want to do instead of focusing on the task at hand, which is probably something you need to remember. They've shown that even having the phone in the room is a distraction. So nowadays when I'm trying to focus on what I'm reading or writing, I put my phone away in another room and I turn it off just in case.

Wylde: Is there anything that you eat or supplement with or that you believe helpful, maybe even a ritual lucky charm? Anything else that you believe enhances your abilities, especially during training?

Wintersoul: I see many studies about the health benefits of what we consume. I would say personally that a lot of the time it feels to me like people are asking for a magic bullet. I don't think there's any magic bullet except being mindful and present and trying to really be there and see what's important in the present moment. Is it more important that my dog is eating leaves right now while we're talking or are the tips that we can give people more important? In this case, I think it's mostly the leaves. No. I'm kidding.

Wylde: I understand that your great grandfather was a Mongolian Buddhist monk. And you mentioned mindfulness a few times. Did he ever share anything related to mindfulness helping the mind and memory?

Wintersoul: He didn't really teach me in the way that we think of teaching now, by drawing on a smart board: This is your mind, this is mindfulness. It was simply the way he was in the world. A lot of us have had this experience with teachers. As a kid, I could really feel which teachers were there just to collect a paycheck, which teachers were there to deal with some kind of weird trauma that they were taking out on us, and which teachers were there there because they enjoyed being there and were really present with us in the moment. In the same way, I think my great grandfather taught me without me even noticing that he taught me. People can feel when you're present or when you're just kind of phoning it in. He was in his nineties when he started showing signs of dementia. There's a famous study called the Nun Study with Buddhist nuns as subjects and showing how their brains barely atrophied. I think it's because they do practice the art of being in the moment and the art of just being still. And that is what memory is. People tell me that they don't remember things. "Oh, we just shook hands," they say, "but I can't remember your name. On some level, it's because they weren't paying attention, because the hardest thing for any of us to remember is something that we never saw at all or never observed at all. And so mindfulness is teaching us how to be in the moment so that we can be there to remember in the first place. Sometimes I think people are quite hard on themselves when they say, "I don't remember that this or that person's name." But it's because they were worried about how they were being perceived or whether their handshake was too firm or too loose or all these other things instead of simply looking to the other person in front of them.

Yanjaa Wintersoul's website is at
www.wintersoul.org

26

DNA COMES TO MIND

From an interview with Dr. Mansoor Mohammed

Genetics is the study of genes as discreet units of inheritance, their expression and the proteins they encode. Genomics is the study of genes in the context of the full genome.

~ ***Dr. Mansoor Mohammed***

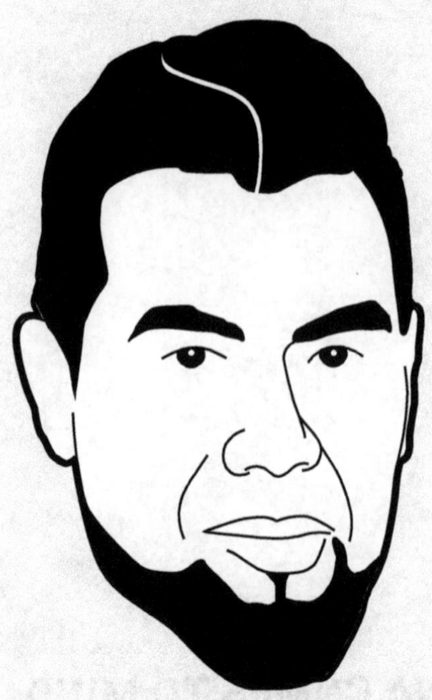

DR. MANSOOR **MOHAMMED**

Dr. Mansoor Mohammed Ph.D. is a recognized authority in the fields of medical genomics and personalized medicine. He is the holder of several patents in the general fields of molecular diagnostics and genomics research. He completed his doctoral dissertation at the University of Guelph, Canada, majoring in both Molecular Immunology and Transgenic Technologies and completed postdoctoral training in Clinical Cytogenetics at both UCLA and Baylor College of Medicine. Mansoor also serves as Chief Science Officer of The DNA Company, one of Canada's most innovative lifestyle and functional genomics companies.

Wylde: I think my readers would be really interested in understanding the difference between genetics and genomics, especially coming from a person whose life work is in this area.

Dr. Mohammed: Of course. It's a nuanced distinction often overlooked in the past. Genetics is the study of genes as discreet units of inheritance, their expression and the proteins they encode. Genomics is the study of genes in the context of the full genome. By way of analogy, the human genome is the whole human operating manual. Genetics is the study of the words or paragraphs in that manual — the genes. To extend the analogy, genomics is not just studying the paragraphs, but understanding that those paragraphs exist in an order and a context. When you read, say, page 22, paragraph 4, what came before it is important and what comes after it is important. The more we study the human genome, the more we understand that how those genes function in the bigger fabric of pathways is what genomics is about.

An expert in a language isn't a guy with a dictionary. Even though he has all of the words in the language, he may not be at all fluent in that language because a language has a context and a grammar. My work as a genomist is to try to understand the language of that human manual and interpret it and derive value from it. For instance. what aspects of this manual inform cellular function? If we really understood the manual's language, we could ask the question, how do micronutrients and neural derivatives impact optimal function? But beyond that, how do nutrients impact optimal function in the context of the individual, given that at the individual level there are unique differences and unique requirements? This is what is being called "functional genomics" or "pathway genomics". Let me give you an example. We'll start at the level of cell function. We know that estrogen and its important sub-type, estrodial, is critical to the development of both the female and male physiology. How does estrogen bring about the changes in the human body from a prepubescent girl to a pubescent teenager to a grown young woman? How does estrogen do this? It does it by binding to particular cells, entering the cells, getting into the nucleus and then causing DNA expression whereby certain "paragraphs" in the genomic manual are expressed and brought into action, changing the cell function or changing the cell environment and allowing prepubescent breast cells, for example, to become something new, and the individual to therefore develop changed external physiology.

That's the hormone estrogen functioning in the human body. Now at the genomic level, is there a genetic instruction that tells the body how to make this important hormone? The answer is yes: the gene CYP19A1 produces a like-named enzyme, the CYP19A1 enzyme, otherwise known as aromatase. Aromatase in turn converts testosterone into estrogen or more precisely, converts testosterone into the estrogen sub-type, estrodial. So here comes the finessed, the nuanced difference between genetics and genomics. At the genetic level, I know that I have the gene CYP19A1 whose function is to produce an enzyme called CYP19A1 and that enzyme metamorphizes testosterone into estrodial. At the genomic level, we learn that there are several versions of the aromatase enzyme that are kinetically faster or slower at doing their job of converting testosterone into estrodial. We typically inherit two copies of every gene. So by looking at the two versions of the CYP19A1 gene that you have inherited, we can determine your "genotype" — the genetic combination of your two copies of that gene. Your version may be a "faster" version or a "slower" version or an "average speed" version. Each of those genotypes expresses its associated enzyme that converts testosterone into estrogen with its characteristic speed. If a young woman had the faster version of CYP19A1, I would expect to see her morphophysiologically manifest greater signs of estrogenisation than the young woman who had a comparatively slower version of it.

But that's genetics. When we move to the perspective of functional genomics, we realize that — hold on — in order to convert testosterone into estrogen via CYP19A1, you have to first make testosterone but it's yet another gene — CYP17A1 — that expresses the enzyme that converts pregnenolone into androgen, which will ultimately make testosterone. And by the way, there are genes and pathways that metabolize and remove testosterone by converting it into DHT and each of these pathways dictates the ability of an individual woman to make testosterone and metabolize testosterone in advance of her ability to make the estrogen sub-type, estrodial. Moreover, after she makes the estrodial via CYP19A1-expressed aromatase, other genes determine how efficiently she metabolizes the estrodial that she just made. So we've now transcended the genetics of CYP19A1 to the functional genomics that traces the fuller story of sex hormone steroidogenesis.

But not the whole story. Let's say we have two different women with the same fast genotype of CYP19A1. If we were only looking at things at the genetic level, we'd assume they had the same phenotype, the same physiology. But from the genomics perspective, we take into account upstream factors. How quickly do they individually convert pregnalone into testosterone via CYP17A1?How quickly do they metabolize testosterone via UGT2B15 genes? How quickly do they convert testosterone into DHT via steroid reductase? All of those differences in these two women will impact their physiologic outcome, even though they both had the same version of CYP19A1.

So there is a distinction to be made between the genetics of CYP19A1 and the functional genomics. The CYP19A1 gene as it relates to steroidogenesis is better understood when interpreted in the context of its fuller genomic story.

27

THINK FITNESS

From an interview with Brent Bishop

Aerobic exercise in particular has been shown to positively impact brain structure, function and cognition, increase oxygen to the brain, enhance neural pathways, increase gray matter and therefore memory, as well as increase in neurotransmitters concentration.

~ Brent Bishop

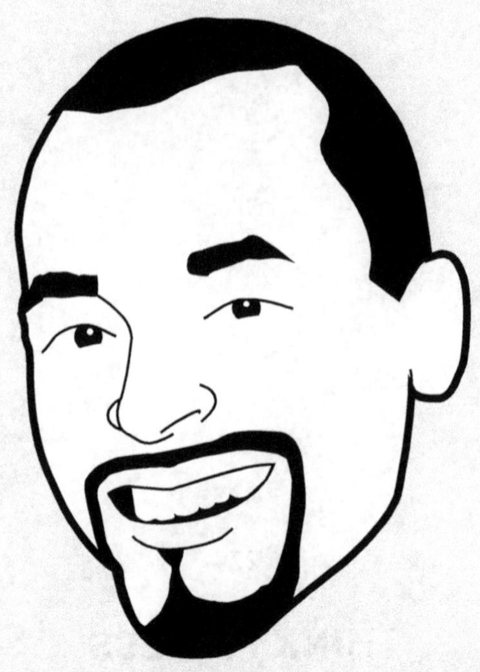

BRENT **BISHOP**

Brent Bishop holds a B.Sc. in Kinesiology from Simon Fraser University, British Columbia and has over 20 years experience inspiring people of all levels to demand more of themselves through fitness and personal development. He has notable fitness career highlights working with Olympians, high level athletes and various film and television personalities. He is a national on-air fitness expert, celebrity trainer, author of strongerstrongly and owner of Think Fitness Studios, performance-inspired conditioning centers in Toronto. He also expands his reach as a trainer on the latest virtual fitness platform, Evolve Functional Fitness. He has made several media appearances on North American networks including KTLA, WFLA Daytime, The Marilyn Denis Show, Global TV, Etalk, ET Canada and Citytv to name a few.

Wylde: Brent, what have you done for your brain today? Did you get a good sleep, nutrition, state of mind, supplementation?

Bishop: Slept for 7.5 hours, with the bedroom dark and cool. Woke up early, completed twenty minutes of meditation and read for twenty minutes. Throughout the day, meal consumption was balanced and consistent. Daily supplementation includes Omega 3s.

Wylde: Why is exercise so important for the brain?

Bishop: Exercise is essential for not just overall health but brain health as well. Exercise is proven to reduce stress and anxiety, enhance mood, increase a positive 'sense of self', and can even help promote new neuron growth in the brain not to mention the feelings of more clarity and focus. Aerobic exercise in particular has been shown to positively impact brain structure, function and cognition, increase oxygen to the brain, enhance neural pathways, increase gray matter and therefore memory, as well as increase in neurotransmitters concentration. Regular exercise can also provide benefits with the aging process by reducing cognitive decline. Physical activity increases levels of brain derived neurotropic factor, which is known to help repair and protect brain cells from degeneration as well as help grow new brain cells and neurons.

Wylde: That's great stuff. I often talk about the importance of BDNF. We are on the same page for sure. How much does psychology play a role in ensuring we get enough exercise? How do you "think fitness"?

Bishop: I believe that fitness and exercise progress is 80% mental. If you have the right mindset, the physical component of exercise comes that much easier as long as it is interest-driven and relative to serving the goals you have for yourself. You can't maintain motivation without inspiration so choosing activities that inspire you – such as going outside or trying a new class – that will help create momentum with your fitness plan. Setting regular benchmarks to evaluate your fitness level in the areas where you wish to achieve goals is also essential for providing direction and motivation to stick to the plan and achieve results. Thinking Fitness is about tapping into what drives you, that internal spark that once ignited compels you to take action. I call this the Think Factor. It is your internal driver that is characterized by inspiration and purpose. Everyone has it and it's different for everyone. One of the best ways to find your Think Factor is to purposely try new activities on a regular basis. For example, re-evaluate your fitness every quarter with some fitness testing, and then re-establish your goals along with a new program for the quarter. Each month plan to try a new workout, a new class, partner up or take things outdoors. Adding something new into your routine each month will do wonders for keeping you engaged with an active lifestyle and enhance program adherence. We all hear about hitting a plateau with fitness; plateaus happen but we can anticipate, prepare and plan for reducing their duration. One of the most significant factors for falling off a fitness routine is actually not so much the physical plateau but the mental plateau. When things become predicable and monotonous, this is when people end up losing interest and momentum in their fitness routine.

Wylde: What do you know about the level of activity centenarians, who live in the various "blue zones" around the world, partake in daily?

Bishop: I do know that there are many people around the world that have regular activity practices that enhance their quality of life, even if that is not their reason for incorporating these activity practices. We were built to move and we are built as social beings. If we keep moving throughout our lives, surround ourselves with positive relationships and focus on this as an integral part of what we do daily, the body and brain respond in such a way that increases health, fulfillment and longevity.

Wylde: From what I've explained to you about the idea behind being a Brainspanner, in an ideal scenario, what would the fitness routine of a Brainspanner look like on a weekly basis in your opinion?

Bishop: The Brainspanner workout should include both a cardiovascular and strength element that is integrated with balance and coordination. The exercise plan would consist of a minimum of 150 minutes per week to produce optimal health and results. An example would be 2 days consisting of 30 minutes of cardiovascular exercise such as jogging, cycling or rowing (i.e. Monday/Wednesday). In addition 3 days of strength-focus exercise, typically completed in a strength circuit (i.e. Tuesday/Thursday/Saturday).

THE BRAINSPANNER CIRCUIT

This is designed to be convenient, time-efficient with minimal equipment and adaptable to all levels. Complete the routine as a circuit with minimal rest between exercises. The idea behind this workout structure is to keep the pace and intensity elevated so you have the cardiovascular benefit within this strength routine. The strength exercises purposely integrate core, balance and joint stability to further increase brain and neuromuscular demand. Complete all exercises in a row then repeat the circuit 3 times.

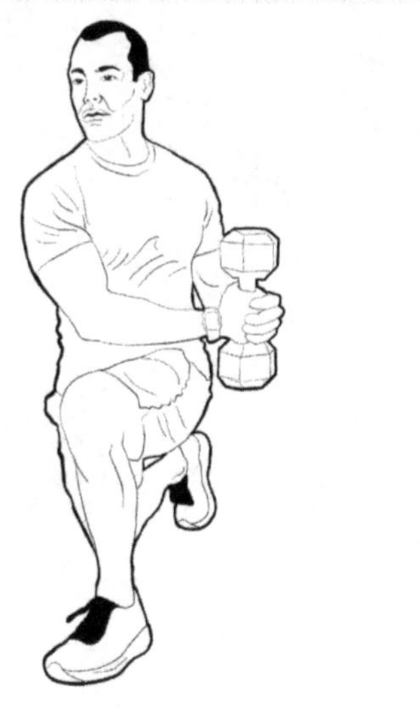

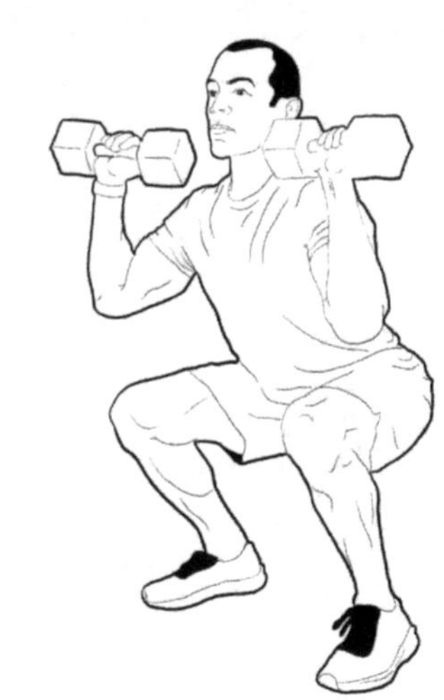

Reverse Lunge with Trunk Rotation

With dumbbell in both hands, step back with the right leg while rotating towards the left.

Keep spine straight and core engaged.Repeat 15 reps then complete the same with the opposite leg.

Squat Press with Knee Drive

With dumbbells at shoulder level, start in a deep squat position.
Drive out of the squat while pressing both weights up and simultaneously driving your right knee up.
Complete for 15 reps then repeat by driving your left knee up.

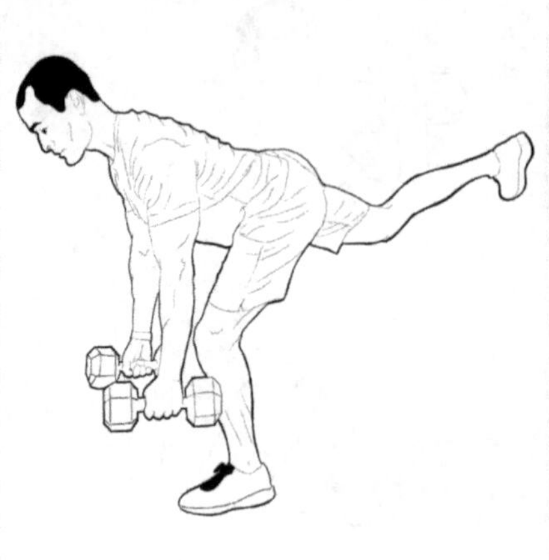

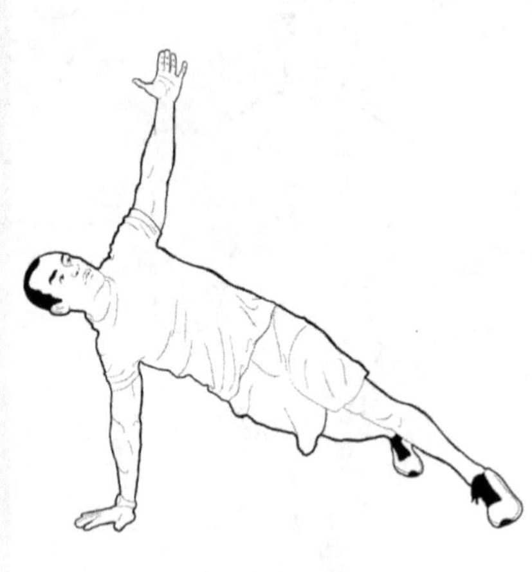

Single Leg Bent Over Row

Standing on one leg with spine straight and parallel to ground and dumbbells held in straight-arm position.

Keeping core engaged, draw shoulder blades together while pulling dumbbells towards your rib cage. Lower dumbbells to starting position and repeat for 15 reps.

Change leg position and complete 15 more reps standing on your opposite leg.

Rotating Push Up

Start in the lower push up position, keeping core engaged and hands directly below shoulder.

Push out of the lower position while simultaneously rotating your body into a side plank position.

Return back to start position and repeat by rotating to the opposite side Complete 20 reps total.

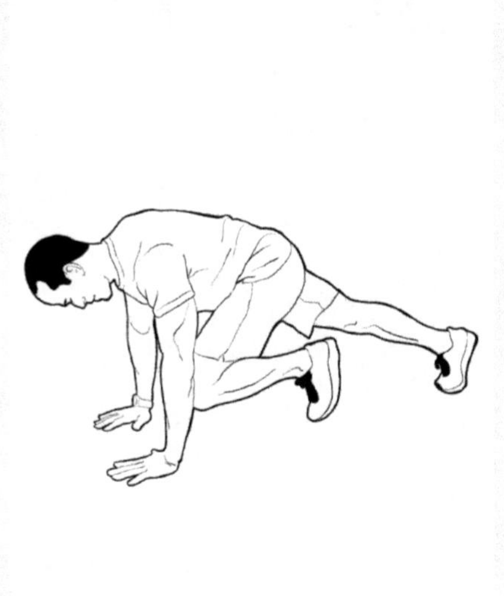

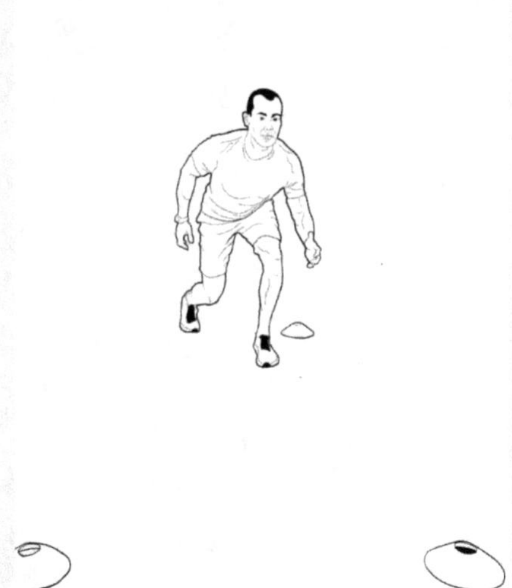

Mountain Climbers

Start in a hand plank position with hands on the ground and shoulders stacked above the wrists.

Keeping your core engaged, alternate driving your knees under your body Complete for one minute.

V-Drill

With three cones (or markers), create a V shape on the ground (approximately 10 feet apart).

Starting at the bottom of the V, quickly run to the right cone and touch.

Quickly run backwards to the base of the V, and then repeat by quickly running to touch the left cone.

Complete this exercise for one minute, aiming to get as many touches as you can.

PART III

THE NUTS AND BOLTS OF THE BRAIN

After many years of research on how the human brain learns to read, I came to an unsettlingly simple conclusion: We humans were never born to read.

~ ***Maryanne Wolf***

28

THE UNIVERSE OF THINKING CELLS

Everything we do, every thought we've ever had, is produced by the human brain. But exactly how it operates remains one of the biggest unsolved mysteries, and it seems the more we probe its secrets, the more surprises we find.

~ Neil deGrasse Tyson

The human body has often been compared poetically to the universe and whatever the merits of such metaphysical flights, there's certainly a sense in which the comparison holds. Viewed from a certain distance, both have appeared simple enough, yet the closer we've approached them, the more we're overawed by their immense complexity. In this chapter, I want to share with you some of that awesome detail but not so much as to drown you or exceed my own depth. I myself, as a clinician, am on a road of discovery and if you can walk with me awhile, I'll have accomplished my mission.

When we talk about the body or the brain, we're accustomed to using and hearing words like "nerve impulses" and "brain cells" and "genes" and "brain chemicals". We hear them so often we can forget that perhaps we don't ***really*** know what they mean. Of course if you're already familiar with these concepts, do skip to the next chapter. But if not, you might want to follow me along as we catch up quickly on a few of the breathtaking advances in brain science.

THE LITTLE PICTURE:
THE CELLS

THEIR SIGNALS

Of course we'll look briefly at the components of our nervous system — the components that anatomists spent the better part of two thousand years sorting out — but before we do, let's review the underlying mechanisms that drive it all.

We're all aware that our system of nerves is all about cells communicating and that nerve cells transmit information to and from our brain and that our brain somehow processes information in some way vaguely analogous to a computer. At any rate, we know it all has something to do with electricity. Perhaps, if we've ever thought about it, we've imagined electricity flowing along the nerves as it does though a copper wire. I've seen several popular science books making that parallel and some of us may even remember how one of the first scientific experiments with electricity involved causing a severed frog's leg to twitch when it was connected to a primitive battery. Case closed, right? Wrong. The nervous systems of living things work on a far subtler principle than household wiring or computer circuits. Let's peer in, using a higher resolution and perhaps manage a better understanding.

I must tell you that it all begins with atoms but, no, I won't be talking about nuclear physics even if I could. However, if we're going to get a better grip on our nervous system and its intricate network of cells, we do need to make a passing reference to ions. Ions, in case you've forgotten your high school chemistry, are atoms. Atoms consist of a nucleus at the centre, surrounded by a zooming swarm of electrons, the basic units of what we call "electricity." Usually there's a proper number of electrons for each type of atom — iron or potassium or sodium as examples — but sometimes there are a few too many and sometimes too few. Then we call the atoms "ions" — a negative ion if there are too many electrons and a positive ion if there are too few.

Phew. That's the limit of my physics. Now back to our brain and its extensions.

Cells are contained within a molecular wall we call a "membrane." In nerve cells — "neurons" — the membrane encloses the cell body and the many feathery "dendrite" extensions that receive signals ***and*** the single "axon" extension that transmits the signals to the neighboring cells. This membrane of a nerve cell, whether it's in the brain or in some remote part of the body, maintains a negative charge — we call it a "negative polarization" — because it contains large resident protein molecules that are comprised of negative ions. Meanwhile, inside the membrane, the cell's fluid is rich in positively-charged sodium ions and the fluid outside the membrane is even richer in positively charged potassium ions. The membrane is pierced by openings called "channels" and there are specific channels for each type of ion. That's the set-up. Now we're ready for action.

So-called "sensory nerve cells" or "sensory neurons" end in various "receptors" that react to our environment. There are receptors sensitive to chemicals, light, touch, sound, changes in temperature, and painful stimuli. Let's travel out to an extreme end of our nervous system and observe what happens when our right forefinger touches a hot element on the stove.

Many sensory nerves — especially those receptive to touch and heat — are immediately excited by the signal from the receptor. Somewhere along the nerve cell's membrane, a cascade of changes begins. A few of those channels tailored for sodium ions open and positively charged sodium ions flow into the cell, which makes the cell interior less negative. Since opposites attract, even more negative sodium ions flow in until the cell is positive in charge. We say it's been "depolarized." This shuts down the flow of positive sodium ions but opens the potassium channels and positive potassium ions now flow out, returning the cell to its normal negative state.

Thanks, you say. But the key here is that this brief disruption — depolarization — in the ionic status of one area of the cell membrane immediately affects the adjacent area, which goes through the same process, as does its neighbour, and ***its*** neighbour. In other words, a chain reaction takes place along the length of the cell and this reaction travels really fast — between 10 and 100 meters per second. This is the "nerve impulse" that lies at the core of not just the signals that travel up the nervous system to the brain and points between, but the signals that travel down other nerve pathways of "motor neurons" to trigger our actions, such as our shouting "Damn!" and snatching our finger from the hot element.

When electricians come to the end of a wire and need to connect it to another, they twist the two wires together and cover the connection with an insulating cap. Electricity surges through a good join with relatively little loss but evolution has not provided living creatures with copper wires carrying raw electricity. Our systems employ a far subtler means for joining one nerve cell to another — and they never actually touch.

At the "sending" terminal of the long axon of a nerve cell, the cell manufactures and maintains a supply of special chemicals called neurotransmitters. Serotonin is a well-known example but other types of nerve cells produce other neurotransmitters such as acetylcholine, norepinephrine, dopamine and gamma-amino butyric acid. When the chain reaction of depolarization/polarization arrives at the terminal, it causes release of the neurotransmitter molecules, which cross the gap — called a "synapse" — that separates the sending cell from the receiving call. Special proteins on the membrane of the receiving cell take up the neurotransmitter molecules. Some of these molecules trigger a new depolarization process and — voila! a new chain reaction signal is on its way — or just as important in other cases — some molecules inhibit further transmission of the signal.

So, it won't surprise you that this same cascade of ionic depolarization and migrating neurotransmitters is what goes on in the 86 billion nerve cells *within* our brain. In other words, a simple shuffling of charged atoms underlies the whole magnificent show.

THE GLIA

With the advancing technology of the microscope and staining techniques in the mid-nineteenth century, a recognition of the neuron as important was growing, if not yet codified. So it was that in 1857, when the German physician and pathologist Rudolf Virchow was searching for whatever connective tissue glued the neurons together to make the organ we call the brain, he discovered a new class of cells he believed to be doing the job and he sensibly named them "glial cells" from the Greek for "glue." Virchow's discovery set in train a hundred and fifty years of productive investigations but unfortunately served to steer those investigations somewhat off the track. It's turned out — and far more recently than we might have expected — that yes, the glial cells hold things together but they are far from being passive scaffolding. With the discoveries of their neurotransmitter and synaptic signalling capacities, we realize that scaffolding may be among the least of their many roles.

We now recognize a number of distinct types of glial cells in the central nervous system (CNS) alone and another sub-set in the peripheral nervous system. Here are some major players in no particular order.

Astrocytes (“***star-shaped cells***”). Like so many components of our central nervous system, the astrocyte cells are formidable multi-taskers and might comprise almost half of all glia cells. I’m going to list a few of the identified or probable roles of astrocytes but we must recognize that at this heady stage in the development of neurological science, so many studies, so many theories, and so many discoveries are in play, we can do little more than touch on the functions of any cell type or molecule.

Like almost all glia cells, the astrocytes help hold the brain together. Remember how the cascade of nerve signals through the neurons involves the expulsion of potassium ions into the surrounding fluid? Like unsleeping janitors, astrocytes soak up the excess potassium so the process can continue. They supplement the supply of glucose fuel in critical brain regions where and when it’s needed. They regulate the flow of ions across the synaptic gaps between neurons and are themselves able to communicate with distant astrocytes through the exchange of calcium ions. They provide vital nutrients to the neurons and seem to play a role in how the neurons regulate blood flow. They’re somehow involved in maintaining the so-called blood-brain barrier that blocks toxins’ access to the brain. They help their fellow glials, the oligodendrocytes, build the insulating sheaths that protect the neurons’ signalling ability. They may facilitate learning and memory in the region of the brain called the hippocampus. They may be an important part of the body’s processes after central nervous system injury. They may act as switches in the circuitry of the nervous system and they certainly have the potential to drive the molecular oscillations that underlie our famous circadian clock. And all that before breakfast.

But maybe the biggest news of all came as recently as 2012, when Dr. Maiken Nedergaard and her colleagues at the University of Rochester Medical Center demonstrated that the brain’s glial cells played a critical role in opening up the interstices between neurons that allowed cerebrospinal fluid

{CSF) to flow more freely through the brain and flush away the accumulated waste products of neural functioning. Since this system of cerebral "canals" mediated by glial cells was seen to be linked to the body's lymphatic system, it was soon being called the "glymphatic" system. In retrospect, it's a wonder that the brain's garbage disposal system had been so long overlooked.

But the implications went deeper — much deeper. Researchers swarmed to the new discovery and confirmed that the glymphatic system (which also appeared to be delivering vital nutrients ***to*** brain cells) is in high gear while the brain sleeps and is largely idle during periods of consciousness. Sleep, in other words, appears to be a prime mechanism for brain health — even survival. We'll see more about this when we get to our chapter on sleep.

Oligodendrocytes ("***cells with only a few branches***" if you don't mind my translation). While you're trying to get your tongue around this glia cell's name, here's a trivia question for you: What relatively common neurological disease do you imagine may be connected to their dysfunction?

While perhaps not such multi-taskers as the astrocytes, the oligodendrocytes are impressively clever. Their most obvious role is wrapping their extensions around the long axons of neurons to create the "myelin sheaths" that both support the axons and provide insulation to protect against ion leakage. Insulated axons, in their capacity as "wires", transmit their ionic signals faster and more efficiently. Oligodendrocytes are also intimately involved in the complex role played by brain-derived neurotrophic factor (BDNF), a protein we're going to meet again and again in this book. Yet other types of oligodendrocytes help regulate extracellular fluid.

The neurological disease? Multiple sclerosis, often devastating and relatively common in northern latitudes. After decades of research, its causes remain mysterious.

Ependymal cells. After the hectic agendas of the astrocytes and the oligodendrocytes, it's something of a relief to turn to the ependymal cells, whose tasks are simple but important. They comprise the ependyma, the thin lining of the fluid-filled ventricles of the brain and the spinal cord's central canal. Their job is to produce the cerebrospinal fluid (CSF) that cushions the central nervous system and allows the brain to regulate its blood flow. They actually have little cilia that wiggle to keep the CSF moving. And it almost goes without saying that, components of the central nervous system as they are, they have other functions understood and not yet understood.

Radial glia. Finally, the central nervous system hosts a population of radial glia cells, which build and support the neurons in the developing brain. As we mature into adulthood, some radial cells — the ***Bergmann glia*** — remain in the cerebellum to regulate the synapses' flexibility in response to varying demands.

That enough glia cells for you? No? Then here's an assortment from the peripheral nervous system that extends outside the brain and spinal cord.

Schwann cells, like the oligodendrocytes of the central nervous system, provide the myelin sheath that insulates the axon extensions of the peripheral neurons. As though that wasn't important enough, they work as nervous system garbage men, disposing of dead neurons. Without this service, there would soon be no room for further neuron growth.

Satellite glial cells function outside the neurons of the peripheral system and use their ability to communicate with one another (just as the astrocytes do within the central nervous system) to regulate the chemical environment — specifically calcium ions. And as we've seen, the chemical environment is what makes the nervous system tick.

Enteric glial cells are multi-taskers that cluster in the ganglia (tight concentrations of nerve cells) that are part of the enormous network of nerves interwoven with our digestive (or "enteric") system. As we go along, we'll have lots more to discover about the enteric nervous system and the connection between the brain and the gut.

We're not done yet, because if we return to the brain itself we encounter the ***microglia***, critical to the functioning of the brain's immune response. They may be small but a deficiency of these tiny cells has been linked to such terrible neurological diseases as Alzheimer's disease, Parkinson's disease, and ALS. There are also the astrocyte-like ***pituicytes*** from the pituitary gland. There are the ependymal-like ***tanycytes*** of the hippocampus. There are in fact some 85 billion glial cells in the human brain, a number almost identical to the number of neurons, which most of us started out thinking constituted our only significant "brain cells."

We didn't know the half of it.

THE BIG PICTURE:
OUR CENTRAL NERVOUS SYSTEM

Let's shift gears. Much of the molecular and cellular story as science now understands is dizzyingly complex and if we travel too far down that path, we'll exceed what I understand and what you can remember. We've glanced at the basic molecular mechanism that underlies our nervous system and some of the cells that comprise it, so let's travel now up through that system to arrive at the monster organ that crowns it.

It's clear to scientists that all the body (and for simplicity's sake, we'll just talk about the contemporary human body} is a single integrated organism. But as an aid to understanding, we talk about the body as consisting of discreet organs: the heart, liver, the skin, the thyroid and so on. This is a little tricky when it comes to the nervous system because its "components" are so obviously and integrally connected to one another. But let's set that observation aside and employ the distinctions that medical science makes.

THE SPINAL CORD

When we follow the "afferent" signals that are headed for the brain and carried by the sensory neurons from, say, the foot, we travel up the leg and smoothly join the huge two-way nerve highway of the spinal cord, cushioned by a channel of cerebrospinal fluid and protected by the bones of the vertebrae. These afferent neurons — along with the "efferent" neurons whose signals descend from the brain to muscle cells, gland cells and other organs, plus a host of other neuron types carrying messages to and from the whole body — are bundled separately in the inner grey matter and the outer white matter of the spinal cord. As we ascend, we pass the 31 places where 31 pairs of nerves servicing others parts of the body join or leave the nerve highway. We think of neurons as extremely tiny, so it's surprising to realize that a signal chain connecting the human foot to the human brain is only four neurons long. A neuron extending from the foot to the bottom of the spinal cord is a few millionths of a metre in diameter but a full metre long. The faster the message travels, the better, and evolution has clearly favoured fewer synaptic gaps.

Even then, some actions can't wait for a message to reach the brain, be processed, and instructions sent down to the appropriate muscles. That's why the spinal cord is more than an information conduit – it's an information processor in its own right. When we're enjoying a beach bonfire and carelessly put a foot down on a hot coal, our spinal cord is equipped to intercept the heat and pain signals and send an urgent message down an efferent nerve to the appropriate foot muscle. Our foot jerks away "reflexively" before our brain can even think about it.

But the human nervous system, in its vast subtlety, does not rely on reflexes alone. The message from the singed toe is destined to do more than a U-turn in the spinal column. The toe will go on to communicate with the brain further up the line, where its unpleasant experience on the beach may perhaps enter the realm of memory, association, and rational planning.

THE BRAINSTEM: **THE BRAIN'S VESTIBULE**

Our journey up the spinal column takes us through a hole in the base of the skull, whereupon the spinal cord expands into the brain stem, the widening organ that anatomists divide into the medulla, the pons and the midbrain. These three sections have been in turn divided into subsections and over the last century researchers have ascribed specific functions to each. That work goes on but the technical detail and taxonomy would soon overwhelm us. For the purposes of this book, the brain's intricate anatomy is only helpful as an introduction to our later chapters on keeping our brain in good health, so let's just summarize the complex role of the brain stem in this way:

1. All neural signals passing to and from the higher (if you're standing up) regions of the brain must pass through the brainstem, which acts as a critical junction crowded with synapses of motor and other neurons.
2. The brainstem integrates brain pathways that govern automatic functions such as breathing, heartbeat, pain sensitivity, sleep, and consciousness.
3. Most of the nerves of the head and face enter the

brain at the brainstem.

By the way, the brainstem is part of what a once-popular theory called the "reptilian brain," that is, a primitive brain upon which evolutionary forces layered later and more complex "brains" such as the cortex, and these late-aboard executives were thought to essentially run the show. It's true that emotions such as fear and pleasure originate in fairly primitive neural circuits but we now understand that emotional experience is seated in many places in the brain, and the brain is not organized in such a hierarchical structure. The brainstem, for example, exercises considerable control over functions located far up in the cerebral cortex.

THE CEREBELLUM: **THE MYSTERY OF THE "LITTLE BRAIN"**

Now we head north in the direction of the giant hemispheres of the cerebrum, whose brilliant rind of cerebral cortex looms above us. That must be our goal since it's there that all the proudly higher functions that make us human reside. Right?

But what's this we pass, just as we're leaving the hindbrain and still behind and below the cerebrum? Another brain, as it appears, smaller but with two hemispheres — the "cerebellum" as Leonardo da Vinci called it — literally, "the little brain" — long slighted as a "motion coordinator" but now the focus of intense brain science research and an explosion of new discoveries.

Throughout the eighteenth century scientists carefully parsed the intriguing anatomy of the cerebellum. As the nineteenth and twentieth centuries progressed, detailed work continued on its unique structure. The cerebellum has turned out to have two principal parts: the folded cerebellar cortex on the outside (don't confuse it with the cortex of the ***cerebrum*** — we haven't got there yet) and the cerebellar nuclei at the core, whose job it is to output the cerebellum's signals to other parts of the brain. The bottom layer of the cerebellar cortex is now known to contain some 70 billion neurons — despite the cerebellum's small size, this is way more than half the total neurons in the whole brain — mostly in the form of tiny "granule" cells. A middle layer of the cortex is only a single cell thick and is comprised entirely of flattened tree-like Purkinje cells. An outer layer of the cortex consists of the axons of the granule cells and the dendrites of the Purkinje cells. It has been estimated that the cerebellar cortex, if it were fully unfolded, would make a sheet one metre long and averaging five centimetres wide – a total surface area of about 500 square centimetres. Clearly there's a whole lot of communicating going on here.

But what does this curious "little brain" do?

At the early stages of scientific study, the examination of patients with cerebellar damage and experiments on animals established that the cerebellum is closely associated with movement. It did not appear to originate voluntary movement – that was believed to be the business of the "higher" motor cortex of the cerebrum – but it did appear to crucially maintain balance and posture and ***coordinate*** the force and timing of voluntary movements that involve many complex muscle groups – keeping your eye on the ball while turning your head, for example. In a related role, it was early recognized to facilitate motor learning of finely-tuned skills such as – in an extreme form – athletes exhibit. In this regard, the cerebellum has been described as an "error-correcting machine." As investigations advanced, the rich neural pathways connecting the cerebellum with the cerebrum's motor cortex have appeared to confirm this relationship.

So, there we have it, the cerebellum and its unconscious coordination of movement. Ho hum.

But not so fast. A few loose ends hung out of the research picture. Damage to the cerebellum meant damage to the capacity for speech. Was this just movement coordination? And then evidence emerged that the little brain played a role in mood, of all things. As Glickstein et al. explain in the September, 2009 edition of ***Neuroscience***, investigators began to ask questions and some of those questions remain to be answered today.

"Do different parts of the cerebellum do different things? The uniformity of the neuronal architecture of the cerebellar cortex suggests that each small region must operate in a similar way, but it is also clear that different regions control different functions. Is there a systematic sensory and/or body representation? What are the functions of the cerebellar hemispheres? Massive in humans and very large in primates, their functions remain in dispute. Because the size of the cerebellar hemispheres parallels the development of the cerebral cortex, some have suggested that the hemispheres in humans and the higher primates may play a role in cognitive functions. ... What are the functions of the two distinctly different [input] systems to the cerebellum: the climbing and mossy fibers?"

Remember, some of those questions remain to be answered today. The "little brain", with its unique circuitry and mechanisms, has become one of the major puzzles of neuroscience. Around the world, laboratories are focusing on cerebellar research with a growing appreciation of the cerebellum's high degree of plasticity and its multiple roles. And what about its vast abundance — apparent overabundance — of neurons? Why are the majority of our brain cells packed into a relatively small sub-section of the brain that, as we've assumed, basically governs movement?

In 2017 — and this is just one experiment among many — a research team at Stamford University was investigating the mouse cerebellum's role in movement using new imaging technology that could focus on activity in the granule cells. To get their mice to move, the scientists had them push a lever to receive a sip of sugary water. The granule cells of course lit up, but to the team's astonishment, the cells also lit up in anticipation of reward, and disappointment when the expected reward didn't materialize. Here was visible evidence that the cerebellum of the mouse was directly involved in "higher" functions than movement. The old assumptions that may have distracted us from this complex organ's true range of roles are wide open to questioning. We don't yet know what new understanding may emerge.

And finally, the "epigenetic clock." Just for now let's say the epigenetic clock is a respected theoretical construct: a biochemical test that can measure age of individuals and of specific organs within individuals based on changes in DNA. I want to talk more about epigenetics later, but for now I want to share this fact: in centenarians the cerebellum is the youngest body part — fifteen years younger, in fact, than would be expected. Not only that, but in recent evolutionary history, the relative size of the human cerebellum appears to have been increasing while the cerebrum has been decreasing. There are respected brain scientists who believe that this correlates to increasing human cognitive abilities. That's the "little brain" for you.

Humbled by what we know and don't know, we move on towards the top and front of the head.

THE CEREBRUM:
THE SHOW IN THE BIG TOP

This is the brain we've been waiting for. In modern mythology, this is the brain that sits at the head of the boardroom table and takes the role of chief executive. This brain we envisage to be the seat of reason, of voluntary action, and probably of consciousness itself. So we tend to believe.

But I've come to realize that the human brain is a staggeringly complex, integrated, dynamic, adaptable organ with functions that are both localized and widely dispersed. For those inquiring into its secrets, it's proven an elusive quarry through more than two millennia. Perhaps it didn't help that the early search was for the soul and later for consciousness, but whatever it was called, searchers recognized that they were searching for something central to who we are as human individuals. In more recent times, the quest, which had wandered around a bit, focused on the massive hemispheres of the cerebrum — the forebrain — and in more recent years still, a shift in our perception of the brain has started to include again the whole organ — and much else beyond the bony case that encloses it. In fact, the profound question that underlies our present quest is this: where do things actually stop being us and start being other?

The natural philosophers of ancient Greece had a pretty shrewd suspicion that thinking was located in the brain, a notion that we would now (wrongly) assume to be intuitive and universal. Aristotle, who may have had the best brain of 300 B.C., was to influence other thinkers for the next fifteen hundred years. Unfortunately Aristotle didn't rate the brain itself too highly, deciding that it was sort of a hot-blood radiator for the heart. Fortunately, other Greeks continued good anatomical investigations and recognized the brain's distinct divisions, though they tended to emphasize the importance of the ventricles — fluid-filled cavities that were certainly an obvious physical feature — and so started brain science down a blind alley it would follow for centuries. Five hundred years after Aristotle, the Roman physician Galen decided that the brain, though he rather chauvinistically thought it to be composed of sperm, was indeed the seat of mental activity. He went further, distinguishing the cerebellum from the cerebrum, our present topic, and observing that the cerebellum was denser, concluded that it must control the muscles, while the larger cerebrum was softer and must therefore process input from the senses. Whatever his reasoning, the man deserved the first-century equivalent of the Nobel prize for medicine. He still got it wrong about the ventricles, though.

By the middle ages physicians generally accepted that physical divisions of the brain handled different functions — a true advance — though old ideas of fluids and humors continued to cause confusion. Leonardo da Vinci — as great an anatomist as an artist — performed meticulous dissections that were followed over the next two centuries by ever more detailed understanding of the brain's anatomy. But as to the more precise functions of these component parts — really, no one could be certain, and in fact a true feature of these advancing studies was the admission of such. The soul was nowhere to be found.

The Renaissance, as we might expect, brought a surge in brain anatomy studies, with men such as Vesalius in 1534 finally dethroning the ventricles, and Thomas Willis in the 1660s recognizing that the cerebral cortex was something far more important that a bunch of blood vessels.

If things moved more slowly over the next two hundred years, they certainly jumped ahead during the nineteenth century, when electrical impulses were observed in the brain, and advancing microscope technology revealed the intricate extensions of billions of brain cells. The door was open to the critical role of the neuron and a detailed linking of brain structure to brain function.

So even if we now allow that the cerebrum shares control with other divisions of a malleable and decentralized brain, we must also allow that it enjoys primacy in many areas. We end our tour by cataloguing in broad strokes what we know about this organ at our literal forefront.

RIGHT BRAIN. LEFT BRAIN.

The cerebrum is divided into the right and left hemispheres, joined by a bundle of fibres that transmits messages from one side to the other. Each hemisphere controls the opposite side of the body. If a stroke occurs on the right side of the brain, your left arm or leg may be weakened or paralyzed.

Not all functions of the hemispheres are shared. In general, the left hemisphere controls speech, comprehension, arithmetic, and writing. The right hemisphere controls creativity, spatial ability, artistic, and musical skills. The left hemisphere is dominant in hand use and language in about 92% of people.

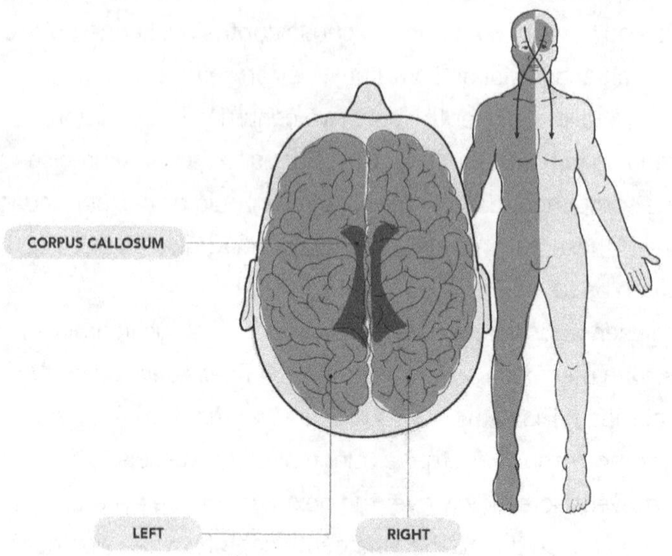

Figure 2.

The cerebrum is divided into left and right hemispheres. The two sides are connected by the nerve fibers corpus callosum.

THE LOBES OF THE BRAIN

The cerebral hemispheres have distinct fissures that divide the brain into lobes — four lobes (frontal, temporal, parietal, and occipital) in each hemisphere —with each lobe divided into areas that serve specific functions. Below, I provide a little catalogue of the functions of the various lobes as we now understand them. But again, the brain is not a collection of distinct organs as their many names might suggest. Scientists for many years to come will be engaged in untangling and understanding the complex relationships between the lobes, the hemispheres, the areas, the glands and all their constituent "parts." Here's a short list of a few major team players and positions played.

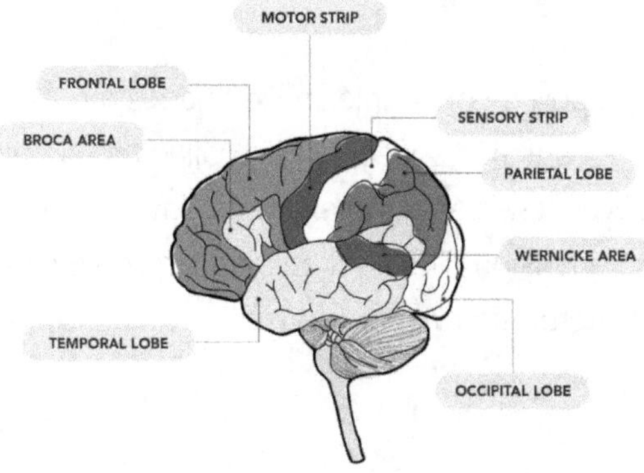

Figure 3.

The cerebrum is divided into four lobes: frontal, parietal, occipital and temporal.

Frontal lobe

◊ Personality, behavior, emotions
◊ Judgment, planning, problem solving
◊ Speech: speaking and writing (Broca's area)
◊ Body movement (motor strip)
◊ Intelligence, concentration, self awareness

Parietal lobe

◊ Interprets language, words
◊ Sense of touch, pain, temperature (sensory strip)
◊ Interprets signals from vision, hearing, motor, sensory and memory
◊ Spatial and visual perception

Occipital lobe

◊ Interprets vision (color, light, movement)

Temporal lobe

◊ Understanding language (Wernicke's area)
◊ Memory
◊ Hearing
◊ Sequencing and organization

THE BRAIN AND LANGUAGE

In the larger proportion of people, the left hemisphere of the brain is responsible for language and speech and is called the "dominant" hemisphere. Broca's area and Wernicke's area, for example, have distinct roles in speech and speech comprehension. The right hemisphere, on the other hand, plays a significant role in interpreting visual information and in spatial processing.

THE CEREBRAL CORTEX

We call the surface of the cerebrum the cortex. The cortex is folded into hills and valleys with 16 billion neurons (the cerebellum has 70 billion for a total of 86 billion) arranged in specific layers. The bodies of the nerve cells color the cortex grey-brown, which is why we like to call it "grey matter". Beneath the cortex are the long nerve fibers (axons) that connect brain areas to one other: these look lighter in color to the eye and we call this inner part of the brain "white matter".

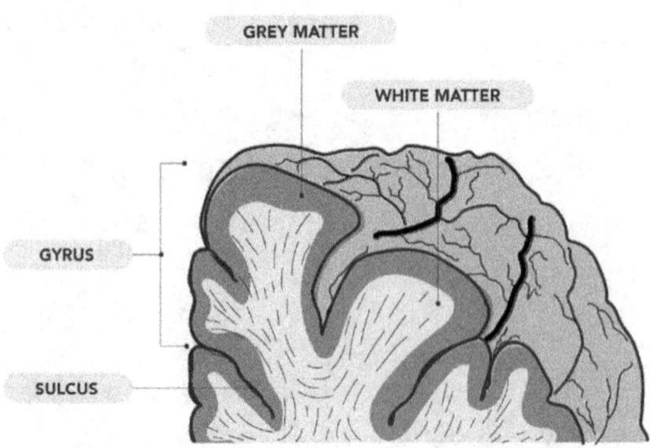

Figure 4.

The cortex contains neurons (grey matter), which are interconnected to other brain areas by axons (white matter). The cortex has a folded appearance. A fold is called a gyrus and the valley between is a sulcus.

The folding of the cortex increases the brain's surface area, allowing more neurons to fit inside the skull. All other things being equal, more neurons is a good thing for intelligence. Each fold is called a gyrus, and each groove between folds is called a sulcus, and each gyrus and sulcus has been given a name that helps anatomists find their way around.

What makes humans different however isn't just the size of our brain. When we compare human brains to those of our primate cousins — we share a common ancestor that lived six to eight million years ago — our brains are only about three times the size but contain about 28 times more thinking cells. For a bit of context, a fruit fly's brain contains 100,000 neurons; a mouse's brain has 71,000,000 neurons; a raccoon's brain has two billion neurons; a chimp's brain has three billion; an elephant has 257 billion neurons and reputedly an incredible memory. Yet clearly elephants, wonderful as they may be, are not as intelligent as, ahem, humans. Some 250.4 billion of the pachyderm's neurons are in its cerebellum and only 5.6 billion in the cerebral cortex. A human has 70 billion in the cerebellum and 16 billion in the cerebral cortex. Where neurons reside and what they do is critical.

HOW MANY BRAIN CELLS?

Earlier attempts to count human brain cells using brain tissue slices and making assumptions looking at the visible cells under the microscope came up with 100 billion neurons. You may still encounter that number. A few years ago, however, Dr. Suzana Herculano-Houzel, a Brazillian neuroscientist, took the time to actually do some counting. She studied multiple whole human brains, stained the nuclei of neurons — the thinking cells in the brain — and then dissolved those brains in detergent that separated the neuronal nuclei. She concluded that on average the human brain contains 86 billion neurons

Our brains feature the most impressive folding of the cerebral cortex in the animal kingdom and this highly evolved prefrontal cerebral cortex is the structure generally regarded as hosting our sense of self, that is, our subjective experience of consciousness. I won't be plunging into an examination of consciousness — one of the thorniest questions in the philosophical universe — except to say that, whoever or whatever may be conscious, our folded cerebral cortex makes us the humans we are.

DEEP STRUCTURES

Again, the cortex — the grey matter — is on the surface and pathways called "white matter tracts" connect areas of the cortex to one other and to structures deep in the brain.

If we'd continued our journey up the fluid-filled spinal canal that cushions the spinal cord, we could have followed the canal until it opened into the cerebrospinal-fluid-filled cavities we call "ventricles" deep in the cerebrum. As we've seen, these are not, for better or worse, the seat of the soul, but their fluid does important work by cushioning the brain and rinsing away waste materials.

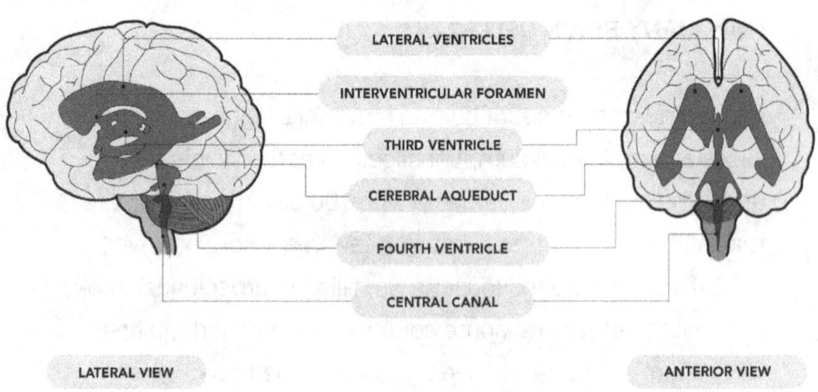

It's beyond the scope of our book to spend too much time in the depths of the brain's anatomy and at risk of the intellectual bends. But since we're down here, let's just look quickly around at one area — say, the region of the third ventricle.

So where exactly are we? Far from the surface of the cortex, the third ventricle is a cavity connected to and just below the large lateral ventricles but on the mid-line between the two halves of the cerebrum. Below it and connected to it is the fourth ventricle which drains down to the spinal canal.

If we picture the third ventricle as a narrow room with four walls, a ceiling and a floor, it turns out that these surfaces are formed by important structures in a part of the brain that controls many autonomic functions and links the endocrine system, the nervous system, and the so-called limbic system. For example, the floor is formed by a number of structures including the ***hypothalamus*** (which is connected to the ***hippocampus***) and the pituitary stalk, which connects the ***pituitary gland*** to the hypothalamus. The side walls are formed by the walls of the left and right ***thalamus***. The back wall is formed by the ***pineal gland.*** But apart from presenting us with a lot of vaguely familiar names, what is the significance of these brain structures clustered around the third ventricle?

To start with, the thalamus that forms the side walls appears to serve as a relay station for almost all the information that comes from and goes to the cortex and is key in pain sensation, attention, alertness and memory.

On the ventricle floor, the hypothalamus, connected to the frontal lobes of the cerebrum above and to the brain stem below, is the master control of the autonomic system governing behaviours such as hunger, thirst, sleep, and sexual response. It also regulates body temperature, blood pressure, emotions, and secretion of hormones. And running close nearby, the pituitary stalk connects the hypothalamus to the pituitary gland, the master gland that controls other endocrine glands in the body and secretes hormones that control sexual development, promote bone and muscle growth, and respond to stress.

On the back wall, the pineal gland helps regulate the body's internal clock and circadian rhythms by secreting melatonin and plays an as-yet-unclear role in sexual development.

So all, all very important. But even more important because these structures and a few others comprise one of the best studied, most controversial, and yet most profound regions of circuitry in the human brain: the so-called "limbic system." The word "limbic" is from the Greek for "border" and here we are in the borderland that bridges between the cerebrum and the brain stem, between our emotional, voluntary and endocrinal responses to our environment. Although there has by no means been total agreement even upon which anatomical strictures comprise it, the limbic region was formerly thought to simply regulate emotional responses. Today, however, when we know much more (and much more about what we don't know), it is regarded as a region of complex circuitry that regulates and integrates visceral autonomic processes — though by no means the only region of the brain to do so — and these processes include not only interpreting emotional responses and regulating hormones but — crucially — processing memories.

In addition to the structures we've already seen in close proximity to the third ventricle, especially the hypothalamus, other major players in the limbic region are the tiny amygdalas, the anterior cingulate cortex, and the little hippocampi.

Various cognitive development theories propose that, starting in childhood, we undergo a socialization process that moves us away from our egocentric conception of self to a more sociocentric one. Freud, Maslow and others agreed that building attachments to groups is a fundamental human motivation that evolved because it supports the survival of our species. These group can be as large as a nation and the emotion as abstract as feelings of patriotism. Whatever the scale, the result is a greater sense of security, feeling of belonging, and prestige. A corollary — and a tested one — is that feeling connected to and cared for and loved by others is correlated to longevity compared to those who feel socially isolated. Improving our social connections improves our neuronal connections and is protective against a range of conditions such as heart disease, cancer, and most notably dementia.

We now know that the brain processes social disconnection in the same way as the threat of physical harm. When a person perceives that their relationship with another person, their community, or their nation is under threat, the brain responds by activating an 'alarm system' in the amygdalas and the anterior (front) cingulate cortex, which set in motion a range of neurophysiological processes. An important point for us is that this alarm is activated whether the threat is in the physical environment, or is simply perceived, based on individual judgment of a threat to social connectedness. The amygdalas and the anterior cingulate cortex, as proper members of the "border" limbic system, play a role in both autonomic functions such as regulating blood pressure and heart rate and such higher-level functions such as attention allocation, reward anticipation, ethics and morality, impulse control (e.g. performance monitoring and error detection), memory, decision-making and emotional responses (including fear, anxiety, and aggression).

The nearby hippocampus (there are two, actually, one on each side of the brain, and so called because they resemble seahorses) has been widely researched and sometimes described as a memory indexing structure that consolidates new memories, connecting them to emotions and senses by filing them away in other parts of the brain. The hippocampus is especially fascinating to me because of a series of learning experiments published in 2013 that employed many different types of mental and physical training and found that, as the subjects learned their tasks, there was an upsurge of new neurons and neural circuits in the hippocampi of their brains. This is compelling evidence of neurogenesis — the birth of new brain cells — in adults.

And when neurons anywhere in the brain signal one another across the synapses between their feathery dendrites and their "transmission tower" axons, those synapses grow stronger. The more often a particular connection is followed, the stronger that connection grows, so new inputs — new experiences — effectively rewire the brain's physical structure. Our brains in fact become what we do with them, and this "plasticity" as it's called, along with neurogenesis such as that in the hippocampi, are clues to the brain's ability to rewire itself if it's damaged.

THE 10% BRAIN AND THE OCTILLIONS

There was long a popular notion that we use only 10% of our brain and the rest remains unused like the empty wings of a shopping mall whose manager can't find the keys for prospective tenants. This was an urban myth that no more applied to the brain than to real estate. There's still a lot we don't understand about the brain, but the physiology of brain mapping suggests that all areas of the brain have a function and we use nearly all of our brain almost all of the time — even when we're asleep.

But some brain truths are stranger than fiction. Our 86 billion neurons, for example, are each connected in a network to about 10,000 other neurons and they're each of them busy passing signals to one another via a total of maybe 1,000 trillion synaptic connections, equivalent by some estimates to a computer with a 1 trillion bit-per-second processor. Now, with the internet available in virtually every corner of the developed world, 56.1% of the world's population has internet access. That means that, as of April 2020, each of us is connected to something like 3.2 billion fellow humans, each of them with 86 billion neurons. So 86 billion neurons multiplied by 10,000 synaptic connections, multiplied by 3.2 billion other brains. means 2,752,000,000,00 0,000,000,000,000,000 neurons have access to one another. Under number naming conventions, that number has a name. It's 2.752 octillion.

Let me go back to individual brains. These vast entanglements of neural connections can in theory be mapped like a wiring diagram or an elaborate river bed over which flows the water of neural activity,. The term for this hypothetical map is the "connectome". An individual connectome would contain a million more connections than a human genome has letters. Creating such a map is the newly-minted discipline of "connectomics". Just as no two people — including twins — are exactly alike, so are no two connectomes. Experiences, thoughts, nutrition, sleep, mental stimuli, and our level of social interaction all influence the map of our connectome. We'll touch on this powerful idea further when we look more closely at memory and at brain trauma and disease.

A DOUBLE FEATURE

It may seem at this point that we've been sitting through a long movie starring our own brain and a cast of billions. When the producers take the stage to announce that we've only been watching the credits — the actual film is head-spinningly richer, more complex and colorful — we look around with concern. Maybe we've seen enough of this one.

But keep your seats. We now know that our brains don't feature just a network of cells, dazzling as their connections are. Yet another production is continually in the works, another cast of billions. Sit back for a second feature. Let *The Story of the Gene* unreel.

30

HOW OUR BRAINS WEAR THEIR GENES

On 28 February, 1955, Francis Crick walked into the Eagle pub in Cambridge and startled its patrons by announcing that he and James Watson had just discovered the secret of life.

I've already mentioned the shock my mother's Alzheimer's diagnosis caused me and how it spurred my growing interest in brain medicine. But the consequences were more personal than that. I'd barely absorbed the truth about my mom when news came that my father-in-law had just received a diagnosis of Alzheimer's. Then my friend Dr. Mehmet Oz disclosed that ***his*** mother had just been diagnosed with the same disease. I recall walking through a Toronto park, dampened by worry and feeling like a World War I soldier trudging up a hill in the face of machine gun fire. Everyone was getting hit. How long could I last? I was my mother's son, after all. What was the role of my genes in this scenario?

Fortunately, the yapping of an excited little dog stopped me and I turned to see a child of perhaps nine approach, almost pulled off her feet by a dachshund's puppyish straining on his leash towards every point of the compass. You don't see dachshunds often, I thought. Perhaps they're temporarily out of fashion. Cute, really. I stopped and let them pass and was still standing there when I noticed a young man in his early twenties coming from the opposite direction, a lanky Afghan hound prancing abreast. I believe Afghans are out of fashion too, but as you might already have guessed, the two dogs experienced an immediate attraction to one another. Everyone within forty feet chuckled or snickered or guffawed at open attraction between two creatures so unalike.

And yet, evidently, the dogs saw one another more clearly than we did. Each recognized the other as ... a dog and their almost comically different appearances are a testimony not simply to nature and her grand workings but to one of humankind's early scientific discoveries: selective breeding — that is, applied genetics.

Today we take for granted that we are somehow the result of interaction between our "genes", whatever those little things are, and our "environment", whatever that is. But how in the modern world can we apply what we know to improve ourselves and enjoy better lives, as our ancestors applied what they knew in order to breed bigger ears of corn, bigger udders, faster horses or smaller dogs?

Before we explore this question, we might want to go back to square one and review what we do know about genetics and how we got to know it. You may already be fully familiar with this remarkable subject, and if you are, please feel free to skip to the next chapter. But if a refresher is in order, don't hesitate to indulge. Because this is one of the greatest stories of modern science — even more important perhaps than the Higgs boson or black holes — and it's a story that's continuing and accelerating today as I write.

THE BEGINNINGS

Genetics is a science, of course, and science for us moderns means an understanding of the world based on empirical observation and reproducible experiment rather than obedience to accepted ancient truths. That's why I began this discussion with selective breeding. Within the limits of what was observable and understood thousands of years ago, humans created an agricultural revolution that transformed cultures from dependency on hunting and gathering to dependency on farming. The realization that something — no one knew exactly what or how — was being passed from generation to generation and that selecting and breeding of plants and animals with desirable characteristics had the effect of enhancing those characteristics in the offspring — this was a key to that revolution. The result in the long run was the creation of civilization — not a bad start for a new science.

For better or worse, that's where things pretty much stood for the next 10,000 years. In 1865, however, two centuries into the Scientific Revolution, an Augustinian friar named Gregor Mendel in the Czech city of Brno delivered a paper on his study of pea plants, a paper whose conclusions are familiar to many of us from our first classroom exposure to genetics. Mendel noticed that pea plants produced pink flowers or white flowers but never a blend. More intriguingly, pink flowers or white flowers were produced on offspring in ratios that could be predicted and described mathematically. Of course it all turned out to be more complicated than it first appeared, but though it was soon forgotten, Mendel's paper made a point that proved an immortal pillar of the as-yet unnamed science of genetics: characteristics of living organisms are inherited as discreet packages, not smooth coffee-and-cream blends of male and female fluids as many wise men had thought. And if Mendel didn't live to see his pea plants make him famous, his writings were rediscovered to influence later nineteenth-century biologists whose ever-improving microscopes were burrowing into the mechanisms of life. By now the cells of living things had begun to give up some of their secrets and even their constituent molecules were being described (if not seen) by a new breed of scientists — the biochemists. But what within these cells transmitted Mendel's discreet "units of inheritance" from one generation to the next?

In the late nineteenth century a series of brilliant experiments and deductions by German biologist Theodor Boveri and others established that structures visible within the nuclei of cells — "chromosomes" they were labelled —were the carriers of inherited information and governed the mysterious process by which a single fertilized ovum could develop into a complex organism. The science of "genetics" was being born, as was its name.

It was soon appreciated that the units of inheritance must lay along the chromosomes and the first half of the new century was devoted to zooming in on these microscopic structures. By 1927, Russian biologist Nikolai Koltsov was able to propose that inherited traits were transmitted via a "giant hereditary molecule" made up of "two mirror strands that would replicate in a semi-conservative fashion using each strand as a template" — a remarkably prescient insight.

No single person can lay claim to the fifty years of work it took to firmly understand the dazzling molecular structure of chromosomes but with time it became apparent that a chromosome did indeed consisted of a "giant molecule" of deoxyribonucleic acid (DNA) bound with packaging proteins that prevented it from tangling. By the 1940s and 1950s, it was accepted that DNA was the molecular code that transmitted genetic information.

A PILLAR OF PRINCIPLES

But how did DNA accomplish that and — still this question — what were the discreet units of heredity? The breakthrough came when the English crystallographers Rosalind Franklin and Maurice Wilkins obtained suggestive images of DNA's structure, and in 1953 Cambridge's James Watson and Francis Crick determined what that structure was, an achievement for which they were awarded a Nobel Prize.

DNA's structure famously consists of two long chains of atoms, the "links" of which are smaller units called "nucleotides." Each nucleotide is composed of one of four "nucleobases" — cytosine [C], guanine [G], adenine [A] or thymine

[T]) — plus a sugar called deoxyribose, and a phosphate group. The two long DNA chains are corkscrew-shaped spirals wound around one another in parallel but head-to-toe and bound together by well-understood forces of molecular attraction. This "double helix" DNA shape immediately suggested the essential mechanism by which living organisms reproduce: if the strands were separated, each could serve as a template for the attachment of new molecular units that would recreate a new double helix.

And the gene, where did it fit in? By the time of Crick and Watson's announcement, there was a general consensus that a gene was simply a specific stretch of the DNA molecule. Genetic information was encoded in the sequence of nucleotides along that stretch — at last, the "unit of inheritance." And this consensus has since been shown to be correct.

But how did this code make itself understood? How did the cells of an organism receive and act on the message that DNA and its genes were carrying? Again, it was a large community of scientists who strove to answer these questions and it was Francis Crick himself who presented a paper in 1957 that summed up what has been called "the central dogma of molecular biology" — a veritable pillar of principles that most molecular biologists could agree upon. We can sum it up like this:

The cell uses a stretch of DNA — a gene — as a template to create a matching molecule we call RNA. This process is termed transcription. The RNA is a messenger that now engages in a second process called translation, whereby a sequence of smaller molecules available in the cell — amino acids — are assembled according to the precise sequence of nucleotides in the RNA. This completed assembly we call a protein — and proteins are the building blocks, the transporters, the messengers, the bureaucrats, and the general gophers of the living body.

THE TORRENT

In the torrent of research and discoveries that followed these breakthroughs — and extended over the next sixty-odd years to the present — one of the most impressive has been the "sequencing" of DNA, that is, the precise mapping of the nucleotides that comprise a complete strand of DNA and finally all the DNA on all the chromosomes carried by a cell. This comprehensive volume of genetic code is called a "genome." In the early years, the genomes of simple organisms such as bacteria and worms were unravelled. But as sequencing technology steadily improved, researchers mapped more and more complex genomes. Finally, in the 21st century, the entire human genome was laid open with ever greater precision.

So what has been the fruit of all this labour? Perhaps the most impressive is our increasingly complete knowledge of the location and role of every stretch of DNA that counts – every gene. (Scientists know many genes so well now, they've given each their own name – DRD2, for example, and ADRA2B, APOE, and the popular BDNF. It might have been easier for laypersons if genes had names like Bill and Roger and Perkins, but bear in mind that there are thought to be in excess of 20,000 genes in the human genome, so names that remind scientists of a gene's function are more useful.) And knowing what a specific gene does has opened the door to exploiting that knowledge for the benefit of humanity.

For example, a certain gene may be slightly different in two individuals. You'll recall those "links" in the DNA chain called "nucleotides" and how each nucleotide is composed of either cytosine [C], guanine [G], adenine [A] or thymine [T] molecules. But occasionally a person may carry a gene that contains a nucleotide in which, say, A is swapped for C. There's normally just a single swap, so these variations are called single nucleotide polymorphisms, or SNPs ("snips"). Since the gene's function is to create a protein through transcription and translation, the protein created will be slightly different – with sometimes negligible or sometimes serious consequences. But knowledge of SNPs can open the door to intervention.

For laypersons who grope their way into the vast field of molecular biology, its immensity and complexity is frankly intimidating, perhaps overwhelming. The countless terms invented to label molecules and their functions stretch away to the horizon. For that reason, I've tried to avoid specific terminology as far as possible and concentrate on the basic mechanisms. But – alas – these basic and critical mechanisms themselves appear ever more complex as our scientists' understanding widens and deepens. One of them arrived on the stage well after the "central dogma" consensus was reached but is still churning the world of genetics and will continue to do so for the foreseeable future. Understanding this "new" mechanism will certainly be the key to advances in human health and medicine.

THE END OF GENETIC DETERMINISM

Jean-Baptiste Lamarck was the pioneering eighteenth-century and early nineteenth-century biologist (he coined the term) who published the first truly cohesive theory of biological evolution. But in the popular scientific imagination, Lamarck is unfairly remembered as the guy who got it wrong. A small part of his theory included the then-familiar concept of "inheritance of acquired characteristics", that is, the notion that what an individual organism does in the course of its life will determine the biological inheritance of its offspring. Simply put, the muscular field worker will tend to produce a muscular son, even if the father is run over by a hay wagon when the son is a week old. Later in the nineteenth century, Charles Darwin's theory of evolution proposed the idea that offspring might differ from parents as the result of naturally-arising mutations and irregularities in the inheritance message, allowing "natural selection" — the survival of the fittest — to have its inevitable way with the variety of offspring. With time, the cool logic of Darwin's mechanism and the growing body of evidence that supported it, persuaded scientists everywhere of its validity. Natural variations and natural selection became the "central dogmas" of biological inheritance.

When Francis Crick summed up the "central dogma of molecular biology" in 1957, he was effectively describing the molecular mechanisms that underlay Darwin's theory. Just as organisms didn't "acquire" inheritable characteristics from their behaviour and environment, so genetic information encoded in DNA didn't change as a result of behaviour and environment. In both cases information flowed in just one direction.

And yet. And yet, experiments and observations had suggested for years that the genetic code — however it worked precisely — didn't determine everything. To make the parallel with evolution again, natural selection was dependent on the environment to favour one variation and disfavour another. It seemed plausible that there might be similar feedback loops in the mechanisms of molecular inheritance.

THE GREAT DISRUPTOR: EPIGENETICS

The phenomenon of gene expression is among the more remarkable discoveries in the modern era of molecular genetics. Every human cell contains *all* 20,000 or so genes in its chromosomes. But that cell has its own specific role in the body, so only the genes in that cell that serve the cell's purpose are activated — the word in biology is "expressed" — while others are "suppressed" — that is, sleep on undisturbed. When the cell needs to produce a certain protein, it wakes up the corresponding gene to express the protein and the protein will go on to play its role in the cell and the body. The chemical mechanisms that signal this expression and suppression of genes are complex and as yet only partially understood. But just by way of illustration, let me mention two. The first depends on the fact that the DNA molecule is wrapped around long chains of proteins called histones and these histones can be modified, changing the shape of the DNA (and thus the expression of a gene on the DNA) without changing the DNA's genetic code of nucleotides. The second, known as "methylation" consists of the addition of large numbers of methyl molecules to certain stretches of the DNA. This methylation tends to suppress gene expression in those areas, again without altering the genetic sequence. There is evidence that both histonic modification and methylation can be to some degree inheritable and this profoundly disrupts the determinism that colored the central dogma of molecular biology.

The implications are clear: the gene is not a passive structure like a step on a staircase or a cookie cutter. It's a dynamic part of a dazzlingly complicated feedback process that we are at last just beginning to understand. Out of a cloud of investigative uncertainty, the field of epigenetics has slowly emerged, "epi" meaning "outside of" and "genetics" referring to the genetic code as it was originally understood — a one-way blueprint-to-building model. Definitions of the word "epigenetics" have proliferated in recent decades as scientists have adapted to new discoveries, but a 2008 consensus has settled on "a stably heritable phenotype resulting from changes in a chromosome without alterations in the DNA sequence."

BACK TO THE BRAIN

So, we ask, what's the relevance of this whole spectacle of molecular genetics to our real subject — the brain and its health? Here's our first clue: of the 20,000 odd genes in the human genome, a full one-third are expressed primarily in the human brain — the highest proportion of genes expressed in any part of the body. If we had any doubts, that fact alone proclaims the amazing busyness inside our heads. But genetics has something much more profound to say about our brains.

During the twentieth century, as our knowledge of the brain grew, we were in awe to discover that our heads contained about 86 billion neurons — "brain cells" — all wired together like transistors in some wonderful way that put our computers to shame. No wonder we were so awfully clever! And we understood that these brain cells were inside our heads from birth or shortly after, and that they gradually died off as we aged until we were gaga if we didn't die first. This confirmed, by the way, why we were all so much smarter than our parents and was quietly supported by the one-way cause-and-effect of classical genetics. But as the discoveries that led to an appreciation of epigenetics undermined the rigid dogma of molecular biology overall, it also undermined its application to the brain. The old model of 86 billion transistors has begun to give way to an appreciation of a two-way relationship between the network of neurons and the genetic codes within those neurons. Learned experience may not simply change the brain by altering the neurons' wiring; it may alter the instructions encoded within our neurons' genes in the long-term. Learned experience might even be passed from generation to generation, an idea that disrupts everything genetic science had believed about the extraordinary organ housed within our skulls.

WHO'S IN THE GENE POOL?

Relax. If there are almost 7,000 genes primarily expressed within the brain (more than any other place in the body), we won't be talking about all of them. But when we recognize how many genes influence the development and functions of the brain, and thus influence how we move, think, feel, behave, and develop diseases — and if we accept on recent evidence that the expression of these genes can in some ways change in response to our environment and experience — we clearly need to meet a few of them in person. However, so many are crowded behind the curtain and waving their little molecular arms, all eager to take their bow, I just can't bring them out in front right now. After the show, they've agreed to appear backstage in the final chapter, the Bookends. Please don't disappoint them.

HOW IT CAME ABOUT

I've taken us on the quickest tour possible through some of the more obvious regions of the human brain, regions that have been observed and studied by anatomists and medical researchers for centuries. In the course of the tour, I followed the path of more recent science, peering close to observe the mechanisms by which the neurons — the basic building blocks of our central nervous system — signal one another. And I led us a little off the trail to look at the work of our marvellous and multi-talented genome, both the architect ***and*** the construction engineer of our bodies. But we can't close this part of our discussion without asking how it all came about. Not ***why*** — that's another subject entirely — but how did our brains happen? Or, to put it more precisely in a scientific era: How did our brain evolve?

A FEW GENES FROM OUR CAST OF THOUSANDS

You'll have met a number of these throughout the book but you won't want to remember every one. Anyway, there's probably some 20,000 in all, with maybe 7,000 expressing in our brains. But I couldn't resist sharing with you a little more of the marvel of modern brain science as it unravels incredible intricacies at the mind's molecular level.

The FADS1 and FADS2 genes

These genes express enzymes that metabolize essential fatty acids (EFAs). EFAs are critical components of the membranes, cell walls, and chemistry of our bodies. Don't confuse them with the saturated fat that we store (especially around our bellies) as on-board energy supplies in case of food emergency.

Our bodies by complicated stages can slowly convert two "parent"

EFAs — omega-3 and omega-6 (found in vegetable and seed oils) — into long-chain fatty acids docosahexaenoic acid (DHA) and arachidonic acid (AA) respectively. (The FADS1 and FADS2 enzymes catalyze that process.) Together DHA and AA make up 60% of the brain and AA does double duty in the vascular system.

Unfortunately there's only so much enzyme to go around at any one time, and if we ingest too much omega-6, our omega-3 conversion process is put on short rations and we have to get by without DHA. This wouldn't be so bad, perhaps, if we hadn't evolved to rely so heavily on this fatty acid, especially for the construction and maintenance of our brain. You'll remember the theory of "shoreline" evolution I mentioned a few pages back. It turns out that marine life — molluscs and fish and the algae at the base of their food chain — are rich in DHA that doesn't require conversion. For reasons I won't go into here, the living world was saturated with DHA for billions of years, years when algae ruled. The upshot of this is that our need for omega-3 and its derivative DHA is no accident — except in the sense that evolution itself is the net result of countless tiny accidents happening to countless opportunistic genes.

The BDNF gene

Once again, the famous BDNF gene, located on the short arm of human chromosome 11, encodes for a neurotrophin (a specialized protein) called BDNF (brain-derived neurotrophic factor), itself an extraordinarily multi-tasking molecule that works in the brain to influence its adaptability (neuroplasticity), the formation of new neurons (neurogenesis), the creation and destruction of the synaptic connections between neurons (synaptogenesis), and the formation of blood cells in the brain. There is evidence that BDNF plays a role in the regulation of mood and behaviour, the enhancement of cognitive processes, and an individual's ability to recover from trauma. Like all genes, the BDNF gene's SNP forms are expressed variously and some have been shown to be linked to such human diseases as schizophrenia, depression, Alzheimer's, epilepsy, addictions, and even aging.

In light of what we're learning from the epigenetic perspective — that genes may be sometimes modified through experience and environment — it's awesome to contemplate what epigenetic changes to the expression of a busybody gene like BDNF might mean for a human being.

The Panacea?

Full disclosure here: I'm a bit of a fan of the BDNF gene and its protein off-spring. It's active in the hippocampal memory region and in the "personality" areas of the cortex. But increased BDNF levels appear to help us lose weight through hippocampal signalling that suppresses appetite. It increases energy metabolism in obese diabetic individuals, partly by activating a protein that creates brown fat easily burned for fuel. In healthy people, the fatter we are, the lower our blood BDNF, which is suspected of being part of a vicious cycle: overweight causing poor sleep over-eating. But when BDNF levels are high, keeping trim comes naturally, acquiring new knowledge comes more easily, and memories are more effectively retained. We feel happier.

Could it be? Could BDNF be a natural weight-loss, mood-boosting anti-depressant, sleep solution?

The COMT gene

The catechol-O-methyltransferase (COMT) gene resides on the long arm of human chromosome 22 and expresses COMT, one of several enzymes that inactivates a class of hormones called catecholamines, produced by the adrenal glands and in the nervous system. Catecholamines such as dopamine, epinephrine, and norepinephrine have several roles in the body but in the brain they function as neurotransmitters, transferring signals from neuron to neuron. A "fast" SNP version of the COMT gene increases enzymatic activity. Dopamine is quickly inactivated, limiting the time it has to bind to the dopamine receptors in your brain. The result is a reduction in the duration of your pleasure response. Conversely, a slow version of the COMT gene results in reduced enzymatic activity where dopamine molecules would not be as readily cleared and remain available longer to bind to their receptors. Said in another way, the variation of the COMT gene determines how long we hold onto thoughts and emotions. For this reason, the variation of the COMT gene you express may predispose you to be a "warrior" or "worrier". If its expression is modified by experience, the effects on our learning and behaviours could be profound.

The IL6 gene

The IL6 gene encodes interleukin-6, a protein involved in the generation of inflammation within the brain and body during immune responses. Variants in IL-6 are also associated with increased risk of certain metabolism-related disorders, specifically obesity and metabolic syndrome, in response to omega-3 fatty acid intake. Many genetic variants are associated with an increased risk of obesity when you don't supplement adequate omega-3 fatty acids

The PEMT gene

The PEMT gene encodes the PEMT enzyme which is responsible for the conversion of phosphatidylethanolamine into phosphatidylcholine within the liver. Phosphatidylcholine is a key component of all 86 billion neuronal cell membranes in our brain. It is also a precursor for the neurotransmitter acetylcholine, which plays a role in memory and other brain functions

The 5HTTLPR & MAOA genes

These two genes are all about serotonin – the happy, feel-good neurotransmitter.

Serotonin is integral to the regulation of mood, neuroendocrine balance, circadian rhythms and eating behaviours. The 5HTTLPR gene encodes for how efficiently the brain recycles serotonin. MAOA is an enzyme that breaks down the neurotransmitters serotonin, dopamine, epinephrine and norepinephrine. This function is very important to our mood balance and how we handle stress.

The DRD2 gene

The DRD2 gene regulates dopamine levels within the brain, which significantly impacts memory, mood, pleasure, reward, and cognition. A pleasure response is initiated when dopamine binds to dopamine receptors. Our DRD2 gene influences the density of our dopamine receptors (literally how many dopamine receptors are present in our brain) and our DRD2 genotype directly correlates to the intensity and readiness with which we can experience pleasure. If we have a high density of dopamine receptors, a pleasure response is often more easily attainable and often more intense. The converse can be expected with a low density of these receptors. If we have the low-density version of the DRD2 gene, we may need more stimuli, or more intense and variegated stimuli, before our pleasure response is triggered.

Let's consider the interaction between just two genes in a single individual. This person has a "fast" COMT gene variation that metabolizes dopamine quickly, and a DRD2 gene that determines a low density of dopamine receptors. That person's pleasure response would be hard to achieve and quite fleeting. This often describes a personality predisposed to pleasure or thrill seeking – even one who is more likely to be disposed to addictions.

The ADRA2B gene

This gene plays a critical role in regulating the neurochemical noradrenaline in the brain. ADRA2B gene variants in individuals are strongly associated with individual differences in processing and recalling emotional memory. What is the underlying mechanism?

The ADRA2B gene encodes the receptor that binds to noradrenaline, so that ADRA2B is to noradrenaline as DRD2 is to dopamine. Noradrenaline is a neurochemical frequently associated with a heightened state of fear or anxiety. When noradrenaline binds to our ADRA2B, a series of neurologic events occur, culminating in heightened vigilance, particularly to negatively arousing events. Variations in our ADRA2B gene strongly influence our ability to process and recall emotionally disruptive or negative events and stimuli. One version of ADRA2B produces a receptor that stays sensitized to negative emotional events for longer and individuals with this gene variant are significantly more likely to retain the imprint of traumatic events (and recall those events) than other persons. They are more sensitive to emotionally

salient stimuli, exhibit a stronger relationship between subjective arousal and memory, and are more likely to suffer from intrusive traumatic memories than others. This variation of the ADRA2B gene has been affectionately referred to as the "drama queen gene". But isn't it interesting that persons with this version are also better able to "read" or detect facial signals of emotional change than others and tend to be much more empathetic?
As with dopamine, the COMT gene plays a central role in neutralizing noradrenaline. Accordingly, the combinatorial impact of the COMT and ADRA2B genes is more telling than either gene on its own. For example, a "slow" COMT genotype paired with a genotype of ADRA2B that remains sensitized to noradrenlaine is likely to exacerbate the depth of negative emotional imprinting and recall experienced by the person who carries this gene combination.. At the risk of oversimplification, these are often individuals who succumb to post-traumatic stress disorder.

The GST genes

The GST family of genes encodes for a very special and powerful antioxidant called glutathione-S-transferase responsible for detoxifying harmful chemicals and metabolic by-products that are dangerous to the human brain. Whichever GST gene variation we happen to have will determine how efficiently toxic compounds are made more water soluble for excretion from the body.

The SOD2 gene

SOD2 is responsible for removing brain-toxic free radicals produced as a result of day to day life. With the aid of the trace mineral manganese, SOD2 facilitates the conversion of free radicals into harmless hydrogen peroxide and oxygen.

The F5 gene

The F5 gene encodes coagulation factor V, a protein which works with other coagulation factors to form blood clots in response to any form of blood vessel damage. Vitamin E (particularly tocotrineols) can act as a blood thinner and can help to manage blood clotting disorders, as well as protect the fragile lining of the cerebral arteries

The MC4R & FTO genes

Our brain is the master centre of appetite and satiety. The MC4R and FTO genes express proteins that play an important role in the regulation of appetite and food intake, and can impact our ability to successfully lose weight and keep it off.

The APOE gene

This gene provides instructions for making a protein called apolipoprotein E, which combines with fats (lipids) in the body to form molecules called lipoproteins. Lipoproteins are responsible for packaging cholesterol and other fats and carrying them through the bloodstream. APOE has three common forms: APOE e2 – the least common – appears to reduce the risk of Alzheimer's. APOE e4 – a little more common – increases the risk of Alzheimer's.

The APP gene

This gene expresses the Amyloid Precursor Protein. Some mutations in this gene (there are over 50) can influence an increase in amyloid beta peptide or a slightly bigger, stickier form of the protein. This can lead to neurons dying, as characteristic of Alzheimer's disease.

PS1, PS2: (Presenilin 1 and 2)

This genes' main job is to cut up APP into soluble or 'dissolvable' pieces. Mutations in this gene can influence the development of Alzheimer's disease.

TREM2

You'll recall the microglia from our discussion of brain cells in chapter __. They're the specialized immune cells that protect the brain and spinal cord from foreign invaders and remove dead nerve cells and other debris. This TREM2 gene expresses a protein called "Trigger Receptor Expressed on Myeloid Cells 2", which interacts with the TYROBP gene and forms a complex that is involved in the development of certain immune cells, particularly microglia cells and dendritic cells. The complex activates these cells, triggering an inflammatory response to injury or disease.

DAP 12/TYROBP

This is the gene that expresses the TYRO (tyrosine kinase binding) protein that forms the complex with TREM 2.

CR1

This gene expresses a protein that is part of the complement activation of the immune system by which immune complexes bind to particles.

NLRP1

This gene's expressed protein participates in the immune system by helping to regulate inflammation. It's involved in assembly of inflammasome, which helps trigger an inflammation process in response to bacteria or virus and apoptosis (that is, the self-destruction of cells). In the course of the inflammation process, the immune system signals white blood cells to the site of injury or disease to fight invaders and repair tissue. The body then stops this response to prevent damage to its own tissue.

LRP1

This gene expresses the LDL receptor protein 1, which functions in the clearance of apoptotic cells and in the alpha 2-macroglobulin-mediated clearance of amyloid precursor protein and beta-amyloid in amyloid plaques in Alzheimer's. It is less expressed as we age and in Alzheimer's disease sufferers.

TFAM

This gene encodes crucial mitochondrial transcription factor functions in mitochrondrial DNA replication and repair. As we've seen, the mitochondria are key to fuelling the brain. For this reason there is much discussion about supplemental support for the mitochondria via this protein.

31

THE EVOLUTION OF THE BRAIN

The very large brain that humans have, plus the things that go along with it - language, art, science - seemed to have evolved only once. The eye, by contrast, independently evolved 40 times. So, if you were to 'replay' evolution, the eye would almost certainly appear again, whereas the big brain probably wouldn't.

~ ***Richard Dawkins***

We begin at the beginning of life and move forward. For several billion years we fail to encounter our quarry. Then finally, a billion years or more ago, there they are: the first living things that possess anything like a brain. These were not the single-celled creatures that had been around since the dawn of life, but if we could only meet them, we'd see how much the constituent parts of these "first-brainers" had in common with the cells that make up our own nervous systems. That is, their cells consisted of a membrane enclosing internal genetic and metabolic material and that membrane would allow the transit of ions in and out through channels with the effect of creating an electrical potential between inside and outside. When single-celled organisms had banned together in working aggregations, molecules emitted by some cells would trigger changes in other cells — the essential basis of signalling. Survival pressures in their watery environment seems to have favored ever more complex organizations and eventually some specialization of cell functions, with certain cells throughout the multi-celled "animal" taking the role of full-time signallers and forming a "neural net" such as jellyfish still possess. Eventually the deficiencies of the net would be solved as the signallers evolved extensions ("axons") that could reach through the organism to almost touch the extensions of other signallers. A nervous system was being born. With the passage a half-billion years or so, "mouths" and "eyes" developed at the "front" end and a concentration of signalling cells would have developed nearby so that external sensations and internal instructions could be coordinated (or "processed"). Voila! The seeds of a brain.

We really have only a hazy idea about the specifics of all this because such delicate, even microscopic cellular structures could rarely fossilize. Still, the appearance of more and more complex organisms didn't mean the disappearance of simpler ones and there are still species in the oceans today that have much to teach us about the first living things, brains included. But skipping lightly ahead to a mere five hundred million years ago, we observe the so-called Cambrian Explosion, when quite suddenly the soup of micro-animals appears to have blossomed into a huge diversity of swimming, stalking, gobbling, and excreting creatures whose descendants triumphed over one another by evolving bigger and better brains. And by the time ever-more-complex fish came on shore as reptiles, they had evolved brains that had parts that were analogous to parts of our own. The future was theirs for the taking.

This is, of course, a thumbnail sketch of the history of evolution itself, in our case starring the brain. But before we press on to the evolution of that most important of brains — our own — let's consider what evolution itself entails. I'm not an expert in evolutionary biology, but like many reading this, I'm familiar with its basic principles as presently understood.

1. Living things are imbedded in their environment and that environment is constantly changing, putting survival pressure on every species.

2. Variations in inheritable characteristics arise naturally in individuals of any species through accidental mutations of sites along the DNA double helix.

3. Some of these variations may be advantageous for the individual; some may be handicaps.

4. Individuals with advantageous characteristics will enjoy a competitive edge, as will their offspring, such that an advantageous characteristic will tend to spread through the population. This is the process dubbed "natural selection".

Earlier, I devoted considerable space to our discussion of genetics, and I hope you'll agree it was worth it, because genes play the central role in human evolution, including the evolution of the brain. Accidental breaks, shufflings and substitutions along the DNA chain — the "mutations" of principle 2, above — sometimes take place within specific genes, stretches of DNA that provide the inheritable code for the creation of specific proteins that in turn play a specific role somewhere in the body. Changes to these genes may entail changes to the individual who inherits them and it's this individual's competitive struggle to survive, thrive, and reproduce that is the basis of natural selection.

So when we speak about a species "evolving", we understand that it is that species' collection of genes that has evolved. Under the pressures of ever-changing environments — and by "environment" we mean everything to which the individual is exposed: climate, food, disease, social changes, new landscapes, everything — some genes have been "selected for", as scientists say, through the survival and reproduction of the individuals that carry them.

Our present suite of genes, then, is our human species' genetic response to environmental pressures — our evolution — and in this chapter, we'll somewhat arbitrarily consider just the evolution of the human brain and just a mere few thousand years of that evolution — or a few million at most. We'll spend most of our time on a quick look at some of the brain-relevant genes we've evolved to this point in our species' history. But before we plunge into that, let's look at a critical but scarcely understood part of the story: the environmental changes that created the conditions that favored the genetic mutations that shaped the brains of our ancestors and that have so far produced us modern humans.

THE ENVIRONMENTAL PRESSURES

We enjoy the advantage of huge hindsight. We know that what was to become the *Homo* line grew gradually more intelligent over several hundred million years, with the various Homo species emerging some two million years ago, their characteristic intelligence accelerating spectacularly in the most recent half million. We can infer this directly from the evidence of their advancing tool technology, and infer it indirectly from their increasing brain size. Applying the principles of evolution by natural selection, we conclude that whatever the environmental pressures were during hominid evolution, they had to be of a type that would favor increased intelligence. Identifying those pressures specifically is more challenging.

It's one of those popular conceptions that probably isn't a misconception, that we started out in the trees. The feet of great apes were and are better suited to grasping than walking. In 2007, researchers at the University of Arizona and the University of California conducted a study that supported the theory that walking on two legs evolved because it used less energy than quadrupedal knuckle-walking. In fact, other researchers have hypothesized many other advantages to bipedalism, including reduced exposure to the sun's rays, wider fields of vision, and hands freed for the better use of tools. Such competitive advantages to walking upright would have been the fuel by which natural selection continued bipedalism's progressive development, inevitably subjecting the human — or humanoid — species to a catalogue of new environments and new forces. The open savannahs and woodlands that may have become their new home would themselves present environmental pressures on which genetic mutations and natural selection could act. And it seems obvious that these mutations and adaptive changes took place in not only the genes that determined the shape, size, and nature of our limbs, but the shape, size, and nature of our brains.

So our ancestors became runners and walkers and, as the fossil record tells us, our running and walking spanned the planet over the last few hundreds of thousands of years. But recent studies have suggested that the two-legged gait wouldn't have taken us so far had we not discovered the control of fire.

This is a subject everybody warms to, and a ton of stuff — scientific and otherwise — has been written on the human relationship to fire. Fire dramatically changed the environment of early humans, and changes in the environment eventually entail changes in the humans themselves — again through natural selection.

Certainly fire improved survivability. All our imaginations are familiar with the sabre-toothed tiger who prowls hungrily beyond the glow of a campfire. Without the fire, it would have been the tiger's work of a moment to drop into the pitch-dark camp for dinner. More important to us, though, is how fire allowed early humans to move north into colder climates, which in due course brought developmental changes to the species, perhaps dietary and metabolic changes.

Most obvious is the effect that fire may have had on nutrition. We can envisage how hominids would have found the flesh of animals caught in grass and brush fires to be easier to chew and digest. With the passing of the millennia would have come the ability to start and control fire and the regular cooking of foods. On this rests the so-called "cooking hypothesis", that the abundance of nutrients necessary for accelerated brain growth had been critically limited by the time available each day for finding and chewing food. When cooking significantly increased the availability of nutrients in both meat and starchy plants, and the effective lengthening of the day by the light of campfires provided more opportunity to eat it, there was relatively suddenly a rich supply of fuel for the growth of brains. Meanwhile, easier chewing — and less of it — would have allowed smaller mandibles and mandible muscle attachments and these would have allowed more room for the brain to grow. And in the tangle of cause and effect that is evolution, it's probable that brain growth was already being selected for by other environmental pressures.

Of course the cooking hypothesis might simply be wrong. Like so much in our knowledge of the evolution of humans, the data is far from complete. There was a linear increase in brain volume of the genus ***Homo*** over time and "species such as ***Homo ergaster*** existed with large brain volumes during time periods with little to no evidence of fire for cooking." But again, the evidence is scant either way and there's something compelling about the idea that early folks who sat around their fires stuffing their mouths with fatty meats were better able to feed their hungry brains than the plant chewers and nut nibblers. Meanwhile paleoanthropology remains in an age of conjecture. The "hunting hypothesis" proposes that the hunting of large and fast animals was the factor that drove the evolution of hominid brains and bodies and led to the development of language and religion. The "savannah hypothesis", not currently fashionable, attributes bipedalism to the shrinking of African forests. Whether that was so or not, few doubt that some early ***Homo*** did end up in the savannahs and woodlands and that these brought their own environmental pressures. And as we know, environmental pressures through the medium of genetic mutation and natural selection can equal evolutionary outcomes for body and brain.

One final hypothesis — and it's been attracting growing attention among paleoanthropologists in recent years — rejects the savannah and similar theories outright. "Early hominids," writes author David Marsh, "apart from Homo erectus (our line) such as Australopethicus, an early savannah dweller, had a far smaller brain than ours (less than half the size of modern brains), and [those brains] stayed the same size for some three million years, whereas Homo erectus, which gave rise to Homo sapiens, developed larger and more capable brains over a fraction of that time — a few hundred thousand years." The explanation, according to March and others, is that our ancestors came out of the trees not to roam the plains, but to become shore dwellers, where they took advantage of endless sea and river food, with its abundant supply of docosahexaenoic acid (DHA), "one of two essential fatty acids which make up 60% of the human brain." From there, mankind followed shorelines around the world, but more important, (since as we've seen, evolution follows environment) our brains evolved to thrive on DHA, which our bodies cannot make.

And finally, we can't leave the question of factors forcing evolution without mentioning the so-called the First Agricultural Revolution. It happened a long time ago — 12,000 years or so — but recently enough, compared to some other factors, that we understand rather more about it. As you'll know, it happened along a crescent — the Fertile Crescent — arcing from the eastern Mediterranean shores north-eastwards and then down into what is present-day Iraq and Iran. The Revolution was characterized by the domestication of plants and animals, such that neolithic hunters and gathers were gradually transformed into farmers. Like all evolutionary influences, it appears as both a cause and an effect: the effect of the developing human brain and human culture, and the cause of dietary and life-style changes that must have acted on the human genome. Indeed, a current stream of opinion has it that our evolution is still scrambling to catch up this revolutionary change in our environment.

THE EVOLVING EFFECTS

I've taken us about as far as I can in describing the pressures that the environments of thousands, hundreds of thousands, or millions of years ago exerted on the human lineage. I hope I've at least made my point that nothing about the evolution of the brain (or any other part) or the human (or any other species) is straightforward. Effects circle back as causes and we end up humbled by the barely understood complexity — very like the complexity of the brain itself. But I want to complete our chapter on evolution by describing some of the ***effects*** of environmental pressures, not just the obvious outcomes — we became taller or stronger or weaker or smarter — but the outcomes for those extraordinary middle-men in the drama of life: the changing genes that make us who we are.

The increase in hominid brain size over time really got underway some two million years ago with ***Homo erectus,*** who sported 800 to 1,100 cm^3 of brain, and peaked perhaps 400,000 or fewer years ago with ***Homo sapiens neanderthalensis, who had*** 1,200 to 1,900 cm^3 of brain, larger even than modern ***Homo sapiens***. This is not necessarily evidence that the Neanderthals were more intelligent than modern humans. First, our pride wouldn't allow such an admission; second, brain size, important as it is, is not the sole determinant of the smarts. Brain structure is just as important, if not more.

For example, we suspect that in the dark, dangerous world inhabited by the Neanderthals, big eyes and large visual processing centers were more important survival factors than abstract reasoning. Similarly, the dramatic earlier increases in brain size from ***Homo erectus*** to ***Homo heidelbergensis*** seem not to have been accompanied by major changes in technology and may instead have produced changes that were "mainly social and behavioural, including increased empathic abilities, increases in size of social groups, and increased behavioural plasticity." And increases in brain size relative to earlier species was most evident after birth and may have allowed for extended periods of social learning and language acquisition in juvenile humans.

And as a final observation to soften the paramountcy of brain size, let's go back to the cerebellum — the little brain — that we met in our chapter on brain anatomy. It turns out that, compared to other primates, hominids and great apes all have a more pronounced cerebellum relative to the neocortex. Researchers have reasoned that this larger cerebellum, with its function of sensory-motor control and the learning of complex muscular actions, and its close coordination with the neocortex, may have underpinned human technological adaptations, including the preconditions of speech. And as Michel A. Hofman writes in the journal Frontiers in Neuroanatomy, "Such a coordinated evolution of the cerebral cortex and cerebellum fits well with the recent clinical and experimental evidence suggesting an important role of the cerebellum in cognitive and affective functions, in close connection with cortical associative areas. Although the cerebral cortex is not the only brain structure which was selected for in evolution for greater growth, as a result of growing environmental pressure for more sophisticated cognitive abilities, it has played a key role in the evolution of intelligence."

It used to be thought that the development of the neocortex alone accounted for the human diversion from the apes. But later research, focusing on the similar behavioural changes in humans and great apes following damage to the frontal lobe, suggested that natural selection was unlikely to have selected the frontal lobe for reorganization. "Instead, it is now believed that evolution occurred in other parts of the brain that are strictly associated with certain behaviors.... The brain volumes were relatively the same but specific landmark positions of surface anatomical features... suggest that the brains had been through a neurological reorganization." (my emphasis)

So it's not enough to talk about a hominid brain that grew larger through prehistory. We also need to take into consideration the growth and development of specific areas of the brain and the functions of those areas. We already know that a disproportionate number of our human genes code for enzymes that play a role in the brain, so it's hardly surprising that we're looking at an organ with many, many moving parts. As Javier DeFelipe wrote at the conclusion of his paper The Evolution of the Brain, the Human Nature of Cortical Circuits, and Intellectual Creativity in Frontiers of Neuroanatomy, "not only the increase in size, and therefore in complexity, of our brains seems to be responsible for our higher or more abstract mental abilities, but also the specialization of our cortical circuits appears to be critical."

GENES AND EVOLUTION

Had enough genes? If I leave you with nothing more than an impression of the overwhelming intricacy of our genome and its expression in our brains, I'll have at least part of my job. But there are also nemerous human genes that speak directly to the evolution of the brain from our hominid and pre-hominid ancestors. So take one more breath and have a peek at these little guys, some of whom may be back here for a second bow.

THE FADS1 AND FADS2 GENES

These genes express enzymes that metabolize essential fatty acids (EFAs). EFAs are critical components of the membranes, cell walls, and chemistry of our bodies. Don't confuse them with the saturated fat that we store (especially around our bellies) as on-board energy supplies in case of food emergency.

Our bodies by complicated stages can slowly convert two "parent"

EFAs — omega-3 and omega-6 (found in vegetable and seed oils) — into long-chain fatty acids docosahexaenoic acid (DHA) and arachidonic acid (AA) respectively. (The FADS1 and FADS2 enzymes catalyze that process.) Together DHA and AA make up 60% of the brain and AA does double duty in the vascular system.

Unfortunately there's only so much enzyme to go around at any one time, and if we ingest too much omega-6, our omega-3 conversion process is put on short rations and we have to get by without DHA. This wouldn't be so bad, perhaps, if we hadn't evolved to rely so heavily on this fatty acid, especially for the construction and maintenance of our brain. You'll remember the theory of "shoreline" evolution I mentioned a few pages back. It turns out that marine life — molluscs and fish and the algae at the base of their food chain — are rich in DHA that doesn't require conversion. For reasons I won't go into here, the living world was saturated with DHA for billions of years, years when algae ruled. The upshot of this is that our need for omega-3 and its derivative DHA is no accident — except in the sense that evolution itself is the net result of countless tiny accidents happening to countless opportunistic genes.

MC AND ASPM

In 2004, researchers at the Howard Hughes Medical Center published a paper that surveyed 214 genes that were associated with brain development in a number of mammals including humans. They found that two genes appeared to control the size of the human brain as it developed: Microcephalin and Abnormal Spindle-like Microcephaly (ASPM). They determined that under the pressures of selection, both of these genes showed significant DNA sequence changes, Microcephalin along the primate lineage and ASPM in the later years of human evolution, once the chimpanzees and human lines had diverged. After a complex comparison and analysis of the DNA of the multiple samples of mammalian species, they came to the conclusion that the differences in the DNA sequences of these genes were due to natural selection and provided the competitive advantage and higher fitness that humans possess relative to other primates. This comparative advantage is a larger brain size, which ultimately allowed the human mind to have a higher cognitive awareness.

ARHGAP11B

Researchers have come to understand that many genes work together to influence the size of the human brain, which is almost three times larger than the brains of our nearest relatives, the chimpanzees. At the Max Planck Institute of Molecular Cell Biology and Genetics in Dresden, scientists introduced the gene ARHGAP11B, which is specific to humans, into the developing brain of ferrets. The human gene caused a significant increase in the number of basal radial glial cells, precursors to neurons, and extended the time window during which the basal radial glial cells produced neurons. The neocortex of the ferret brains grew larger, suggesting that ARHGAP11B plays that very role in our own brains.

FOXP2

One of the earliest stars in a galaxy of discoveries about genes and the human brain is FOXP2, discovered by Simon Fisher and colleagues at Oxford in 2001, just a year or so after the mapping of the human genome. They were studying a family with distinctive language difficulties that extended to fifteen members across three generations. From the generational pattern of the affliction, the Oxford group could determine that it was caused by a dominant gene, with a single copy being enough to produce the condition. The researchers couldn't identify the precise gene until by chance they encountered an unrelated child with a similar problem, enabling them to pinpoint the FOXP2 gene and the specific mutation on that gene that gave rise to the condition. From there, they went on to identify FOXP2 as a master controller that regulated gene activity elsewhere in the brain including the growth and connectivity of brain cells during learning — language learning in the case of the unfortunate family.

For us, perhaps the most important lesson of the FOXP2 story is that this gene is "conserved" — that is, remains very similar in sequence — through many species. Only a couple of amino acids separate the mouse FOXP2 from the human — even fewer between chimpanzee and human. Its ultimate job description is a facilitator of sequence of movements. In the case of humans, that would be the complex sequences of movements necessary for speech, but in other species, the gene manages other movements entirely. As T. M.

Powledge observes on the Genetic Literary Project, even forty years ago scientists had proposed that those dramatic differences in appearance and behavior between humans and chimps came about largely because humans evolved new ways of regulating our similar genes

This is one of the core secrets of evolution in the brain and elsewhere: nothing is invented from scratch; everything is an improvisation on something that already exists.

NOTCH2NL, *SRGAP2, TBC1D3 AND ALL THE REST*

We won't extend our little catalogue of brain-related genes much further: it's too vast and complex for our purposes. The NOTCH2NL gene encodes a protein — notch homolog 2 N-terminal-like — that appears to increase the number of cortical stem cells and delays the generation of neurons, ultimately leading to a greater number of neurons and larger brains. The SRGAP2 gene plays a critical role in synaptic development, brain mass, and the number of cortical neurons.

Sometimes brain genes don't do their work by directly increasing the number of neurons. If there's something almost everyone knows about brains, it's that they're wrinkled. Or wait a minute, is that right? Are snake brains wrinkled? Mouse brains? Dog brains? Monkey brains? If you haven't looked this up already, I won't keep you in suspense. Human brain wrinkling (or cortical folding or gyrification) is impressive; in fact, it's gone about as far as it can go, since the thicker (and so more "intelligent") the neocortex, the harder it is to fold. Dolphins too are impressively folded and even baboons get a B+. Monkeys, cats, camels, and raccoons are still in the running, though squirrels and frogs don't cut it, nor do snakes, though there's significant gyrification of their cerebellums. From this random selection we can draw the broad but not entirely unfair conclusion that at this stage in the evolution of the planet's living creatures, only the more intelligent have more folded cortices. The reasons are reasonably well understood.

All other things being equal, size counts, and the size of the neocortex, the multi-layered rind of neurons that comprises the grey matter at the top front of our brain, accounts for a good deal of our brain and a good deal of what we regard as our humanity. Lose your legs if you must, but by all means hang on to your neocortex. As a sheet that could be hypothetically flattened to perhaps 1200 cm^2, the cortex presents a storage problem to which gyrification is the solution. This still begs the question of how the developing brain folds the cortex. I don't intend to answer that question, except to say that of course, genes are involved. I will however provide us here with the abstract of a paper that may identify one of these genes.

The hominoid-specific gene TBC1D3 promotes generation of basal neural progenitors and induces cortical folding in mice

Xiang-Chun Ju, Qiong-Qiong Hou, Ai-Li Sheng, Kong-Yan Wu, Yang Zhou, Ying Jin, Tieqiao Wen, Zhengang Yang, Xiaoqun Wang and Zhen-Ge Luo

"Cortical expansion and folding are often linked to the evolution of higher intelligence, but molecular and cellular mechanisms underlying cortical folding remain poorly understood. The hominoid-specific gene TBC1D3 undergoes segmental duplications during hominoid evolution, but its role in brain development has not been explored. Here, we found that expression of TBC1D3 in ventricular cortical progenitors of mice via in utero electroporation caused delamination of ventricular radial glia cells (vRGs) and promoted generation of self-renewing basal progenitors with typical morphology of outer radial glia (oRG), which are most abundant in primates. Furthermore, down-regulation of TBC1D3 in cultured human brain slices decreased generation of oRGs. Interestingly, localized oRG proliferation resulting from either in utero electroporation or transgenic expression of TBC1D3, was

> often found to underlie cortical regions exhibiting folding. Thus, we have identified a hominoid gene that is required for oRG generation in regulating the cortical expansion and folding."

I don't quote this paper to cause either of us to feel scientifically illiterate, but to make two points:

> (1) the brain and its evolution is about genes; and
> (2), as Rodney J. Douglas and Kevan A.C.Martin of the Institute for Neuroinformatics, Zürich, Switzerland, wrote in 2012, "The complexity of the brain is so overwhelming that at every level investigators have been forced to focus only on particular aspects of its evolution and development, or its structure and function, or the behavior it generates."

PART IV

THE BOOKEND

I think that you're supposed to know when it's time to say goodbye.

~ Judy Sheindlin

MY FAVORITE THINGS

If we learn we have liver disease as a consequence of excessive alcohol use, or become obese because we couldn't resist eating pastries with every meal, or develop a lung problem because we once smoked two packs a day, or develop back problems because of continual heavy exertion at our work, or have chronic digestion problems for unknown reasons — and whether or not we change our habits — we at least understand that our liver, our adipose tissue, our lungs, our back, and our bowels are physical parts of our body that respond to our behavior. It's not surprising maybe that it's hard to think of our brain in that way. After all, we can't see it and we can't feel it and its main product isn't something like bile or poop, but "mind" — and largely unconscious mind at that. Nonetheless, our brain is a physical organ like the others, and for all its almost indescribable complexity, it's at least as vulnerable as our heart or our kidneys. For me, these factors explain why until very recently we had so rudimentary an understanding of how to look after the thing. My hope is that this little book will offer encouragement to do just that.

In the course of researching and writing, I inevitably developed my favorite topics and themes. If you've come this far, you'll be familiar with them by now: the BDNF gene and its expressed factor that fosters neuroplasticity and neurogenesis; the omega-3 fatty acids that are no less than the very building blocks of our brain; the elimination of the subtle toxins that are potent destroyers of our brain structure and chemistry — and one other topic — The True Brainspanners — which I've hardly mentioned until now.

This book and the years that have preceded it have been a journey of discovery for me. I hope, if you've read this far, that it's been worthwhile for you too. But I can assure you of this, based on my own experience: A breathtaking horizon for health has opened up for all of us, a horizon perhaps as broad as that offered by the germ "theory" in its day and the discovery of antibiotics. For the first time, with a strong tailwind of knowledge behind us, we can begin to take personal control of the care and feeding of our most personal organ.

Thank you.
Bryce Wylde
2020

THE TRUE BRAINSPANNERS

The concept of brainspan is about both quantity and quality. A wonderfully productive life that ends at twenty-nine is less that ideal. An extraordinarily long life that is mostly spent in poor mental and physical health is hardly better. That's why I've found it so inspiring that there are many people with exceptional brainspans. They got old and they stayed smart. They're the centenarians.

Over the years I've made it a habit to take note of centenarian studies and statistics. Call it a sort of hobby. It's still too early to make dogmatic statements about the centenarian phenomenon, but I expect that you find stories of these "oldies but goodies" intriguing, even compelling.

In 2009, author Dan Buettner published a book called ***The Blue Zones***, which examined centenarian "hot spots" around the world and noted their life styles. He writes that many centenarians, in order to avoid weight gain, regularly stop eating before they feel completely full. They tend to the smallest meal of the day in the late afternoon or evening. They eat mostly plants, especially beans, and eat meat rarely, in small portions of three or four ounces. They drink alcohol moderately but regularly, perhaps the equivalent of one or two glasses of wine a day.

The Greek island of Icaria appears to have the highest percentage of 90-year-olds on the planet, with nearly one out of three people making it to their nineties. They eat a diet rich in goat's milk, honey, legumes (especially garbanzo beans, black-eyed peas, and lentils), wild greens, fruit and fish. They attribute their sharp minds to their consumption of feta cheese, lemons, and herbs such as sage and marjoram. Meanwhile, the famous centenarians of Okinawa attribute their mental sharpness to bitter melons, tofu, garlic, brown rice, green tea and shitake mushrooms. Not to be outdone, Sardinian centenarians eat sharp pecorino cheese made from the milk of grass-fed sheep, which contains high levels of omega-3 fatty acids. They enjoy their cheese with a moderate amount of flat bread, sourdough bread or barley, with plenty of fennel, fava beans, chickpeas, tomatoes, almonds, milk thistle tea and locally produced wine. There are a disproportionate number of centenarians on the Nicoya peninsula in Costa Rica. Their staple diet consists of beans, corn and squash plus papayas, yams, bananas and peach palms, a small Central American oval fruit high in vitamins A and C. As it happens, researchers in Italy have shown that healthy centenarians have high levels of vitamins A and E.

The Seventh-day Adventists in Loma Linda California are particularly interesting to me because their proven longevity appears to be the consequence of deliberate lifestyle choices. They shun smoking, drinking and dancing and avoid TV, movies and other media entertainments. Their diet is plant-based, focused on grains, fruits, nuts and vegetables. They drink only water. Some eat small amounts of meat and fish. Sugar is taboo.

One of the largest studies done on sleep quality in centenarians was published in the journal Sleep. It looked at nearly 2,800 people over 100 and was the first to examine sleep issues in such a large sample of exceptionally old adults. Results showed that about 65 percent of the sample reported that their sleep quality was good or very good, and the weighted average daily sleep time was about 7.5 hours including naps. Centenarians were 70 percent more likely to report good sleep quality than younger participants aged 65 to 79, after controlling for variables such as demographic characteristics, socioeconomic status and health conditions.

I could add so many more but I think my point is made. There appears to be a common thread that runs through the studies of these old, sharp-minded individuals. If you're a stressed-out smoker and drinker who tends to over-eat and go to bed late, possibly with the help of sleep medications, you may find the 100-year challenge a daunting one.

THE TAKE-AWAY

I know only too well how difficult it is to retain so much information, never mind apply it to our lives. So without slighting the importance of whatever else I've written, I'd like to include in this final section a "take away" — something I'd like you to remember and try if you don't remember and try anything else.

As I've had several occasions to talk about already, omega-3 fatty acids — eicosapentaenoic acid (EPA) and docosahexaenoic acid (DHA) — are recognized as providing significant health benefits. But I find it especially empowering that there's abundant evidence to suggest a direct link between an individuals' omega-3 index (O3i) score and longevity. Research has demonstrated that O3i levels are inversely associated with total mortality across multiple studies including the Cardiovascular Health Study, the Heart and Soul Study, and the Women's Health Initiative Memory Study. A recent meta-analysis that included over 27,000 subjects concluded that O3i is a better indicator of longevity than one of the best-known markers of wellness, cholesterol. Consistent with these observations, a higher O3i is associated with larger total normal brain volume, improved brain function, with an inverse relationship existing between O3i and telomere attrition, a marker of biological aging.

A 2004 study at the Lipid and Diabetes Research Center of the University of Missouri demonstrated that the optimal O3i is greater than 8% while an index of less than 4% may be regarded as a risk factor. To optimize our O3i, we need to increase our consumption of both DHA and EPA. Studies suggest that although you can obtain omega-3s from a whole food diet, most U.S. adults are not meeting their recommended needs. In fact, the average O3i in the U.S. is estimated to be around 4%, which is significantly lower than the desirable O3i level of 8%. Additionally, with the low consumption of Omega-3s, there is an imbalance towards the intake of Omega-6 fatty acids, which may increase inflammation and disease. Due to the significant health benefits of omega-3s, and the low consumption in the Western diet, the intake of dietary supplements has greatly increased over the years.

Fish oil is a common form of supplemental omega-3, yet many of us have wondered if this the most effective form. The tissues and livers of oily fish, though rich in omega-3s, often contain high levels of mercury and other environmental contaminants that can end up in fish oil supplements and ultimately in consumers. If that doesn't worry you, it probably concerns you that overfishing has led to a decline in global catches since the late 1980s. The same holds for another popular omega-3 source, krill, the tiny crustaceans that bigger fish eat. And with the increased demands on aquaculture production and fish farming, the nutritional value of the finished products has decreased, EPA and DHA levels having declined over time and represent only 18% and 12% respectfully of naturally occurring fish oils. Omega-3 fatty acids derived from fish and krill actually go through a transesterification process to concentrate the DHA and EPA.

Amidst this bad news, the good news is that marine microalgae have emerged as a more sustainable, and potentially more bioavailable, source of omega-3. Remember our discussion of the FADS1 and FADS2 genes, DHA, and algae's role in the brain's evolution back in the chapter on that subject? Microalgae are and always have been the primary producers of omega-3 fatty acids in the marine environment and are the source of supply of DHA and EPA to the marine food chain. Microalgae can naturally reach much higher EPA and DHA content than other sources, and can be controlled to ensure they are pollutant free. As a spin-off, if marine algae were to become the primary source of omega-3s in the nutraceutical arena, it would lower the industry's catch of fish by 30%, contribute to the restoration of the marine ecosystem, and eliminate multiple processing steps required for the fish-derived supplement. Many of my patients are now aware of the importance of these nutrients. Their vegetarian origin, improved taste and more agreeable scent are obvious appeals.

WHY I'VE CHOSEN TO SUPPORT A SPECIFIC PRODUCT

In 2015 a U.S. company called Brain Armor entered the brain supplement picture and I have since agreed to serve on the medical advisory board of that company. Their product, also called Brain Armor, became well known to NFL teams, in part through the company's association with Dr. Julian Bailes (see our conversation in Part II, Talking to the Thinkers), who previously served as the team physician for the Pittsburgh Steelers and on various NFL medical advisory boards. Division 1 NCAA football programs began using Brain Armor as part of their concussion protocol.

Brain Armor's advisors advocated daily dosing that would enable the healing process to begin immediately for contact sport players subjected to repetitive sub-concussion blows during practices and games. Meanwhile, in Fort Worth, Texas, Dr. Jonathan Oliver was conducting a double-blind placebo study with 81 players of the TCU football team. The findings from this study, the first large-scale study examining potential prophylactic use of DHA in American football athletes, included identification of the optimal dose of DHA and attributed a neuroprotective effect to DHA supplementation.

As further confirmation, Brain Armor initiated its own study employing 64 participants over 90 days to monitor the effects of daily dosing with its Omega-3+ formula, which includes algal-derived DHAs identical to those in the TCU study, plus other clinically-proven brain-supporting nutrients with their product. The study monitored the effects on individual O3i levels and on inflammatory markers. Over the 90 days of supplementation there were significant changes in outcome measures, with an average increase in O3i of 65.79%, bringing the group average beyond the desired 8% O3i to 8.8% O3i. At the end of the trial, 100% of the participants who supplemented with Brain Armor appropriate to their age showed an increase in O3i, including those subjects who were supplementing with different sources of omega-3s prior to the start of the study. Similar results were obtained for two other health outcomes: the ratio of omega-6 to omega-3 and the AA: EPA ratio.

I include the study report in this section ("The Living Brain Project") because its language is straightforward and I feel that no other recommendation I could make is more likely to be effective for my readers' brain health. You'll find other details of this formula there too, under "Brain Armor".

BRAIN ARMOR:
THE SUPPLEMENT

Since joining the board, I've worked with Brain Armor's team to create strict product criteria that are, as far as I can determine, matched by no other brain supplement. We've adopted the acronym STEP to describe these criteria: Safety & Sustainability, Transparency & Traceability, Evidence & Efficacy, Purity & Potency.

SAFETY & SUSTAINABILITY

Fish oils are extracted from wild fish. There is no control over their diet or exposures. Oils derived from wild fish have unpredictable and varying levels of many known (and unknown) toxins such as mercury, PCBs, dioxins, and furans.

Algal oil has been certified as generally recognized as safe (GRAS) by the United States Food and Drug Administration (FDA) and is an efficient, environmentally friendly, and sustainable source of DHA and EPA. As we know, omega-3s are originally formed within algae, mainly in the form of DHA, and are the base of the food chain for fish. Fish consume algae and metabolically concentrate high amounts of EPA and DHA in their tissues. One kilogram of omega-3 of the type included in Brain Armor has the potential to replace as much as 12 kilograms of wild fish, fish that won't need to be caught to make fish oil.

TRANSPARENCY & TRACEABILITY

The history of the Brain Armor product begins in outer space, when in the early 1980s a NASA program was exploring the use of microalgae as a food supply, oxygen source, and waste disposal catalyst on long-duration interplanetary missions. A group of scientists continued work independently after the completion of the NASA program, founding Martek Biosciences, which was to become a leader in microalgae research and development. The company went on to identify a special type of Crypthecodinium cohnii algae that produces high levels of DHA omega-3 fatty acid.

In 2011 Martek was acquired by DSM, the leading global supplier of both marine and uniquely vegetarian omega-3 ingredients, who then launched the Brain Armor product line. Brain Armor's formula incorporated DSM's micro-algal oil, supplied as Life's OMEGA™ 60, and containing a higher proportion of DHA omega-3 than EPA omega-3.

Life's OMEGA™ 60 the first high potency, vegan and non-GMO omega-3 fatty acid product on the market. It is grown in closed fermenters, under sterile conditions, and FDA inspection in Maryland, USA. The microalgae is harvested and processed to extract the clear, amber-colored oil that is rich in DHA. The final product is free from sugar, gluten, artificial flavors, and artificial sweeteners

EVIDENCE & EFFICACY

Omega-3 is the most researched nutrient in the world, with well over 25,000 published papers to date testifying to the positive health benefits of a diet rich in omega-3 essential fatty acids. DHA accounts for approximately 97 percent of the omega-3 fats in the brain. Dietary omega-3 fatty acid supplements, especially DHA, have been shown to significantly improve brain health and neuronal development, as well as enhance cognitive function. Brain Armor contains the only non-fish source of both EPA and DHA on the market, delivering twice the natural potency of the highest omega-3 levels in oils derived from any species of fish.

The product also contains medium chain triglyceride (MCT) oil. All fats are made up of strings of carbon and hydrogen. Short-chain fats have fewer than 6 carbons (e.g. butyric acid); long-chain fats have 13 to 21 (e.g. omega 3s) and medium-chain fats have 6 to 12. The goMCT® oil formulated in Brain Armor contains C8 and C10 MCTs, the oil molecules that most effectively convert to ketones, a potent alternative energy source for the brain. Evidence strongly suggests that MCT oil enhances the ability to think clearly and process information effectively. The Brain Armor formula includes supplemental vitamin D3, associated with a wide range of benefits, including increased cognition.

PURITY & POTENCY

Fish do not enhance the EPA and DHA they incorporate from ingested algae; they simply bioaccumulate it. It is now known that the purest and most potent form of EPA and DHA is obtained by going straight to the algae source, bypassing further "processing" by fish

During the Brain Armor fermentation process, algae cells are fed only pure, food-grade (or better) nutrients from certified suppliers. The omega-3s so derived are free of toxins.

BRAIN ARMOR INGREDIENTS

Omega-3 DHA/EPA. Life's OMEGA™ 60 supplied by DSM is derived from the marine algae Schizochytrium sp and contains 60 per cent total omega-3, with a minimum content of 300 mg/g DHA and 150 mg/g EPA in a natural triglyceride form for optimum bioavailability. Rosemary extract. ascorbyl palmitate and tocopherols are added as antioxidants to provide stability. Life's Omega (DSM) is prepared in North Carolina and compounded in Texas.

Medium chain triglycerides. Compound Solutions Inc.'s goMCT® enhances ketone production, which has been shown to enhance alertness, awareness and focus.

Vitamin D. Brain Armor uses DSM's vitamin D3 (dl-alpha-tocopherol) liquid, consisting of crystalline cholecalciferol in medium chain triglycerides.

TESTING YOUR BRAINSPAN

The Brainspanner Assessment Platform

During the last decade, the scientific understanding of human brain function shifted dramatically from a perceived static functioning organ to one that was, in fact, dynamic and capable of daily change. Alas, we are neuroplastic, however the assessment of brain function has remained 'dated'. The assessment of neurologic function to date has focused on "snapshot" assessments. This lack of development in assessment failed to match the rapid evolution in the understanding of function.

The Brain Armor research group sought to address this gap and to do so capitalizing on another evolving trend; the prevalence of mobile medical technology and game culture. The Brainspanners Assessement Platform (BAP) was developed as a means of measuring neurological function in a manner that is clinically relevant, scientifically accurate and technologically contemporary. The data that it captures and presents provides a clinical perspective of the user that is a 'movie'; a movie of the function of the mercurial organ that is the human brain.

BAP is a game changer in computerized neurocognitive assessment

COMPUTERIZED NEUROCOGNITIVE ASSESSMENT

The software found on the BAP was developed in the laboratory of Dr. Adrian Owen, Excellence Research Chair in Cognitive Neuroscience and Imaging (owenlab.org), over the course of his 30-year career. The tasks assess core aspects of cognition that are key to quality of life, including reasoning, memory, attention, and verbal ability. We use these cognitive domains every day to effectively make good decisions, learn from experiences, concentrate on important tasks, and communicate intelligently with other people. Over 300 scientific studies using the CBS tasks have been conducted, many published in leading academic journals, yielding important discoveries about how the brain works and how to improve it.

Tasks found in the BAP are based on classic neuropsychological batteries, and are closely related with tests of intelligence. However, BAP emphasizes that the brain cannot be summed up in a single number, and tests measuring each cognitive domain provide individuals with important information about the strengths of their particular brains. Indeed, each cognitive domain is associated with different brain networks, as revealed by fMRI studies. The BAP tasks were also designed from the ground up to take as little time as possible, and to be accessible on a wide variety of devices. Furthermore, they're very engaging and gamified—this is one cognitive assessment you might actually enjoy completing!

The flexibility of BAP has enabled large-scale studies involving participants from all over the world. As a result, over 75,000 participants have contributed to a normative database representing the population. Your results are presented as scores relative to people of the same age range.

Information about how an individual's brain is functioning can be invaluable. The first assessment reveals which cognitive abilities may be strongest, then repeatedly tracking performance over time reveals which brain health efforts are working, and which efforts require adjustment. The tasks are designed to be fun and repeatable, yet retain the scientific validity of 30 years of research to provide meaningful results, quickly.

The Brainspanner Assessment Platform using Computerized Neurocognitive Assessment can be accessed at: **www.brainspanners.com**

WAIST TO HIP RATIO

When these numbers are ideal, the risk of inflammatory conditions caused by belly fat – high cholesterol, high blood sugar, high blood glucose – are significantly less.

All you need to measure your WHR is a measuring tape. Hip circumference is measured over your hip bones and waist circumference over your belly button. Simply divide the number you get for your waist by your hip. Male brainspanners should have a WHR of less than 0.85 and female brainspanners should have less than 0.75.

Another number to keep in mind is that your waist size (your current pant size) should be one half your height or less in inches.

MAGNETIC RESONANCE IMAGING OR SINGLE-PHOTON EMISSION COMPUTED TOMOGRAPHY

MRI (with hippocampal and cortical volume) or SPECT done every few years can help ensure your percentiles are steady or even increasing for age.

SLEEP STUDY

We have come to learn how important a deep sleep is to reset and detox the brain. Anyone can conduct a sleep study, but you need to rush to have one done especially if you snore to assess your apnea-hypopnea Index

VIDEONYSTAGMOGRAPHY

VNG is a test that measures a type of involuntary eye movement called nystagmus. These movements can be slow or fast, steady or jerky. Nystagmus causes your eyes to move from side to side or up and down, or both. It happens when the brain gets conflicting messages from your eyes and the balance system in the inner ear due to trauma like mTBI. The vestibular system works together with your eyes, sense of touch, and brain. Your brain communicates with the different systems in your body to control your balance. An abnormal VNG could indicate areas of concern in the brain.

BIOELECTRIC IMPEDANCE ANALYSIS

BIA is a way to accurately assess fat tissue and muscle mass percentages in your body. Keeping an optimal muscle mass will help you thwart frailty – the number one killer of all eclipsing diabetes, heart disease and cancer combined. Keeping an optimal fat tissue percentage will reduce inflammation in your body and keep hormones in check – two key elements of becoming a brainspanner. For optimal reference ranges see page 75 at this link: https://www.biodyncorp.com/pdf/clinician_desk_reference_bio.pdf

LABORATORY ANALYSIS

One fundamental aspect of practicing functional medicine is to leverage comprehensive laboratory science to develop patient profiles that help to determine the underlying causes of disease. I believe strongly that everyone should have their genetics evaluated. The DNA Company (**www.theDNAcompany.com**) offers the best and most functional testing available. Besides genomic evaluation, a few of my favorite functional tests that I use in a clinical setting on a regular basis are called the NutrEval and GI Effects (**www.gdx.net**). The former is a blood and urine analysis and the latter a stool microbiome test both offered by Genova Diagnostics, a leading functional medicine laboratory in Asheville, North Carolina.

Laboratory test results are not meaningful by themselves, rather their meaning comes from comparison to reference ranges as well as considering their levels along with other tests. Values that are well outside expected ranges can provide clues to help identify possible conditions or diseases. "Normal" reference ranges are the values expected for a healthy person. The difference between "normal" and "optimal" is often vast.

While accuracy of laboratory testing has significantly evolved over the past few decades, some lab-to-lab variability can occur due to differences in testing equipment, chemical reagents, and techniques. It is important to know that you must use the range supplied by the laboratory that performed your test to evaluate whether your results are "within normal limits."

"Optimal" target values will vary depending on your gender, genetics, and environment. Work with a clinician well versed in functional medicine to decide the appropriate laboratory investigation and optimal levels for you. The list below is a comprehensive list of laboratory tests and target values I consider optimal on ***average*** based on my training in functional medicine and personal clinical experience.

A GUIDE TO OPTIMAL LAB VALUES

Laboratory Analysis	Target Values	Comments
		HORMONES
Progesterone	5-20 ng/mL or 16-63.5 nmol/L	Optimal levels will vary depending on genetics, whether you are male or female, the time of day, and for females the day of their menstrual cycle. Regulates cognition, mood, inflammation, mitochondrial function, neurogenesis and regeneration, myelination and recovery from traumatic brain injury
Testosterone	1000-1500 ng/dL or 34.7-52.05 nmol/L (M)	Optimal levels will vary depending on genetics, whether you are male or female, the time of day, and for females the day of their menstrual cycle. Testosterone plays a key role in spatial cognition tasks and overall mood.
Free Testosterone	7-15 pg/mL (M)	Optimal levels will vary depending on genetics, whether you are male or female, the time of day, and for females the day of their menstrual cycle. More important than Testosterone, the bioavailable Free Testosterone plays a key role in spatial cognition tasks and overall mood.
Estradiol (E2)	100-250 pg/mL or 367-915 pmol/L (F)	Optimal levels will vary depending on genetics, whether you are male or female, the time of day, and for females the day of their menstrual cycle. Estradiol is involved in functions such as fine motor control, learning, memory, sensitivity to pain and motor coordination, as well protecting against stroke damage and Alzheimer's disease

Laboratory Analysis	Target Values	Comments
Pregnenolone	50-100 ng/dL	Pregnenolone is a neurosteroid because it is also made in the brain and carries out several cerebral functions such as neuroprotection, neuroplasticity and neurogenesis. It also regulates mood and memory.
DHEA-S	400-500 (M) 350-400 (F) ug/dL or 10.8-13.5 (M) 9.5-10.8 (F) umol/L	Also a neurosteroid, it increases dopamine (by up-regulating tyrosine hydroxylase levels, the enzyme responsible for its production)
Cortisol	12-16 ug/dL or 330-440 nmol/L	High levels of cortisol can wear down the brain's ability to function properly. Stress can kill brain cells and even reduce the size of the brain. Chronic stress has a shrinking effect on the prefrontal cortex, the area of the brain responsible for memory and learning
TSH	1-2.5 mU/L	Thyroid hormones regulate metabolism in every organ of the body, including the brain and when they are imbalanced, this can affect mood, memory span, ability to concentrate, and contributes to the feeling of brain fog
Free-T3	3.2-4.2 pmol/L	See TSH
Free-T4	1.3-1.8 pmol/L	See TSH
Reverse-T3	10-20 ng/dL	See TSH
Vitamins B6	75-100 nmol/L	Helps the body make the hormones serotonin (which regulates mood) and norepinephrine (which helps your body cope with stress)

Laboratory Analysis	Target Values	Comments
Vitamin B12	1000-1500 ng/mL	Deficiency has been associated with memory loss, especially in older adults. The vitamin may play a role in preventing brain atrophy, which is the loss of neurons in the brain and often associated with memory loss or dementia
Vitamin B9 (Folate)	20-25 ng/mL	Very active in the brain and central nervous system necessary for making DNA and neurotransmitters, aids in cellular detoxification, and crucial to the proper formation of the nervous system during development
Vitamin C	1.5-2.5 mg/dL	Low levels are implicated in anxiety, stress, depression, fatigue and low mood
Vitamin D (25OHD)	100-150 nmol/L	Aids in the function of neuronal and glial tissue. A deficiency affects a type of brain "scaffolding" that supports the neurons, increases risk of developing dementia, and is linked to depression and the development of autism and schizophrenic-like disorders, hypoxic brain injury, and other mental illnesses.
Vitamin E	15-20 ug/mL	Elevated levels of oxidative stress in the brain has been shown to contribute to Alzheimer's disease. Vitamin E (particularly tocotrienols) protects the brain from oxidation.

Laboratory Analysis	Target Values	Comments
RBC Magnesium	2.0-2.5 mmol/L	Magnesium (especially in the form of Magnesium Threonate) has been shown to improve memory. It plays an essential role in nerve transmission. There is strong data to suggest a role for magnesium in migraine and depression, and emerging data to suggest a protective effect for anxiety and stroke
Calcium	8.5-10.5 mg/dL	Involved in memory, regulates several neuronal functions such as neurotransmitter synthesis, release, and neuronal excitability. An imbalance may trigger Alzheimer's Disease.
Copper:Zinc	Ratio of 0.8-1.2	An imbalanced ratio has been linked to several neurological disorders including Alzheimer's and Parkinson's. This ratio has also been identified as critical to the enzymes that activate the brain's neurotransmitters in response to stimuli.
Selenium	110-150 ng/mL	Key ingredient for motor performance, coordination, memory and cognition.
Potassium	4.5-5.5 mEq/L	Although low levels of potassium is rare, it can interrupt electrical signals that drive the brain causing confusion, sluggish thoughts, and brain fog, and is linked to mild cognitive impairment
Coenzyme Q10	0.46-1.72 ug/mL	Important for mitochondrial function. The brain is highly dependent on mitochondria. Optimal levels show benefit in cognitive decline

Laboratory Analysis	Target Values	Comments
		BLOOD SUGAR
Fasting insulin	<20-40 pmol/L	Affects feeding behavior and body energy stores, the metabolism of glucose and fats in the liver and adipose, and various aspects of memory and cognition. Elevated levels can influence the development or progression of Alzheimer's disease, other forms of dementia, and brain trauma recovery time.
Hemoglobin A1c (HbA1c)	4.0-5.5%	Elevated blood sugar over time and type 2 diabetes are associated with cerebral atrophy, cognitive impairment and dementia. When HbA1c is out of range, lowering it by 1% reduces mortality from diabetes and complications by 20%
Fasting Glucose	3.5-6 mmol/L	See HbA1c
		LIPIDS
LDL-p	700-1000 nmol/L	LDL-P measures the actual number of LDL particles and may be a better predictor of risk than standard LDL-C
Oxidized LDL (Ox-LDL)	<45 U/L	A sensitive biomarker of atherosclerosis, coronary artery disease, and acute myocardial infarction. High Ox-LDL has also been associated with metabolic syndrome, impaired glucose tolerance and insulin resistance, and untreated overt hypothyroidism.
Lp(a)	<30 mg/dL	Elevated "low-density lipoprotein little a" in Alzheimer's disease correlates with brain amyloid beta but also help regulate neurobehavioral function and energy balance.

Laboratory Analysis	Target Values	Comments
Cholesterol	150-200 mg/dL or 5 – 5.2 mmol/L	This is a goldilocks scenario but it is important to note that low blood cholesterol does not cause low brain cholesterol (the brain makes its own). Low total blood cholesterol levels may contribute to depression, violent behavior, and suicidal thoughts. Too much on the other hand, can contribute to thickening of artery walls (if inflammation is also high) and negatively affects blood supply to the brain. This increases the risk of heart disease, stroke and dementia.
Triglycerides	<150 mg/dL or <1.7 mmol/L	As opposed to cholesterol, TGs do cross the blood brain barrier into the brain and central nervous system. Once inside the brain they influence the hypothalamus, the part of the brain that regulates energy expenditure and the "set point" of your weight and metabolism and are negatively correlated with cognitive function
HDL	60-70 mg/dL or 1.55 -1.80 mmol/L	Anti-oxidant, anti-inflammatory, endothelial health, anti-thrombotic, and modulation of immune function in the brain.
	INFLAMMATION	
hs-CRP	<0.9 mg/L	As opposed to CRP, hs-CRP is "high sensitivity" and more accurately depicts inflammation in the body
Omega 3 index	>8%	The omega-3 fatty acids EPA and DHA are critical for normal brain function, development, and disease prevention throughout all ages and stages of life. They are abundant in the cell membranes of brain cells, preserving cell membrane health and facilitating communication between brain cells.

Laboratory Analysis	Target Values	Comments
*Cytokine IL-6	<=5 pg/mL	Quantitative Multiplex Bead Assay. Precise reference ranges vary greatly depending on age, sex, etc. and need to be interpreted along with other tests that measure inflammation including Hs-CRP
*Cytokine TNF-a	<=22 pg/mL	Quantitative Multiplex Bead Assay. Precise reference ranges vary greatly depending on age, sex, etc. and need to be interpreted along with other tests that measure inflammation including Hs-CRP
Homocysteine	<7 umol/L	Elevation may indicate damage to arteries and helps determine need for B-vitamins
C4a	< 2830 ng/mL	Inflammatory marker of greatest significance to innate immune responses in those with exposure to mold and water damaged buildings. Traumatic brain injuries, Lyme disease, and mold infections have very similar symptoms.
8-OHdG	<=15 mcg/g Creat (urine)	When elevated, it's important to identify the sources of oxidative stress and test glutathione. Reducing oxidative stress is valuable in optimizing brain health and longevity.
TOXINS		
Glutathione (whole blood)	>700mmol/L	Essential for the cellular detoxification of reactive oxygen species in brain cells. Low levels are directly associated with the oxidative stress that occurs in neurological diseases
RBC thiamine pyrophosphate (TPP)	100-150 ng/mL	Maintains glutathione in red blood cells (ability to manage toxins that affect the brain)

Laboratory Analysis	Target Values	Comments
Zonulin (pre-Haptoglobin 2	<4 ng/mL	Good indicator of leaky gut and leaky blood-brain barrier
Diamine Oxidase & Histamine	<10 ng/mL & <1 respectively	Good indicator of histamine intolerance which can lead to brain fog and/or depression as well as sinus problems
Mercury	<dL	Mercury should be less than detectable limits (dl). Studies show that there is no safe levels of mercury in the body.
Lead	<1 ug/dL	Can damage the prefrontal cerebral cortex, hippocampus, and cerebellum and can lead to brain damage, behavioral problems, nerve damage, Alzheimer's, Parkinson's, and schizophrenia.
Arsenic	<2.5 ug/dL	Toxic effects on neurotransmitters involved in cell-to-cell signalling within the brain
Cadmium	<0.5 ug/dL	Elevated levels play a role in neurodegenerative diseases including Parkinson's, Alzheimer's, and Huntington's disease

*https://www.mayocliniclabs.com/test-catalog/Clinical+and+Interpretive/75139

THE LIVING BRAIN PROJECT

– report on an ongoing research study –

Nick Pili, author

METHOD

PARTICIPANTS

The original study group consisted of 67 participants. Between day 1 and 90 of the study there were 9 participants who dropped out or stopped taking the supplements for various reasons, and 2 additional participants delayed their start date and are currently in the process of their 90-day dosage. The current study sample consisted of 56 human volunteers (46 male, 10 female) aged 3 to 66 years old. Participants were recruited from the general community, resided throughout the United States of America, and exhibited different health histories, daily food intake, and physical activity practices.

PROCEDURE

Each participant took an initial **Omega Quant** Omega-3 Index test to establish baseline outcome levels. Each participant was then provided with, and instructed to take, a daily dose of **Brain Armor's Omega-3+** supplement that was compatible for their age, and to remain consistent with other variables of their diet and exercise routine. Some participants were already supplementing with Omega-3s from other sources prior to the start of the study. Those participants were asked to stop current supplementation and take only Brain Armor for the duration of the study. Participants consumed their assigned supplement daily for 90 days, then a second **Omega Quant** Omega-3 Index test was performed to assess any changes in outcome measures.

Brain Armor supplements are created to deliver DHA & EPA at a 2:1 ratio in amounts required to best support different life stages that include; Adult, Active Adult, 50+ Senior, and Pro NSF Certified for Sport. Each daily dose includes:

YOUTH

_1833mg Omega-3; 1000:500mg DHA:EPA; 1200IU Vitamin D; 30IU Vitamin E; 1100mg Medium Chain Triglyceride Oil

ACTIVE ADULT

_2292mg Omega-3; 1250:625mg DHA:EPA; 1800IU Vitamin D; 45IU Vitamin E; 4500mg Medium Chain Triglyceride Oil

50+ SENIOR

_2750mg Omega-3; 1500:750mg DHA:EPA; 2400IU Vitamin D; 60IU Vitamin E; 4000mg Medium Chain Triglyceride Oil

PRO NSF CERTIFIED FOR SPORT

3667mg Omega-3; 2000:1000mg DHA:EPA; 3600IU Vitamin D; 90IU Vitamin E; 2250mg Medium Chain Triglyceride Oil

SUPER OMEGA-3 VEGAN SOFTGELS

_1283mg Omega-3; 700:350mg DHA:EPA; 800IU Vitamin D; 20IU Vitamin E; 45mg Medium Chain Triglyceride Oil

This was not a clinically controlled study. All participants were given the supplementation to take under instruction with regular check ins to ensure best consistency and compliance. A smaller cohort of participants continued supplementation to assess 180 days of supplementation voluntarily. The average number of days between the baseline and follow up testing was 113 days.

OUTCOME MEASURES

The outcome measures for this study were the Omega-3 Index, Omega-6: Omega-3 ratio, and AA:EPA ratio. All measures were assessed using the Omega Quant Omega-3 Index Test. **Omega Quant** Analytics, LLC, is an independent, CLIA-certified lab that offers Omega-3 Index testing to researches, clinicians, and the public, and sets the standard for fatty acid testing. Their assays have been validated per FDA Guidelines for the industry and are able to run validation studies specific to work if required.

The O3i test is sent in the mail directly to the participant. The test service provides a sample collection kit with instructions to collect the sample via finger prick from the comfort of home. The kit is then sent back in the mail with the provided return label and individualized results are received within 1-2 weeks.

RESULTS

OVERALL OMEGA-3 INDEX (O3I)

For the study group, the average baseline O3i was 5.59% which is significantly higher than the average O3i of individuals in North America. Over the 90 days of supplementation there were great changes in outcome measures with an average increase in O3i of 65.79% bringing the group average beyond the desired 8% O3i to 8.8% O3i.

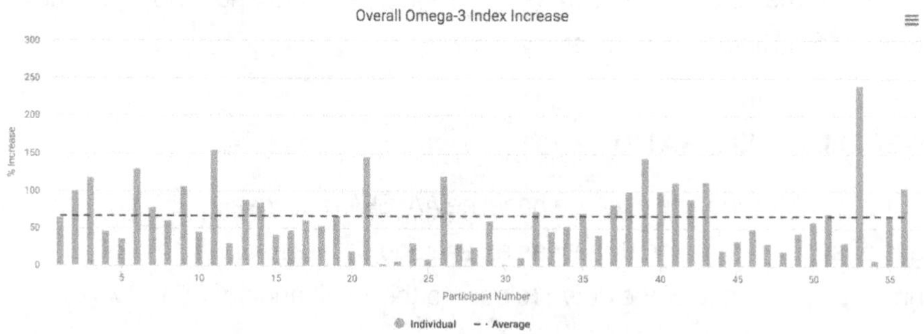

Overall, every single participant demonstrated an increase in O3i levels using Brain Armor's new formula for 90 days, even those who were taking Omega-3 supplements from another source prior to the start of the study. By the end of the 90 days, 71.42% of all participants had reached, or exceeded, the optimal O3i level of 8%.

The average Omega-3 Index increase has been calculated by taking the sum of the percentage increase for each participant and dividing by the number of participants in the study.

OVERALL OMEGA 6: OMEGA 3 RATIO

For the study group, the average baseline Omega6: Omega 3 ratio was 7.35:1. Over the 90 days of supplementation there was an average decrease in Omega6: Omega3 ratio of 35.31% bringing the group average down to 4.5:1 which is closer to the ideal range of 3:1. 9% of the study participants reached or exceeded the optimal Omega 6: Omega 3 ratio of 3:1.

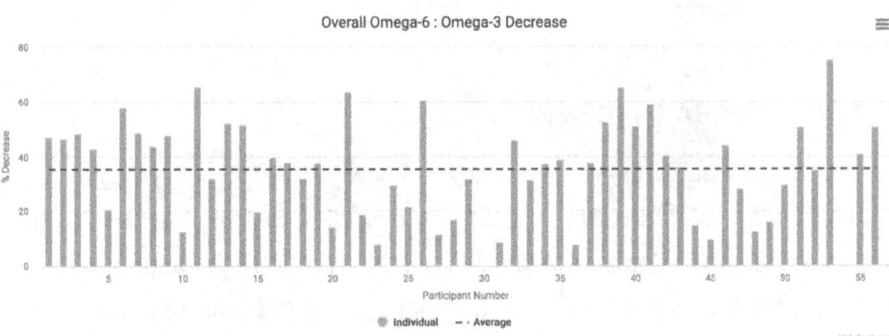

The average Omega-6 : Omega-3 decrease has been calculated by taking the sum of the percentage decrease for each participant and dividing by the number of participants in the study.

OVERALL AA: EPA RATIO

For the study group, the average baseline AA: EPA ratio was 21.8:1. Over the 90 days of supplementation there was an average decrease of AA: EPA of 51.46% bringing the group average down (closer to the ideal range of 3:1) to 7.76:1.

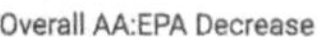

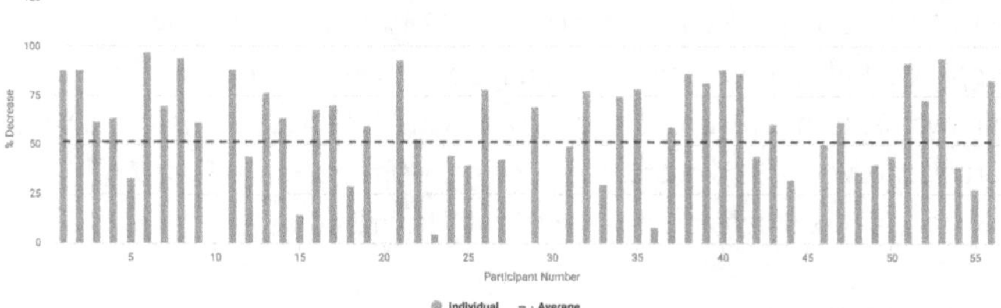

The average AA : EPA decrease has been calculated by taking the sum of the percentage decrease for each participant and dividing by the number of participants in the study.

YOUTH

The Youth participants demonstrated an average increase in O3i of 70.8% from a baseline average of 5.23% O3i to an average of 8.85%. The Youth participants also showed a decrease in their Omega6: Omega 3 ratio of 28.5% from a baseline average of 7.5:1 to an average (closer to the desired range of 3:1) of 4.5:1. Additionally, there was an observed decrease in AA: EPA ratio of 39.8%, from baseline average values of 21.4:1 to an average (closer to the desired range of 3:1) of 7.6:1.

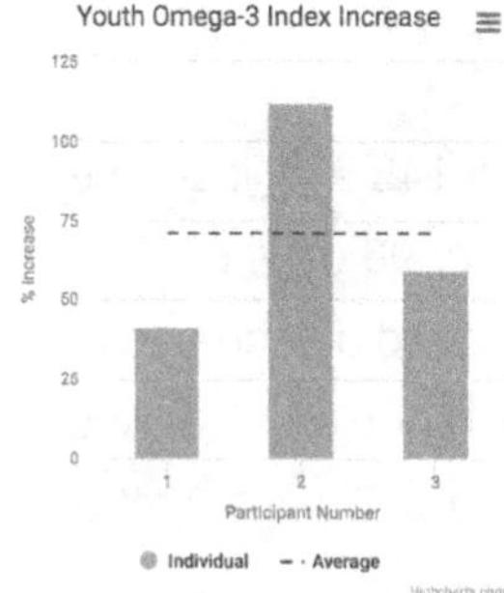

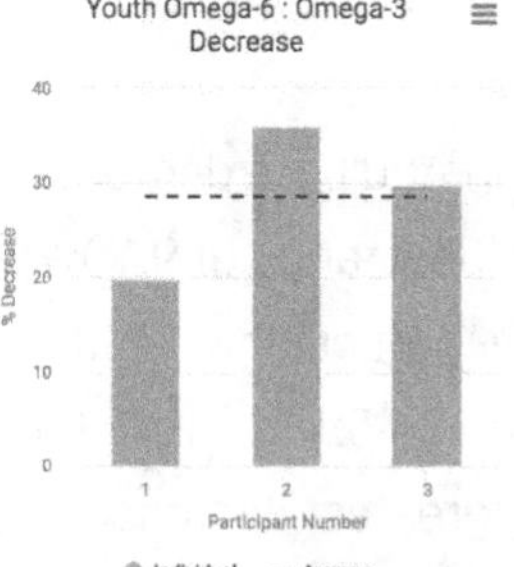

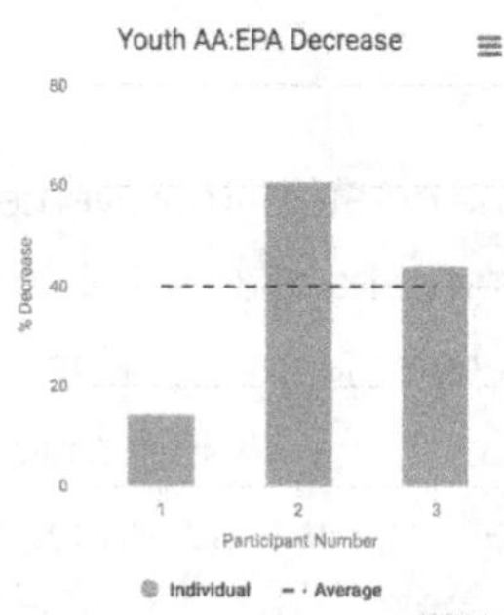

The greatest improvement in Youth O3i demonstrated a 112.2% increase from 4.10% O3i to exceed the ideal range at 8.7% O3i after 90 days of supplementation. This same participant also experienced the greatest improvements in Omega 6: Omega 3 ratio and AA: EPA ratio among the Youth participants with a 36% decrease in Omega 6: Omega 3 ratio from 7.5:1 to 4.8:1, and a 60.9% decrease in AA: EPA ratio from 24.6:1 to 9.6:1.

ACTIVE ADULT

The Adult participants demonstrated an average increase in O3i of 60.88% from a baseline average of 5.67% O3i to an average within the ideal range at 8.74% O3i. The Adult participants demonstrated a decrease in Omega6: Omega 3 ratio of 34.01% from a baseline average of 7.15:1 to an average (closer to the desired range of 3:1) of 4.52:1. There was also an observed decrease in AA: EPA ratio of 49.9%, from a baseline average of 21.0:1 to an average (closer to the desired range of 3:1) of 7.91:1.

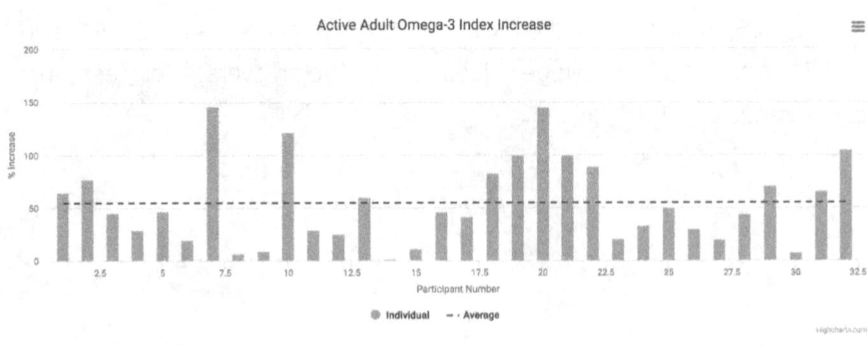

The greatest improvement in Adult O3i demonstrated a 145.95% increase from a base 3.7% O3i to an ideal range of 9.10% O3i after 90 days of supplementation. This same participant also demonstrated a decrease of 93% in the AA: EPA ratio from 24.5:1 to within the ideal range of 1.7:1. Another participant experienced the greatest decrease in Omega 6: Omega 3 ratio of 65.22% from 9.2:1 to of 3.2:1.

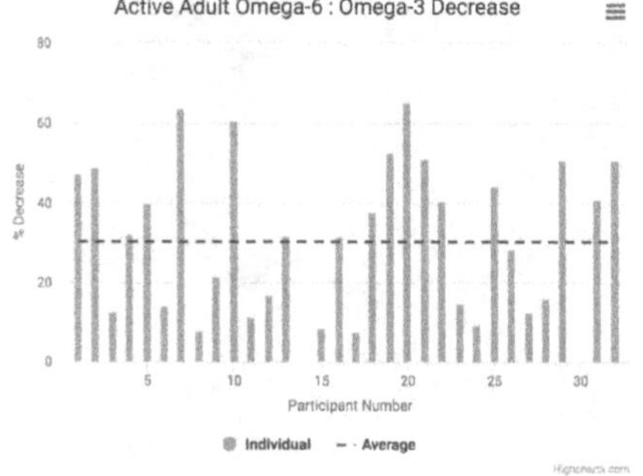

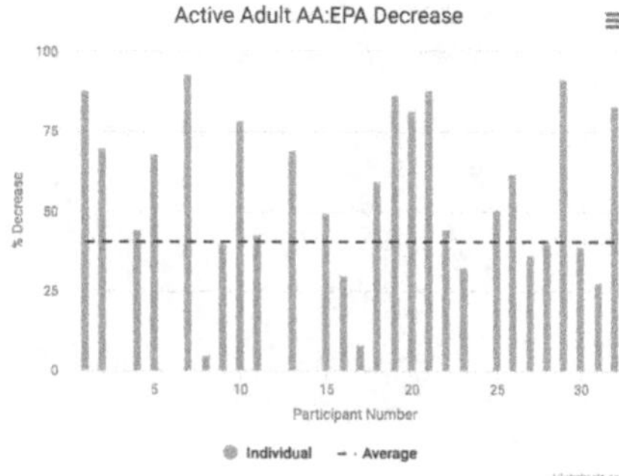

OVER 50

The 50+ Adult participants demonstrated an average increase in O3i of 66.96% from a baseline average of 5.49% O3i to an average within the ideal range at 8.75% O3i. The 50+ adult participants also demonstrated a decrease in Omega6: Omega 3 ratio of 36.02% from a baseline average of 7.43:1 to an average closer to the ideal range at 4.53:1. There was also an observed decrease in AA: EPA ratio of 52.68% from a baseline average of 22.1:1 to an average closer to the desired range at 7.79:1.

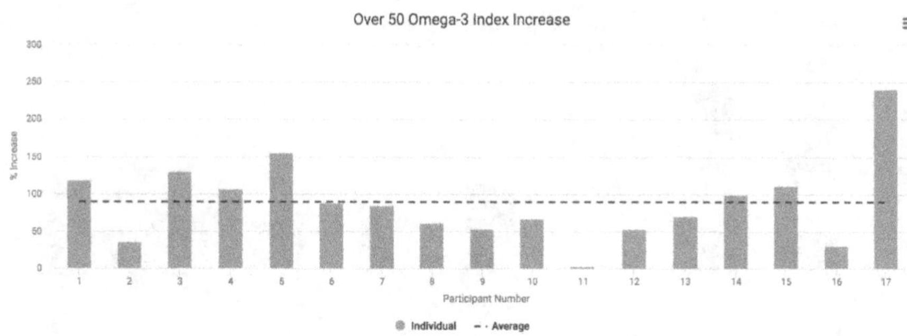

The greatest improvement in 50+ Adult O3i demonstrated a 241% increase from 3.4% O3i to well within the ideal range at 11.6% O3i after 90 days of supplementation. This same participant also demonstrated the greatest decrease in Omega 6: Omega 3 ratio of 75.41% from 12.2:1 to within ideal range at 3:1. Another participant demonstrated the greatest decrease in AA: EPA ratio of 97% from a baseline average of 150.1:1 to an average closer to the ideal range at 4.4:1.

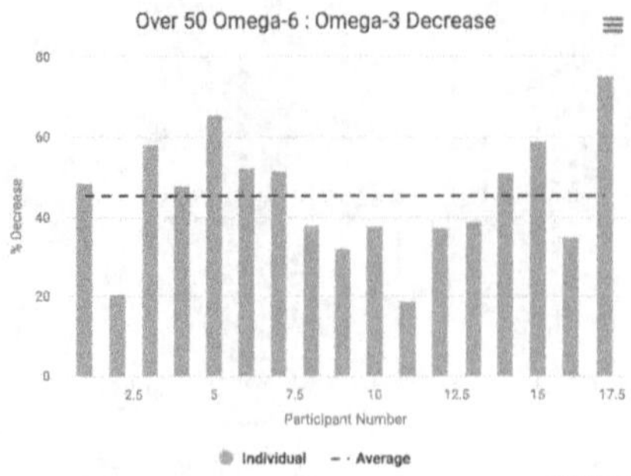

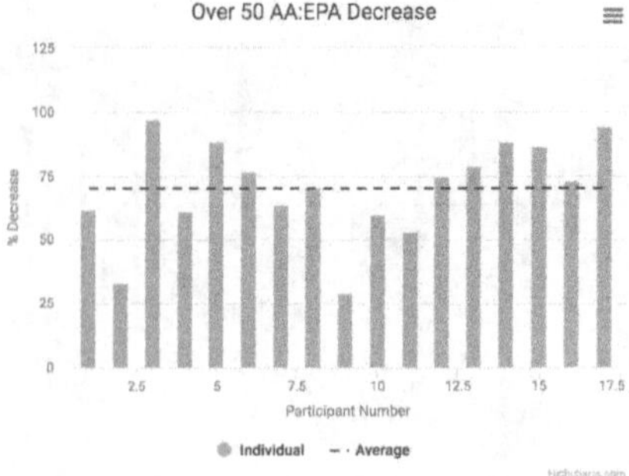

PROFESSIONAL

The Pro NSF Certified participants demonstrated an average increase in O3i of 69.36% from a baseline average of 5.43% O3i to an average within the ideal range at 9.02% O3i. The Pro NSF Certified participants also demonstrated a decrease in Omega 6: Omega 3 ratio of 38.12% from a baseline average of 7.2:1 to an average closer to the desired range at 4.38:1. There was also an observed decrease of AA: EPA ratio within this group of 54.47%, from a baseline average of 19.9:1 to an average closer to the ideal range at 7.4:1.

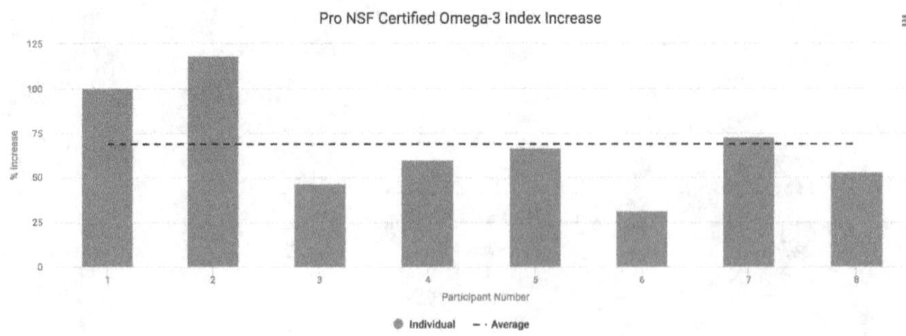

The greatest improvement in Pro O3i demonstrated a 118.37% increase from 4.9% O3i to 10.7% O3i. This same participant demonstrated the greatest decrease in Omega 6: Omega 3 ratio of 48.48% from a baseline of 6.6:1 to closer to ideal range at 3.4:1. Another participant in this group demonstrated the greatest decrease in AA: EPA ratio of 88.06% from a baseline of 20.1:1 to within ideal range at 2.4:1.

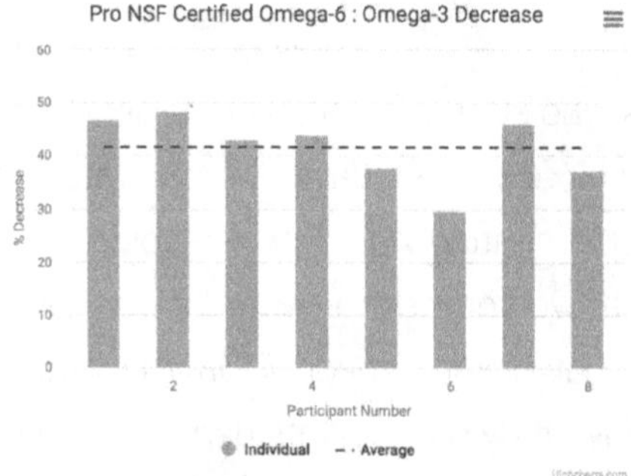

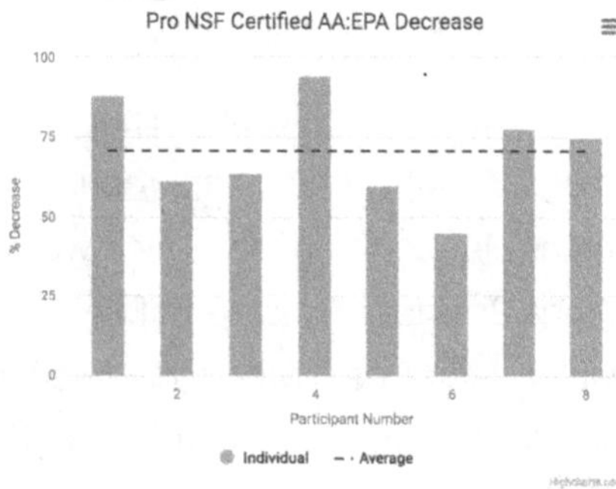

GENDER DIFFERENCES

Although some studies suggest that males (M) and females (F) respond differently to Omega-3 supplementation across different clinical outcomes, this was not observed in this case. In the current study when separated by gender the average increase in O3i levels were 63.11% for F, 65.709% for M, the average decrease in Omega-6: Omega-3 ratio was 35.02% for F and 35.31% for male, and the average decrease in AA: EPA was 51.20% for F and 51.46% for males.

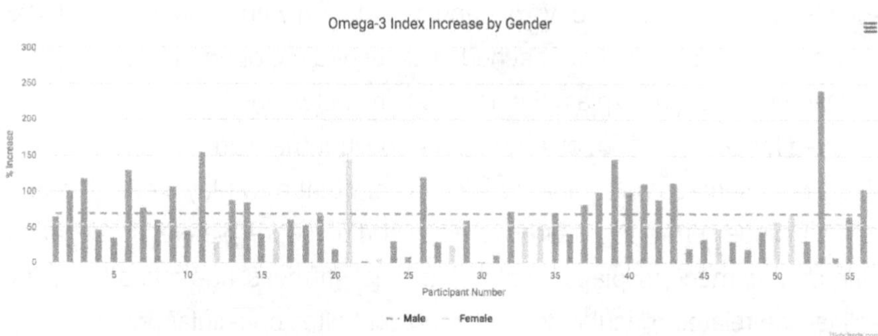

CONCLUSION

In this study 100% of the participants who supplemented with Brain Armor Omega-3+ supplements appropriate for their age for 90 days demonstrated an increase in O3i. Even those who were supplementing with different sources of Omega-3s prior to the start of the study showed great improvement. Similar results stand true for the other two health outcomes, Omega 6: Omega 3 ratio and AA: EPA ratio. In this study 96.4% of the study participants demonstrated improvements in their Omega 6: Omega 3 ratio, and 91% of the study participants demonstrated improvements in their AA: EPA ratio. Since each participant was asked to remain consistent with other variables of their diet and exercise routine, the differences in the measured health outcomes were influenced primarily by Brain Armor supplementation daily for 90 days.

Several previous studies have concluded that there is a direct link between an individuals' Omega-3 Index score and longevity. O3i levels were found to be inversely associated with total mortality across multiple studies including the Cardiovascular Health Study, the Heart and Soul Study, and the Women's Health Initiative Memory Study. Research indicates that the optimal O3i is >8%. At the start of the study 10% of the study participants were at or exceeded 8% O3i. After 90 days of supplementation with Brain Armor, 71.42% of the study participants had reached or exceeded the optimal level of 8% O3i.

Mechanisms that explain the associations between higher O3i and improved longevity are not clearly understood, but there are beneficial effects of Omega-3s on a variety of risk factors that may play a role. These factors include serum triglyceride levels, blood pressure, platelet aggregation, inflammatory markers, plaque build-up, arterial stiffness, age-related cognitive decline, age-related macular degeneration, and rates of cellular aging.

It is of interest to determine the most effective source and quantity of Omega-3s needed to optimize O3i, and therefore, decrease risk for all cause mortality. This study observed an increase in O3i in every participant by providing Omega-3s in a 2:1 DHA: EPA derived from marine algae, in combination with other clinically proven brain supporting nutrients, Vitamin D, Vitamin E, and Medium Chain Triglyceride oil. Since a number of participants were regularly taking an Omega-3 supplement derived from fish or krill oil prior to the start of the study, it can be concluded that the combination of ingredients found in Brain Armor Omega-3+ supplements are more effective at raising O3i levels than obtaining them from a whole food diet or obtaining them from another type of supplementation.

Along with improvements in O3i with Brain Armor Omega-3+ supplements, 96.4% and 91% of the study participants experienced improvements in the Omega 6: Omega 3 ratio, and AA: EPA ratio. When the ratio between Omega-6 and Omega-3 fatty acids is excessively high, which is typical in the Western diet, it can create a pro inflammatory state which promotes many disease conditions. A ratio of 4:1 Omega 6: Omega 3 is associated with a 70% decrease in total mortality. Overall, a lower ratio of Omega 6: Omega 3 fatty acids is desirable in reducing the risk of many chronic diseases of high prevalence in Western Countries. Similarly, Arachidonic Acid (AA) is a type of Omega 6 fatty acid that is found primarily in plants and plant oils, and the higher the AA: EPA ratio, the higher the levels of cellular inflammation and risk of chronic disease. Both the Omega 6: Omega 3 ratio, and the AA: EPA ratio, can be improved through diet, and results show that intake of Omega-3s of approximately 2.5g per day is sufficient to bring the AA: EPA ratio into the desired range for optimum wellness.

In conclusion, our observations show that supplementing with Brain Armor Omega-3+ supplements daily can improve O3i, Omega 6: Omega 3 ratio, and AA: EPA ratio in a few as 90 days.

Study details here: (includes graphs outlined above)
https://thelivingbrainproject.com/study

Results:
https://thelivingbrainproject.com/results

Participant Feedback:
https://thelivingbrainproject.com/feedback

Living Brain Project Video Testimonials:
https://brainarmor.com/testimonials/

To participate in your own Living Brain Project,
visit: TheLivingBrainProject.com

CPSIA information can be obtained
at www.ICGtesting.com
Printed in the USA
BVHW050230120122
625987BV00003B/219